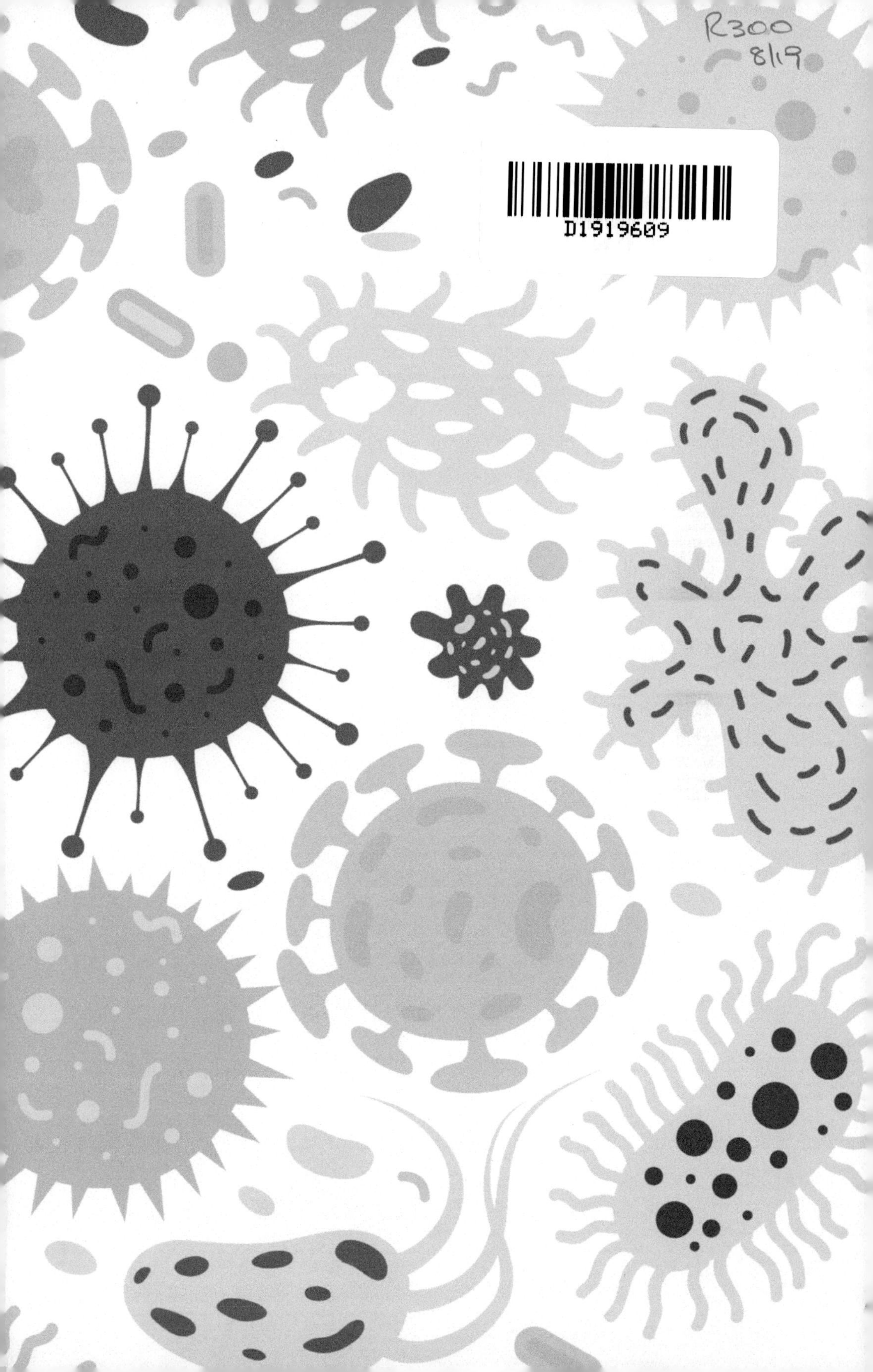

Epidemics and the Health of African Nations

EDITED BY

Zamanzima Mazibuko

THIS RESEARCH PROJECT WAS SUPPORTED BY:

science & technology

Department: Science and Technology REPUBLIC OF SOUTH AFRICA

First published by the Mapungubwe Institute for Strategic Reflection (MISTRA) in 2019
142 Western Service Rd
Woodmead
Johannesburg, 2191

ISBN 978-0-6399955-9-5

Production and design by Jacana Media, 2019
Editor in chief: Joel Netshitenzhe
Text editor: Alison Lowry
Designer: Alexandra Turner
Set in Stempel Garamond 10.5/15pt
Printed and bound by ABC Press
Job no. 003560

Please cite this publication as follows:
MISTRA. 2019. *Epidemics and the Health of African Nations.* Zamanzima Mazibuko (ed). Johannesburg: Mapungubwe Institute for Strategic Reflection.

Contents

SECTION THREE: CONTENDING WITH CHRONIC CONDITIONS IN AFRICAN HEALTH SYSTEMS

SECTION FOUR: THE FUTURE OF HEALTH SYSTEMS IN AFRICA

Preface

Africa bears an inordinate proportion of the world's diseases and epidemics. Recent outbreaks of cholera and Ebola caught several countries off guard and without the strategies needed to combat them.

The rate at which devastating diseases emerge, spread, and re-emerge has generated much discussion about the efficacy of African countries' health systems. This pertains to such issues as health policy, infrastructure, staffing, funding, and management models.

However, across the continent there have been both failures and successes in dealing with epidemics.

The manner in which the threat of Ebola was swiftly contained and eliminated in Nigeria in 2014 and the encouraging outcomes in managing malaria in southern Africa bear positive appraisal. Despite resource constraints, some countries, such as Ghana and Rwanda, are progressively introducing forms of national health insurance. On the other hand, Zimbabwe has over the past decade experienced two major outbreaks of cholera, which resulted in a combined death toll of over four thousand residents.

Establishing a direct correlation only between the sturdiness of health systems and success in dealing with epidemics can, at times, be a thankless exercise. For instance, Nigeria's health system is not much different from those of Guinea, Sierra Leone, and Liberia which bore the brunt of the 2014 Ebola crisis. South Africa's maternal mortality rates are far higher than in countries with much fewer resources and weaker health infrastructure.

These experiences underline the need to approach epidemics from a much broader perspective. The Ebola episode in Nigeria, it is argued in this volume, speaks to the professionalism of health workers such as Dr Ameyo Stella Adadevoh, who stood her ground in the face of pressure, given the diplomatic status of Patient Zero. Mobilisation by government and other sectors of society to prevent a disaster of monumental proportions in as heavily a populated a city as Lagos was also fundamental. Dr Adadevoh, who had come into contact with Patient Zero after he had been misdiagnosed, herself succumbed to the disease.

The collapse of governance and the neglect of sanitation and water infrastructure in Zimbabwe's capital city of Harare was in large measure responsible for the outbreak of cholera and the resulting high fatality rates. This was also a consequence of the dire economic situation and the monstrous disjuncture between national government and the opposition-led urban municipality.

Herein lies the relevance of a syndemics approach to the management of disease, which informs much of this volume. It is an approach that proceeds from the perspective that political dynamics, socio-economic issues as well as environmental factors do contribute to the outbreak and management of disease. Combined with these are internal and cross-border migration, quality of nutrition rather than just food security, and a myriad of cultural and other factors. In other words, the biosocial complex has an important bearing on the outbreak of diseases and interactions among them.

Authors in this book also draw attention to the organisational hierarchies in health facilities and the workloads borne by doctors, the mass of frontline health workers, and the communities of care. How the health professionals are managed, including striking the right balance between paperwork and clinical duties, is crucial in determining the quality of care. This calls for multidirectional empathy between patients, health workers, and communities.

In the recent period, non-communicable diseases have started to take their toll on larger numbers of African populations. Ironically, the rise of the middle strata – combined with the chaotic manner in which sections of the population are urbanising and adopting new lifestyles – is largely responsible for this.

The central message of this book is that strengthening health systems and countering outbreaks of diseases require an integrated, inclusive, and transdisciplinary approach. A critical element of this is the need for African countries to forge partnerships in developing research capacity that is responsive to the lived experiences and health needs of their populations.

The Mapungubwe Institute hopes that by examining the challenge of epidemics in Africa from a broad, biosocial perspective, this book will encourage panoptic reflections and integrated policy development and implementation.

MISTRA wishes to thank the authors, peer reviewers, and other partners – across the continent – who worked with us in conducting this research. Profound gratitude is also due to the Department of Science and Technology and the extended family of funders who render such work possible.

– Joel Netshitenzhe
Executive Director

Acknowledgements

The Mapungubwe Institute for Strategic Reflection (MISTRA) would like to express its gratitude to Zamanzima Mazibuko, who was project leader and editor of this volume, and Wandile Ngcaweni, who provided valuable support and assisted with the co-ordination of the project. Thanks also go to Salimah Valiani and Nolwazi Mkhwanazi, who assisted with the conceptualisation and initial direction of the project.

Thank you to the other MISTRA staff who contributed to the successful outcome of this project: the project management directorate led by Xolelwa Kashe-Katiya, supported by Dzunisani Mathonsi and Towela Ng'ambi; the operations directorate led by Barry Gilder, supported by Terry Shakinovsky, and the fundraising and financial management department led by Lorraine Pillay, with support from Magati Nindi-Galenge. We thank all in the research directorate who contributed to this body of work and helped pull the volume together: the researchers, including Anelile Gibixego, who provided all-important assistance with the manuscript, and Director Research Susan Booysen for her efforts to ensure that this publication meets the highest standards. MISTRA also extends its appreciation to Alison Lowry for editing the manuscript and to Jacana Media who are responsible for the design, layout and production of the book.

PROJECT FUNDERS

Intellectual endeavours of this magnitude are not possible without financial resources. The Department of Science and Technology (DST) deserve our special thanks for their support of this project.

MISTRA FUNDERS

MISTRA would also like to acknowledge the donors who were not directly involved with this particular research project but who support the Institute, and make its work possible. They include:

- ABSA
- Airports Company of South Africa Limited (ACSA)
- Albertinah Kekana
- Anglo American Platinum
- Anglo Coal
- Aspen Pharmacare
- Batho Batho Trust
- Belelani Group
- Discovery
- Exxaro
- First Rand Foundation
- Friedrich-Ebert-Stiftung (FES)
- Goldman Sachs
- Harith General Partners
- Jackie Mphafudi
- Kumba Iron Ore
- National Institute for the
- Humanities and Social Sciences (NIHSS)
- Oppenheimer Memorial Trust (OMT)
- OSF - SA (Open Society Foundation for Southern Africa)

- Phembani Group
- Power Lumens Africa
- PEU
- Robinson Ramaite
- Royal Bafokeng Holdings
- South Africa Breweries
- Safika
- Shell South Africa
- Simeka
- Standard Bank
- Vhonani Mufamadi
- Yellowwoods

Contributors

Zamanzima Mazibuko, editor of this volume, is the Senior Researcher in the Knowledge Economy and Scientific Advancement Faculty at The Mapungubwe Institute for Strategic Reflection (MISTRA) in Johannesburg, South Africa. She obtained her MSc (Med) in Pharmaceutics cum laude and has published on nano-enabled drug delivery systems.

Samuel Adu-Gyamfi is a lecturer in the Department of History and Political Studies at the Kwame Nkrumah University of Science and Technology (KNUST), Ghana. His research focus is on evolutions in health, public health, and health policy, environment, policy in science and technology, traditional and integrative medicine research, as well as social and political development of Africa.

Miriam Di Paola is a PhD candidate at the University of the Witwatersrand and a Research Fellow at the Tricontinental Institute for Social Research. She has participated in international research projects and authored several publications on the South African labour market, labour migration, and on the contribution of nurses to public health.

Kenneth Juma is a researcher at the African Population and Health Research Centre, Kenya. Kenneth is a doctoral student in Clinical Epidemiology and Biostatistics at Makerere University, Uganda. He holds an Erasmus Master in Public Health in Disaster Settings from the University of Oviedo and Catholic University of Louvain, an MSc in Epidemiology, and a Bachelor of Science from the University of Nairobi.

Pamela A. Juma works as a health systems and policy research and capacity building consultant. Pamela holds a Master's in Community Health and Development, and a PhD in Nursing with a focus on Health Systems and Policy from the University of Ottawa, Canada.

Bill H. Kinsey holds three postgraduate degrees from Stanford University, including a PhD from Stanford's Food Research Institute. He has done extensive fieldwork on southern Africa, particularly in Zimbabwe. He is currently a Visiting Fellow at the African Studies Centre at Leiden University in The Netherlands.

Farai D. Madzimbamuto is an anaesthesiologist and associate professor at the University of Zimbabwe. Prof. Madzimbamuto is the Chair of the Department of Health Professions Education and a founding Chair of the Zimbabwe Association of Doctors for Human Rights.

Kaka Mudambo is a malariologist and public health specialist employed as the Focal Point/Regional Coordinator of the RBM Partnership to End Malaria for East, Central, Southern, and West Africa. Brigadier General (Dr) Mudambo is also the regional coordinator of the SADC 16 Member States Military Health Services (MHS), of which he was a founder member, and responsible for all Military Health programmes. He is a board member of the Malaria Elimination Eight (E8) and Chairperson of the E8 Board oversight committee (OC).

Steven Mufamadi is the founder and managing director of Nabio Consulting (Pty) Ltd, a start-up company that provides consulting services on nanotechnology, biotechnology, and pharmaceutics, since 2015. His PhD is in Pharmaceutics from University of the Witwatersrand, Johannesburg.

Sunanda Ray is a medical doctor and public health physician. She is also a Fellow of the Faculty of Public Health (UK) and is currently employed by the Department of Community Medicine, University of Zimbabwe College of Health Sciences, Harare, Zimbabwe. Dr Ray has 35 years' experience of working in public health in Zimbabwe, Botswana, and England and as an activist for social justice in health.

David Sanders is Emeritus Professor and founding Director of the School of Public Health at the University of the Western Cape, Cape Town, South Africa, and is a paediatrician qualified in Public Health. He was awarded an Honorary Doctorate by the University of Cape Town for his contribution to the global policy of Primary Health Care. He is a founder and currently Global Co-chair of the Peoples' Health Movement.

Nathaniel Umukoro is senior lecturer and head of the Department of Political Science and Public Administration, Edo University, Iyamho, Nigeria. He obtained a BSc degree from the University of Benin before proceeding to the University of Ibadan, Nigeria, where he obtained MSc, MA, and DPhil degrees.

Beth Vale is an independent researcher and writer. Her research interests span youth sex and body politics, nocturnal cities, health and illness, and the everyday production of sociality, power, and privilege in South African society. Dr Vale holds a DPhil in Social Policy and Intervention from Oxford University, an MA in Sociology from the University of Cape Town, and a BA Honours in Philosophy and Political Studies from Rhodes University.

Alex van den Heever presently holds the Chair of Social Security Systems Administration and Management Studies at the University of the Witwatersrand, Johannesburg. He is an adjunct professor and has a Master's degree in Economics from the University of Cape Town. He has published extensively in the field of health policy, the implementation and review of health public private partnerships, and the regulation of health systems.

Gerald Yonga is the President of the NCD Alliance in East Africa and a Visiting Professor at the NCD Research Thematic Unit, School of Medicine, University of Nairobi, Kenya. He is founder chair of the NCD Alliance Kenya, the East Africa NCD Alliance and the Africa NCD Alliances Network, and is a board member of the NCD Alliance (Global).

List of abbreviations

AAAS	American Association for the Advancement of Science
ACT	artemisinin-based combination therapy
ADCA	Alcoholic Drinks Control Act
AESA	Alliance for Accelerating Excellence in Science in Africa
AHIA	Advancing Healthcare Innovation in Africa
AHS	Africa Health Strategy
AIDA	Accelerated Industrial Development of Africa
AIM	Action and Investment to defeat Malaria
ALMA	African Leaders Malaria Alliance
AMS	aluminium-magnesium silicate
ANDI	African Network for Drugs and Diagnostics Innovation
ART	antiretroviral treatment
ARV	antiretroviral (drugs)
ASTIF	African Science, Technology and Innovation Fund
AU	African Union

BDP	Botswana Democratic Party
BITRI	Botswana Institute for Technology Research and Innovation
BMI	body mass index
BRICS	Brazil, Russia, India, China, South Africa
CA	communal area
CADRI	Capacity for Disaster Reduction Initiative
CARI	Coalition for African Research and Innovation
CBHI	community-based health insurance
CCHF	Crimean-Congo haemorrhagic fever
CCM	Chama Cha Mapinduzi
CEO	chief executive officer
CERF	Central Emergency Response Fund
CFR	case fatality rate
CHAG	Christian Health Association of Ghana
CHPS	community-based health planning and services
CHW	community health worker
CMS	Council for Medical Schemes
COHRED	Commission on Health Research Development
COPD	chronic obstructive pulmonary diseases
CPMR	Centre for Plant Medicine Research
CPP	Convention People's Party
CSHERCC	Civil Society Health Emergency Response Coordinating Committee
CSIR	Council for Scientific and Industrial Research
CT	computerised tomography
CUF	capillary ultrafiltration
CVD	cardiovascular disease
DALY	disability-adjusted life years
DELTAS	Developing Excellence in Leadership, Training and Science
DG	director-general
DID	Department of Infrastructure Development
DMHIS	District Mutual Health Insurance Scheme
DMP	Direction du Médicament et de la Pharmacie
DoH	Department of Health

DRC	Democratic Republic of Congo
DRG	diagnostic related grouper
DST	Department of Science and Technology
E8	Elimination 8
ECOWAS	Economic Community of West African States
EDA	Egyptian Drug Authority
EDL	essential drugs list
EED	environmental enteric dysfunction
EEOC	Ebola Emergency Operations Centre
EMS	emergency medical services
EOC	emergency operation centre
EPR	epidemic preparedness and response
EVD	Ebola virus disease
EWARN	Early Warning Alert and Response Network
FCMC	First Consultants Medical Centre
FCTC	Framework Convention on Tobacco Control
FDA	Food and Drug Administration
FMH	Federal Ministry of Health
GDP	gross domestic product
GOARN	Global Outbreak Alert and Response Network
GoZ	Government of Zimbabwe
GTFCC	Global Task Force on Cholera Control
GTS	global technical strategy
HA	height-for-age
HAART	highly active antiretroviral therapy
HIV/AIDS	human immunodeficiency virus and acquired immunodeficiency syndrome
HMI	health market inquiry
HOD	head of department
HPTDG	Health Professions Training and Development Grant
HRW	Human Rights Watch
ICDDR	International Centre for Diarrhoeal Diseases Research
ICT	information communication technology
ID	identification
IDC	Industrial Development Corporation

IHD	ischemic heart disease
INH	isoniazid
IHR	International Health Regulations
IMF	International Monetary Fund
IP	intellectual property
IPD	In-Patient Department
IPTp	intermittent preventive treatment in pregnancy
IRS	indoor residual spraying
IV	intravenous
JRC	Joint Research Centre
JRC-EURO	Joint Research Centre of the European Commission
KNUST	Kwame Nkrumah University of Science and Technology
LEAP	Livelihood Empowerment Against Poverty
LIC	low-income country
LLIN	long-lasting insecticide-treated bed nets
LMIC	low- and middle-income country
LNCPP	National Laboratory for the Control of Pharmaceutical Products
LSM	larval source management
MCO	managed care organisation
MDA	mass drug administration
MDC	Movement for Democratic Change
MDG	Millennium Development Goal
MERS-CoV	Middle East respiratory syndrome coronavirus
MLI	medium- to low-income
MLIC	medium- to low-income country
MMR	maternal mortality ratio
MoH	Ministry of Health
MOSASWA	Mozambique–South Africa–Eswatini
MPP	medicines patent pool
MSAB	Medical Schemes Amendment Bill
MSF	Médecins Sans Frontières
NAFDAC	National Agency for Food and Drug Administration and Control
NANOAFNET	Nanosciences African Network

NCAA	Nigerian Civil Aviation Authority
NCCE	National Commission for Civic Education
NCD	non-communicable disease
NDC	National Democratic Congress
NCDC	National Centre for Disease Control
NEMA	National Emergency Management Agency
NGO	non-governmental organisation
NHI	National Health Insurance
NHIB	National Health Insurance Bill
NHIF	National Health Insurance Fund
NHIP	National Health Insurance Policy
NHIS	National Health Insurance Scheme
NIC	Nanotechnology Innovation Centre
NLC	National Liberation Council
NM	nanometer
NMCP	national malaria control programme
NMEP	national malaria elimination programme
NP	nanoparticle
NPEP	Nanotechnology Public Engagement Programme
NPP	New Patriotic Party
NR	natural region
NRF	National Research Foundation
NT	National Treasury
NTSG	National Tertiary Services Grant
OCV	oral cholera vaccine
OHSC	Office of Health Standards Compliance
OOP	out-of-pocket
OPD	Out-Patient Department
PC	primary care
PCR	polymerase chain reaction
PES	provincial equitable share
Pf	Plasmodium falciparum
PHC	primary health care
PHEIC	public health emergency of international concern
PLG	poly(lactide-co-glycolide)
Pm	Plasmodium malariae
PMB	prescribed minimum benefit

PMHI	Private Mutual Health Insurance Scheme
PMTCT	prevention of mother-to-child transmission
Po	Plasmodium ovale
PS	permanent secretary
PSM	procurement and supply management
Pv	Plasmodium vivax
PZA	pyrazinamide
R&D	research and development
RA	resettlement area
RBM	Roll Back Malaria
RDT	rapid diagnostic test kit
RHD	rheumatic heart disease
RMoH	Rwanda Ministry of Health
RMP	rifampin
RPF	Rwandan Patriotic Front
RVF	Rift Valley fever
SAASTA	South African Agency for Science and Technology Advancement
SADC	Southern African Development Community
SAHPRA	South African Health Products Regulatory Authority
SAP	Structural Adjustment Programme
SARN	Southern Africa Regional Network
SARS	severe acute respiratory syndrome
SARS	South African Revenue Service
SBU	strategic business unit
SDG	Sustainable Development Goal
SDN	solid drug nanoparticle
SHI	social health insurance
SMEs	small and medium enterprises
SOE	state-owned enterprise
SSA	sub-Saharan Africa
SSNIT	Social Security and National Insurance Trust
STISA	Science, Technology and Innovation Strategy for Africa
TB	tuberculosis
TES	tax expenditure subsidy

THRiVE	Training Health Researchers into Vocational Excellence
TIA	Technology Innovation Agency
ToR	Terms of Reference
UFS	University of the Free State
UHC	universal health coverage
UK	United Kingdom
UN	United Nations
UN-IASC	United Nations Inter-Agency Standing Committee
UNCDA	Uganda NCD Alliance
UNICEF	United Nations International Children's Emergency Fund
USD	US dollars
VISET	Vendors Initiative for Social and Economic Transformation
WA	weight-for-age
WASH	water, sanitation and hygiene
WFP	World Food Programme
WH	weight-for-height
WHO	World Health Organization
Wits RHI	Wits Reproductive Health and HIV Institute
YLL	years of life lost
ZANU-PF	Zimbabwe African National Union-Patriotic Front
ZDHS	Zimbabwe Demographic and Health Survey
ZINWA	Zimbabwe National Water Authority
ZRDHS	Zimbabwe Rural Demographic and Health Survey
ZUNDAF	Zimbabwe United Nations Development Assistance Framework

Section One

Epidemics and Syndemics in Africa: Disease in Context

THIS FIRST SECTION OF THE BOOK provides a context for epidemics and health conditions in Africa. It initially offers a brief history of some of the world's deadliest epidemics, showing how far the global health status has come – from a time when an outbreak would cause millions of deaths to the present time when control of epidemics means mortality is limited. Although there has been great improvement in health conditions across the globe and in Africa, there remains a disproportionate burden of disease in sub-Saharan Africa. This section explores the reasons behind the imbalance and also offers alternative frameworks for understanding the prevalence of epidemics in Africa.

Chapter 1, which is the introductory chapter of the book, argues that epidemics do not occur in a context-free vacuum. Zamanzima Mazibuko shows how underlying structural drivers have rendered certain populations, especially African women, vulnerable to disease. This argument is further supported by Bill Kinsey's chapter, which describes how diseases often interact with one another and are exacerbated by the social, economic, environmental, and political situations of affected populations (Figure 1). This interrelationship is referred to as 'syndemics', and is drawn on throughout the book to help understand the extent to which social conditions and health are synergistic.

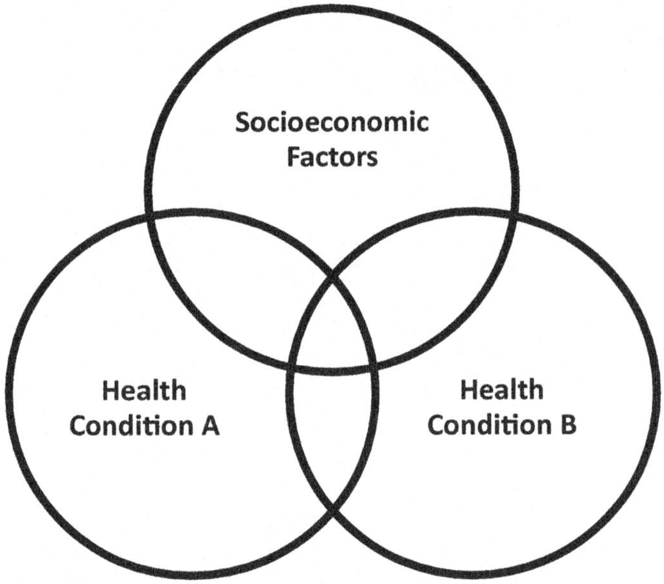

Figure 1: Syndemics Model

Chapter 1 also explores so-called 'zoonotic' diseases, namely those diseases which are transmitted between humans and animals. Mazibuko points to the World Health Organization's (WHO) call for greater resources, including research, to fight these emerging diseases, and warns of the danger of these becoming the diseases of the future. She argues for the importance of taking into account the factors that promote zoonotic diseases when analysing how best to counter epidemics and strengthen health care systems in Africa.

In Chapter 2, Kinsey uses the syndemics perspective and examines undernutrition in Zimbabwe to show the multifactorial issues that result in worsened health conditions. Kinsey argues for broader conceptual frameworks that take account of varied factors in order to better address health concerns.

This first section lays the foundation for the rest of the volume and for a comprehension of how and why the African continent is vulnerable to disease. The two chapters challenge conventional thinking and medical understanding to push for a more multifaceted understanding that acknowledges the context of illness on the continent. The authors argue that this syndemic approach will assist in the development of inclusive public health policies and will improve the probabilities of effective interventions.

ONE

Introduction

Epidemics and Health Systems in Africa

ZAMANZIMA MAZIBUKO

'Epidemics do not just happen.
They are not random events. They have histories.'
(Barnett & Whiteside, 2006: 65)

THESE WORDS ARE EMINENTLY true for epidemic outbreaks that have occurred in Africa. Often details of these outbreaks are presented without the relevant backdrop, or reference to the chains of preceding triggering and facilitative events and conditions. As De Waal (2017) notes, it is as if an epidemic disease 'simply arises from the miasmas of Africa's forests, in a context-free vacuum'. Africa's vulnerability to disease can be attributed to several factors which influence both the spread and prevalence of disease, as well as to the effectiveness or lack thereof of measures for prevention, reduction, or elimination (Fonn, 2018). These factors are a function of historical, political, environmental, and economic forces (Dzingirai et al., 2017; Fonn, 2018). It is important that the underlying foundation and structural drivers of Africa's vulnerability to diseases be stated clearly. Disease occurs commonly because of political and economic influences. These factors have a strong bearing on the way diseases are managed and controlled and on what happens to the affected populations (Mackey et al., 2014; De Waal, 2017; Dzingirai et al., 2017).

Historical interventions such as exclusionary urbanisation, in forcing certain populations out of their homes and displacing them into areas where they are vulnerable to disease, are described by Dzingirai and colleagues (2017), underpinning their argument: conditions that are ripe for the spread of disease among poor and marginalised people are commonly created by the state (through poor governance) and by the private sector (in its quest for accumulation and industrialisation). Poverty, low status, and inequality, together with forced migrations (Farmer, 2004), have been linked to vulnerability to infection.

Syndemics is a conceptual framework used to describe and understand the impact of the above phenomena by highlighting the effect of macro-level social factors on disease clustering, and the effects of this on both entire population groups as well as on individuals (Mendenhall et al., 2017). Adopting a syndemics approach, and so interrogating such phenomena, would enhance comprehension of the connection between disease and society. It would lead to a more exhaustive understanding of the foundational drivers of disease, and equip societies and decision-makers for their better prevention and control. Going further, mainstream medicine and its framework for disease, which is often preferred over alternative ways of understanding and practising medicine, should also be interrogated as these have implications for how treatment is given and, in turn, received.

This is the basis for the reasoning – now widely accepted – that efforts to counter outbreaks of disease and epidemics in sub-Saharan Africa need to be expanded beyond the biomedical approach. More valuable would be to integrate the biomedical approach with understanding and incorporating structural factors closely associated with susceptibility to disease.

It is important to emphasise that diseases do not occur in isolation. Diseases interact with one another, as well as with multiple social and/or environmental factors (Singer et al., 2017). Often, co-infection occurs with two or more pathogens and this affects the pathway of each infection, causing them to deviate from their natural courses (Corbett et al., 2003). This is commonly observed with HIV infections where exposure to other pathogens, particularly tuberculosis, exacerbates infections and increases transmission of both pathogens (Corbett et al., 2003). In recent years the burden of epidemics has been worsened by a significant increase in non-communicable diseases (NCDs) such as heart disease, stroke, cancer, and diabetes. Previously thought of as diseases of the more affluent, NCDs are on the rise in sub-Saharan Africa (Ezzati et al., 2018). Mental illness, which is often neglected, is another NCD that needs to be addressed. There is thus an increased risk of the interplay of diseases (both communicable and non-communicable); the impact of this interplay is aggravated by the social, economic, environmental, and political conditions in which a population finds itself (Sharma, 2017).

HISTORY OF EPIDEMICS IN THE WORLD AND IN AFRICA

Medical research, technology, and innovation have improved health across the globe. Throughout history, epidemics of diseases that are now (mostly) under control have caused the deaths of millions of people globally within short periods of time. Epidemic diseases, which can be viral or bacterial, are highly communicable and they rapidly infect large numbers within a population. The number of cases reported in one area is generally higher than expected (Newman, 2002; Wilke, 2017). Outbreaks of some of the worst and deadliest epidemics in history impacted permanently on the population at the time that they occurred (Pariona, 2018). One of the earliest recorded was the Antonine Plague, which killed about 2,000 people a day in Rome, totalling 5 million deaths over the period 165–180 AD (Wilke, 2017). The Plague of Justinian, which struck from 541–542 AD, is recorded as an epidemic in which the highest number of lives was lost, with an estimated 20–25 million deaths in the Roman Empire (Horgan, 2014; Wilke, 2017). This plague was carried across the world by rodents on trading ships, resulting in the infection spreading rapidly from China to Northern Africa and throughout the Mediterranean (Pariona, 2018).

Today, influenza is far from being the deadly disease it was a century ago when the Great Flu Epidemic of 1918 took its punishing toll. Spread by soldiers returning from around the world at the end of World War 1 (Wilke, 2017), it killed between 20 and 40 million people. Among other epidemics which caused millions of deaths were The Black Death (1334); the Cocolitzli Epidemic (1576); the Third Cholera Pandemic (1852–1860); the Third Plague Pandemic (1855); Typhus fever in the later years of World War 1 (1917); the Asian Flu Pandemic (1957); and lastly, the HIV/AIDS global pandemic (1960s–present), which has killed an estimated 25 million people and infected 65 million people since it was first reported in 1981 (Wilke, 2017).

A comprehensive history of epidemics in Africa is not easy to compile because data prior to 1970 is inadequate. Table 1 provides a summary of the epidemics in the WHO African region from 1970–2016, along with the number of times they have occurred. Cholera outbreaks have occurred the most frequently (476 times), closely followed by polio (439). Both diseases are now preventable, although a few cases of polio reappear now and then in inaccessible areas or conflict zones where efforts to vaccinate and to maintain disease surveillance are thwarted (Polio Eradication, 2017). Cholera outbreaks remain persistent in sub-Saharan African countries with areas in which conditions of poverty – contaminated water, inadequate sanitation, lack of hygiene – prevail (Lessler et al., 2018).

Table 1: Summary of outbreaks or epidemics reported in the WHO African region period 1970–2016 by known disease

Disease Total disease types: 38; unknown conditions: 2	Frequency
Acute Flaccid Paralysis	1
Acute Jaundice Syndrome	1
Acute Neurological Syndrome	3
Acute Respiratory Syndrome/Infection	7
Aflatoxicosis	1
Anthrax	46
Chickenpox	1

Chikungunya	13
Cholera	476
Crimean-Congo	20
Dengue Fever	23
Diarrhoeal Disease	42
Ebola	31
Fever with Jaundice (Febrile Icterus)	1
Hepatitis (undefined)	1
Hepatitis A	1
Hepatitis B	2
Hepatitis E	8
Influenza	17
Lassa Fever	28
Leishmaniasis	2
Leptospirosis	1
Malaria	60
Marburg Disease	12
Measles	75
Meningococcal Disease	99
MERS-CoV	3
Monkeypox	16
Nodding	1
O'nyong-nyong Fever	2
Plague	47
Polio	439
Rift Valley Fever	17
Schistosomiasis	1
Typhoid Fever	27
West Nile Fever	4
Yellow Fever	131
Zika Virus	1
Unknown Epidemic	96
Unknown Haemorrhagic Fever	22
Total	**1,779**

Source: WHO, 2016a

LEADING CAUSES OF DEATH IN AFRICA

In Africa, epidemics and endemics[i] remain a public health challenge. Over the years, a plethora of diseases have attacked the continent and some still persist, causing a significant burden of illness, disability, and mortality. These diseases range from periodic outbreaks, such as malaria and cholera, to endemics such as HIV, and even outbreaks of uncommon diseases like listeriosis.[ii] Of the ten leading causes of death in Africa as shown in Graph 1, the first seven are epidemics (infectious diseases and NCDs), the two afer those relate to maternal deaths, and the last stems from injury (in this graph, road injury) (WHO, 2016b).

If one puts the above statistics into context, it becomes clear that while infectious diseases remain the leading cause of death in Africa the mortality rates in this category are declining, while deaths from NCDs are on the increase. In 2015, out of a total of 9.2 million deaths in Africa, 5.2 million (56.5 per cent) were from infectious diseases. This figure was down from 5.7 million (61.4 per cent) in 2010. In 2015, the deadliest infectious diseases were lower respiratory diseases, HIV/AIDS, diarrhoeal diseases, tuberculosis, and malaria. NCDs accounted for 3.1 million deaths (33.5 per cent), which was an increase from 2.7 million (29.4 per cent) in 2010. The leading causes of death in this group were stroke, ischaemic heart disease, and cirrhosis of the liver. The last category, which is death caused by injury, accounted for 930,000 (10.1 per cent) in 2015, an increase from 841,750 (9.1 per cent) in 2010. These statistics show that, although infectious diseases are still the leading

---

i The constant presence of a disease or infectious agent in a particular geographic area or population group is an endemic. This differs from an epidemic in that epidemics are outbreaks of diseases that attack a large number of people at the same time and spread through one or several communities (http://www.fao.org/wairdocs/ilri/x5436e/x5436e04.htm).

ii A listeriosis outbreak took place in South Africa in 2017–2018 and has been the largest recorded globally (Chersich et al., 2018). The source of the outbreak was identified in March 2018, when traces of a food-borne pathogen – Listeria monocytogenes – were found in a food production facility that produces ready-to-eat processed meat products in Polokwane, Limpopo Province (Department of Health, 2018). It took more than a year for the source of the outbreak to be identified from the time of the first case being reported. By that time, approximately 950 cases of the disease had been reported, with a total of 180 deaths. In early April 2018, a total of 1,011 laboratory-confirmed cases of the disease had been documented, with a mortality rate of 28 per cent among cases with a known outcome (Dramowski et al., 2018).

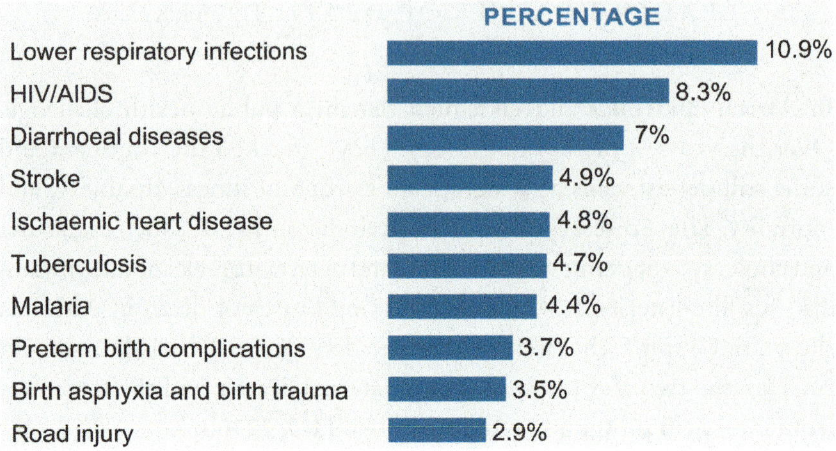

Graph 1: Top 10 leading causes of death in Africa

Source: WHO, 2016b

cause of death in Africa, the percentage of cases is decreasing, while that of NCDs (and to a lesser extent, injuries) is growing. This trend is projected to continue: expectations are that Africa will see a rise in NCDs previously associated with the developed world, especially with increasing urbanisation.

Health issues are a global concern. When compared to the rest of the world, however, sub-Saharan Africa carries a disproportionately high disease burden. In 2015, 90 per cent of global malaria cases and 92 per cent of malaria deaths (WHO, 2016b) were in the sub-Saharan region; and between 2000 and 2015, 83 per cent of global cholera deaths occurred in sub-Saharan Africa (Lessler et al., 2018). In addition, sub-Saharan Africa has some of the widest gender income disparities in the world and African women are among the poorest people. This makes African women even more vulnerable to infections (see UNESCO, 2015; UNESCO, 2017).

This book aims to explore the reasons behind this imbalance. It focuses on a selection of epidemics from which lessons can be drawn on the importance of a strong health system in preventing, detecting, and responding to calamitous diseases, thereby preventing outbreaks from becoming epidemics. The cases cited also highlight the effects of political interference and governmental neglect on the occurrence and prevalence of epidemics. They are a basis for policy analysis. Included in the selection, based on the immensity of its impact, is Ebola, which devasted the West African region in 2014–2016 and provided key lessons for addressing epidemics.

Sections in this book thus use specific cases of epidemic outbreaks to explore how structural and/or political-economic factors play a role in the vulnerability to disease. In their individual chapters the authors demonstrate that at the core of this vulnerability are weakened or weak health systems. At a second level, they show how the interactions between diseases and with socio-economic factors further exacerbate the occurrence and spread of epidemics – the implications being support for a multifaceted approach to addressing epidemics.

THE BURDEN OF EPIDEMICS

Together, communicable and non-communicable disease outbreaks cause millions of deaths throughout sub-Saharan Africa yearly (WHO, 2016b) and although the status of health care has improved over the years (WHO, 2014), the burden of disease still afflicts the continent disproportionately (WHO, 2016b). In many parts of the world, diseases that cause epidemics have been eradicated or brought under control (Tatem et al., 2006). Sub-Saharan Africa, however, continues to battle outbreaks and endemics. This is not due to either simple bad luck or purely medical reasons. Rosenberg (1992) argues that epidemic diseases should be regarded as a 'configuration' because of the structural and relational characteristics necessary for the transmission of pathogens between persons. This approach moves away from the notion of 'contamination', which is the reductive, technical mechanism of transmission; in that framework epidemics are not viewed as a result of the intersection of pathogens and social factors.

Africa was exploited by colonialists, with populations left in poverty and in areas of disrupted ecologies (De Waal, 2017; Dzingirai et al., 2017). Post-colonial development has not made sufficient progress in addressing inequalities and systemic underdevelopment (Obeng-Odoom, 2015), and nor have resilient health systems been established (Dzingirai et al., 2017; Olu, 2017).

Through a few case studies – the 2008–2009 cholera outbreak in Zimbabwe, the 2014–2016 Ebola outbreak in West Africa, the HIV endemic in South Africa, malaria in the Southern African Development Community (SADC) region, and the ever-increasing rise of NCDs on the continent – the authors show how structural drivers affect health services and outbreak response. The aim is to help inform health practitioners, policy makers, and researchers about ineffective as well as successful approaches to disease containment and health care provision in Africa.

Cholera in Zimbabwe: political-economic drivers

The worst cholera outbreak in Africa, which took place in Zimbabwe in 2008–2009, resulted in 98,531 recorded, suspected cases and 4,282 deaths (Youde, 2010). Political and economic choices, more than health-related decisions, were what led to this crisis. A combination of the large-scale collapse of the water and sanitation infrastructure, a weakened health care system, and a struggling economy contributed to the outbreak.

In the years prior to the outbreak, government policies and actions resulted in the disintegration of Zimbabwe's water and sanitation infrastructure and the incapacity of the health care system to provide even the most basic services (Muzondi, 2014). The ZANU-PF-led national government took over the municipal water supply from the opposition MDC party in order to weaken the latter's position and to gain more political power (Musemwa, 2008). The Zimbabwe National Water Authority (ZINWA) was established in 1998 to head the development and management of national water resources and associated infrastructure throughout the country (Bulawayo resisted the ZINWA takeover and had very few cholera cases). However, instead of reinforcing the country's water infrastructure and increasing access to clean and safe water, ZINWA was used as a political tool and a source of funding for ZANU-PF (Youde, 2010). Consequently, the water and sanitation infrastructure deteriorated and access to clean and safe water decreased considerably (Musemwa, 2008; Youde, 2010). The politicisation of water by ZANU-PF thus played a big role in creating conditions for the outbreak of cholera and for the disease to flourish.

A decade later, in 2018, Zimbabwe experienced another cholera outbreak. Questions arose regarding the reasons behind the recurrence of a preventable disease. What became apparent was that the water and sanitation infrastructure was still dilapidated, with burst pipes gurgling sewage onto the streets (Nyoka, 2018). Water supplies were contaminated by blocked sewers that had been left unattended (Mutsaka, 2018; Nyoka, 2018). The emergence and re-emergence of cholera in Zimbabwe goes far beyond the field of public health. It has to do with a government making political decisions which have a ripple effect, leaving its citizens dying from avoidable infections. This is discussed in more detail in Chapter 3.

Ebola in West Africa: weak health care systems

Weakened health systems underpinned the unprecedented spread of the Ebola virus in West Africa in 2014. Calamitous civil wars experienced by Guinea, Liberia, and Sierra Leone led to the collapse of those countries' health system infrastructures. They were left with the weakest health care system infrastructures in the world, with the lowest human development indices (WHO, 2000; UNDP, 2014). Therefore, when they were hit with the Ebola outbreak, their public health systems were not equipped to control it; in addition to this those countries also lacked a strong health care workforce. Table 2 depicts the poor health systems in the three countries and how they lacked the necessities required to manage an outbreak.

Table 2: State of health care systems in Guinea, Sierra Leone, and Liberia

Country	Health workforce density (per 10,000 population)	Number of hospital beds (per 10,000 population)	Per capita government expenditure on health per year (US$)
Guinea	< 1.5	3	9
Sierra Leone	2.2	4	12
Liberia	< 3.7	8	13
Minimum required to provide most basic health coverage	22.8	No standard	44

Source: Shoman et al., 2017; WHO, 2012; WHO, 2014

The Ebola outbreak further weakened these countries' health systems by significantly limiting the availability of health care workers, and decreasing financial resources and medical equipment (Save the Children, 2015). A study by Shoman et al (2017) revealed that Ebola claimed more lives among health care workers than any other viral haemorrhagic fever. Because health care workers were in direct contact with symptomatic patients, not only were they at a high risk of infection and death, but they were stigmatised and rejected by communities. This placed additional strain on the remaining health care workers; nurses became the frontline of the outbreak. An expert who was interviewed as part of the study reported that a lack of investment was the biggest problem: in training health care workers, in infrastructure, in supply chain management, and in community engagement (Shoman et al., 2017). The lack of resources meant that treatment of, and vaccinations against, other infectious diseases were not a priority, which led to additional outbreaks. People suffering from any condition other than Ebola were not provided with adequate health care. Moreover, the stigma attached to health care workers resulted in patients opting out of receiving treatment for other conditions out of fear of becoming infected by the health care workers (Shoman et al., 2017). Inevitably, the weakened health workforce enabled the Ebola virus to cause devastation in Guinea, Liberia, and Sierra Leone.

Nigeria, on the other hand, which managed to swiftly contain the 2014 Ebola outbreak, succeeded in rallying the country's health workforce to prevent the disease spreading. Expeditious and meticulous control measures were required to avert the disastrous effect of an Ebola outbreak on Nigeria's two large cities – Lagos, with approximately 20 million people, and Port Harcourt (> 1 million people). These were successfully implemented, thereby limiting the number of cases (Musa et al., 2016). The accurate and swift diagnosis of the index case by a female physician at the First Consultants Medical Centre (FCMC), Dr Ameyo Stella Adadevoh, allowed for implementation of a much more strategic process and for the virus across the country to be contained (DRASA, 2018). Health care workers were mobilised and deployed to carry out fast and thorough tracing of all potential contacts, to monitor all these contacts continuously, and immediately to confine potentially infectious contacts (Courage, 2014). The Ebola outbreak in Nigeria clearly illustrates the crucial role of the health workforce in containing a potential epidemic as detailed in Chapter 5.

Chronic diseases: implications for health systems

Non-communicable diseases (NCDs), such as cardiovascular diseases, cancers, diabetes, and chronic respiratory diseases, are predicted to become the leading cause of death in sub-Saharan Africa by 2030 (Marquez & Farrington, 2013). These diseases are caused by modifiable behaviours[iii] such as tobacco use, high consumption of alcohol, a sedentary lifestyle, and an unhealthy diet, which lead to metabolic changes like increased blood pressure, obesity, increased blood glucose levels, and increased levels of fat in the blood (Naik & Kaneda, 2015). As with the previously mentioned health conditions, prevalent social and economic conditions determine a population's vulnerability to NCDs and associated health outcomes (WHO, 2010a). The rise in cases of NCDs in low-income countries is influenced by such consequences of globalisation as inequitable trade and reckless marketing, as well as hasty and haphazard urbanisation (WHO, 2010b). NCDs are closely linked with poverty. Because they require long-term treatment, household costs that are related to health care increase, and often they result in the loss of breadwinners (WHO, 2010b). Here, too, women bear an inordinate share of the burden of disease. According to the WHO (2010b), women in less developed countries are extremely vulnerable to NCDs, which affect them in their productive years and often cause their premature death. Also, where household or family illness occurs it is women, disproportionately, who assume responsibility for care.

It has already been established that many African countries have weak health systems. Yet these systems need to be robust enough to address the above gender matters and to manage the growing and long-term burden of NCDs. The efficiency of a country's health system has commonly been evaluated by determining the number of patients who frequent its health facilities (Tapela, 2017). This measure has usually not considered chronic care, but has been based on short-term outbreaks of

iii Modifiable behaviours are commonly developed during adolescence or young adulthood, creating optimal conditions for NCDs later in life (Naik & Kaneda, 2015).

diseases (Tapela, 2017). The double burden of communicable diseases and NCDs indicates that an integrated approach to addressing health care is required. The prevention and management of NCDs is best implemented at the primary health care level (Temu et al., 2014), where symptoms of NCDs should be diagnosed and controlled.

The management of NCDs has suffered from the insufficient collection of data about successful NCD interventions in African primary health care settings. In developing countries one typically encounters weak mortality surveillance systems; underdeveloped information technology for data collection and analysis; insufficient data on health care quality, cost, and outcomes; and minimal technical capacity to conduct NCD surveillance (Krishnan, 2016). NCDs need to be recognised and prioritised as a public health issue, one that requires decision-makers, programme planners, and policy makers to develop and implement policies and strategies aimed at managing these illnesses.

HIV/AIDS was described as a 'long-wave disaster' by Barnett and Blaikie (1991) long before antiretroviral therapy (ART) was widely available.[iv] ART became increasingly available in parts of Africa in the mid-2000s, and this changed the course of the illness. By the end of 2009, 37 per cent of people who required ART in sub-Saharan Africa were receiving treatment, compared with only 2 per cent in 2002 (Nixon et al., 2011). In 2016, 60 per cent of people living with HIV in East and Southern Africa (an estimated 11.7 million) were on ART (UNAIDS, 2017) and the number of AIDS-related deaths dropped from 760,000 in 2010 to 420,000 in 2016 (UNAIDS, 2018.). The introduction of ART has gradually shifted HIV from being a terminal disease to a chronic illness and this has implications for the capacity of health systems already burdened with other infectious diseases. While people with HIV are now living far longer lives, they are also having new experiences of disability caused by HIV and its related conditions (Nixon, et al., 2011). These range from physical, mental, and intellectual disabilities to sensory impairments (Banks et al., 2017). The side-effects of medications may also lead to a range of impairments,

iv Barnett and Blaikie (1991) described HIV/AIDS as a long wave disaster because it did not take the form of a distinct event, with recognisable stages and responses, and because it was a long time in the making. This was before antiretroviral therapy was widely available.

including musculoskeletal weakening, which may restrict activities (e.g. self-care, mobility) and access to health care (Banks et al., 2017).

This chronicity of HIV thus requires health systems designed to efficiently implement HIV-specific programmes while integrating other components of the health system (Doherty et al., n.d.). Disease-specific programmes, such as providing access to ART and the prevention of mother-to-child HIV transmission programmes (PMTCT), can only be effective with the support of a strong health system (Doherty et al., n.d.). It is imperative that in the context of the under-resourced and overburdened health systems that are found widely in Africa, the routines of care for chronic patients are given due consideration.

STRENGTHENING HEALTH CARE SYSTEMS

Building resilient health systems should be a priority in all African countries. This is borne out by the two different cases discussed above: one a crisis situation, the other chronic. The West African Ebola outbreak demonstrated how a crisis is exacerbated by a weak health system. The care for patients living with chronic NCDs or HIV exposes how an under-resourced health system affects the health outcomes of patients. According to Olu (2017), the health sector encompasses all activities – in the home, the community, and the formal health sector – that directly enhance health outcomes. Extensive investment into these elements by national governments would contribute towards building a strong health system. Corruption, delayed responses, and neglecting to assign funding to fundamental and strategic national entities are all barriers to well-functioning systems. If strong health systems are to be realised, national governments need to be proactive. They need to allocate appropriate budgets to health care, not just to address outbreaks but also to meet the day-to-day health needs of their citizens. Governments need to do the necessary strategising and planning. And the plans that are made then need to be implemented. This is the underlying message of this book and of all its contributors.

Another theme that runs through this book is the role of the international community (including regional networks and other African initiatives), historically and currently. Organisations such as the

United Nations (UN), World Health Organization (WHO), and African Union (AU) all bear a responsibility and a humanitarian obligation not only to intervene when disaster strikes, but also to assist with building resilient health systems. Often delayed responses to public health emergencies of international concern (PHEICs) result in the spread of disease, a situation that could have been contained had there been a more timely response. National governments as well as the international community need to rethink short-term the mobilisation of resources. This mobilisation generally occurs when an emergency calls for it (Hoffman & Silverberg, 2018), but this leaves no resources for building stronger public health systems at a national level, which is the first-line defence against potential outbreaks (Sands, 2017). Greater investment in long-term health system preparedness is required instead of quick solutions. The latter may be effective at the time but the health system will remain vulnerable to epidemics. Dzau and Sands (2016) argue that in fact greater investment in mitigating infectious-disease risks should be seen as a fundamental part of responding to PHEICs, and that outbreaks should not only be viewed as a health issue, but as human dignity and economic security issues as well.

Furthermore, Dzau and Sands (2016) argue that acting early in managing outbreaks and building strong defences limits the spread of epidemics. In fact it is much more cost-effective, they conclude, to invest in preparedness than to spend in response. An investment in systems of effective surveillance and contacts at the local level, for instance, would help to identify cases of infections, leading to timely responses (André et al., 2017). In many parts of Africa epidemics and disease outbreak surveillance systems are weak, which makes it difficult to determine the true scope of the problem. If surveillance systems were to be upgraded, this would allow for quicker identification of diseases in communities and the immediate implementation of primary control measures (Wassilak et al., 2017).

According to the WHO, 'a well-functioning health system working in harmony is built on having trained and motivated health workers, a well-maintained infrastructure, and a reliable supply of medicines and technologies, backed by adequate funding, strong health plans and evidence-based policies' (WHO, 2016c). These factors are what the

WHO refers to as Health System Building Blocks. There are six main ones. They are: (1) service delivery, (2) health workforce, (3) information, (4) medical products, vaccines and technologies, (5) financing, and (6) leadership and governance (WHO, 2010). Strengthening the health system (Table 3) involves 'improving the six health system building blocks and managing their interactions in ways that achieve more equitable and sustained improvements across health services and health outcomes' (WHO, 2007: 4).

Table 3: The health system building blocks

Building blocks	Priority areas addressed	Intended results
Service delivery	Packages of essential health services; service delivery models; health infrastructure; management of health services; safety and quality of care; and demand creation for health care.	Ensuring delivery of effective, safe, and quality personal and non-personal health interventions to those who need them, when and where needed, with minimum waste of resources.
Health workforce	Ministry of health to show leadership for human resource issues through developing good policies and investment plans, advocacy, setting of norms and standards and intelligence. Creating, motivating, and sustaining a productive workforce tackling the priority health needs.	Ensure that the health workforce works in ways that are responsive, fair, and efficient to achieve the best health outcomes possible for the available resources and circumstances. Availability of health workforce in sufficient numbers, skills mix, fairly distributed; competent, responsive, and productive to ensure access to care of good quality.
Information	Facility and population-based information and surveillance systems; research; global standards; tools; quality and completeness of data.	Availability of a well-functioning health information system that ensures the production, analysis, dissemination, and use of reliable and timely information on health determinants, health systems performance and health status.

Building blocks	Priority areas addressed	Intended results
Medical products, vaccines and technologies	Norms, standards, policies, and regulations; reliable procurement, distribution, and rational use of essential medicines and technologies; equitable access; quality.	Ensure equitable access by all citizens to essential medical products, vaccines, and technologies of assured quality, safety, efficacy, and cost-effectiveness, and their scientifically sound and cost-effective use.
Financing	National health financing policies; tools and data on health expenditures; costing.	Raise adequate funds for health in ways that ensure people can use needed services, and are protected from financial catastrophe or impoverishment associated with having to pay for services; efficient use of resources.
Leadership and governance	Health sector policies; harmonisation and alignment; oversight and regulation; co-ordinating prioritisation of investments.	Ensuring strategic policy frameworks exist and are combined with effective oversight, monitoring and evaluation; stewardship role at all levels; coalition building, the provision of appropriate regulations, incentives and accountability; co-ordinating operational planning.

Source: WHO, 2007

As illustrated in Table 3, each building block is important and contributes to strengthening the health system in different ways. All these components work to ensure effective policy and regulation, enough resources (including human resources), and distribution of care (WHO, 2010). It should be remembered that the building blocks are not exhaustive or all-inclusive; additional sectors are often needed to contribute to a resilient health system.[v] Communicable diseases and NCDs both have an adverse impact on national income, productivity,

v Health outcomes are determined by several factors beyond the health system. These include socio-economic conditions, patterns of consumption associated with food and communication, demographic patterns, learning environments, the cultural and social fabric of societies, and socio-political and economic changes, including commercialisation and trade and global environmental change (Kumar & Preetha, 2012). This means sectors involved in the mentioned factors are implicated in ensuring good health outcomes.

and household expenditure, and both, therefore, influence economic growth (Temu et al., 2014). Health is a crucial factor in economic development, which in turn must be based on an all-encompassing approach that takes cognizance of the role of health in development (Temu et al., 2014). Although the building blocks are a good place to start to monitor and evaluate developments in the health system, the blocks exclude the social and economic factors that affect health outcomes. An analysis of the building blocks would therefore benefit from a syndemics approach, which considers all the interactions of the various factors and their effect on health conditions. Further considerations should be the origins of diseases and the impact of their pathogenesis on future epidemic outbreaks (an adjunct focus of the book) as a fundamental part of preventing and managing epidemics.

Understanding the origins of diseases is a necessary aspect of strengthening health systems; this knowledge will affect how diseases are handled and how epidemic outbreaks are contained. The origins of the disease-related epidemics highlighted in this volume – malaria, cholera, HIV, and Ebola – and of the NCDs discussed have implications for how the epidemics are managed and/or treated. Investigation into pathogenesis assists in developing preventive measures against disease, as well as treatments and/or vaccines.

Epidemic diseases with ancient histories, like malaria, which possibly dates back to 3200 BC (Institute of Medicine, 2004), and cholera, which may go as far back as the 1st century (History.com, 2018), have been studied for many years and their transmission and symptoms are understood. Continuous research improves their management. With malaria, mosquitoes (female Anopheles species) ingest malaria parasites from infected humans through bites and then subsequently transmit malaria parasites when feeding on an uninfected host (Cox, 2010). Therefore, the most widely promoted (and consequently adhered to) malaria preventive measure is the introduction of insecticide-treated nets in malaria-endemic regions; this measure also takes into account that the female Anopheles species bites at night (Malaria Consortium, 2016). With cholera, toxic strains of Vibrio cholerae – a bacterium found naturally in aquatic ecosystems – are responsible for transmission (Reidl & Klose, 2002). Infections occur through ingesting contaminated water and/or improperly prepared food, resulting in the cholera toxin that causes cells lining the intestines to release increased amounts of water, leading to diarrhoea and rapid loss of fluids and electrolytes (Reidl & Klose, 2002; History.com, 2018).

Infectious diseases like HIV/AIDS and Ebola, on the other hand, are not in the category of ancient and well-understood diseases. HIV was first identified in 1981 (Sharp & Hahn, 2011) and Ebola in 1976 (WHO, 2018a). Unlike ancient eminent diseases, HIV and Ebola are far from being under control and they still require extensive research. Of the two, however, HIV has received the most attention over the years. Numerous research and development (R&D) programmes have been put in place and funding made available for learning more about this virus, searching for treatments, and thus decreasing mortality rates. Ebola has not yet received the same attention. The 2014 outbreak in West Africa caught the region and the international community off guard and unprepared. The epidemic had many people questioning the origin and rapid transmission of the outbreak. Various other 'new' diseases such as Lassa fever, Legionnaires' disease, and hantavirus pulmonary syndrome have been identified in the last few decades (Morse, 1995), and archaic diseases (such as tuberculosis, malaria and cholera – including new strains) are re-emerging. This is an indication that the battle against infectious diseases, known and unknown, is far from over.

THE FUTURE OF EPIDEMICS IN AFRICA

Rapid human development, involving a series of changes in demographics and the environment, has led to the emergence of new infectious diseases and also the re-emergence of old ones (Mackey et al., 2014). Migration, travel, and trade are all common features of human development, but increased globalisation has led to their acceleration and escalation. With the growth of the human population and intercontinental migration, and with the mingling and breeding of different animal species for trade, comes the transferral of microorganisms to new locations (Brown, 2004) and thereby prospects for triggering infectious diseases. Industrialisation and the invasion of wildlife terrain have led to an increase in the contact between humans and animals (Mackey et al., 2014). An example of this can be seen in the study 'Wildlife–human interactions: from conflict to coexistence in sustainable landscapes', which aimed to analyse wildlife–human interactions in Indian multi-use landscapes (and one Norwegian landscape) with a view to understanding conflicts and sustaining mechanisms of co-existence (Nandini, 2010). The shift in the ecology of human–animal interactions caused by an expanding, increasingly urbanised global population has given rise to zoonoses (or zoonotic diseases). These are infectious diseases that can be transmitted between animals and humans (CDC, 2017). Examples are anthrax, Rift Valley fever, Ebola, Chikungunya, Zika, and severe acute respiratory syndrome (SARS), but many others are also in evidence (Halliday et al., 2015; Kemunto et al., 2018).

In a recent study by the World Health Organization the top diseases listed that are likely to cause severe epidemics in the current global health landscape are zoonotic diseases (WHO, 2018b), the reason being the lack of efficient drugs and/or vaccines to counter a public health emergency (WHO, 2018b). The following diseases were identified for accelerated research and development:

- Crimean-Congo haemorrhagic fever (CCHF)
- Ebola virus disease and Marburg virus disease
- Lassa fever
- Middle East respiratory syndrome coronavirus (MERS-CoV) and severe acute respiratory syndrome (SARS)
- Nipah and henipaviral diseases
- Rift Valley fever (RVF)
- Zika
- Disease X

ZOONOTIC DISEASES AROUND THE GLOBE

Some infectious diseases that have historically affected humans, such as the Black Death (or bubonic plague) and typhoid fever, are of zoonotic origin. The continuing growth of human populations and urbanisation since prehistoric times has led to ensuing invasions of human populations by increasing numbers of different pathogens

(Dobson & Carper, 1996). Bubonic plague is a disease of wild rodents in which the bacterial pathogen, Yersinia pestis, is spread by infected fleas (Duncan & Scott, 2005). Typhoid fever is caused by the bacterial pathogen Salmonella, which is commonly found in chickens, pigs, turkeys, and cows, although various species of wildlife – birds, reptiles, frogs, and fish – can also carry the bacteria (Meštrović, 2018). Meat and other animal products that have not been cooked thoroughly are the main vehicle of transmission (Meštrović, 2018). Emerging diseases are incessant and the emergence of diseases such as AIDS, SARS, avian influenza (H5N7), swine flu (H1N1), West Nile virus, and Ebola (EVD) is an indication that infectious diseases remain a global threat. In regions where the population is dense and expanding rapidly, the risk of these diseases spreading is increased.

Over 1,400 species of parasites and microbes have been recorded as pathogenic in humans and more than 60 per cent of these originate from animals (Cleaveland et al., 2001). As has been mentioned above, humans are susceptible to a greater number of pathogens as a result of animal domestication and increased proximity to wildlife. Closer proximity means that person-to-person transmission, subsequent to animal-to-human transmission, is increased.

Globalisation has also had a large impact on the rate, pattern, and geography of epidemics (Morand, 2018). It is estimated that endemic zoonotic diseases will cause more than 2.2 million human deaths and 2.4 billion cases of illness annually (Kemunto et al., 2018). More than 25 per cent of the disability-adjusted life years (DALY) lost to infectious diseases in low-income countries has been reported to be attributable to zoonotic diseases, compared to less than one per cent in high-income countries (Grace et al., 2012). As with other conditions on the disease spectrum, investigations into zoonotic diseases have neglected zoonoses affecting the most vulnerable and disease-burdened populations (Fèvre, 2015; Kemunto et al., 2018). Knowing about and understanding the advent of zoonotic diseases, including their pathogenesis and development, symptoms, diagnostics, and treatment, as well as how to approach their prevention and control, is crucial to managing diseases and containing epidemic outbreaks.

Africa is especially vulnerable to zoonotic diseases, in part because of its rapid population growth. The continent is projected to have the largest population increase globally, with an estimated 1.68 billion people in 2030, which is 42 per cent larger than the 2015 population of 1.19 billion, which is 25 per cent of the world's population (Canning et al., 2015; UN, 2015). It is estimated that in 2060 Africa's population will have grown to 2.8 billion people. The risk in Africa of encountering, contracting, and subsequently spreading infections through population movement and resultant concentration in urban areas is already high, and it is increasing.

This pattern gives zoonotic pathogens continual opportunity to infect new hosts and for new hosts to interact with each other and transfer their infections. Specifically, zoonotic diseases are transmitted to humans in these ways: through scratches or bites from animals; through the ingestion of the meat of an infected animal or dairy products made from the milk of infected animals; by inhaling dust that has been exposed to the faeces, urine, or milk of an infected animal; or through the bite of an infected rodent or flea (Moleko, 2018).

The proximity of humans to animal habitats and animals to human habitats has stemmed from ecological disturbances such as deforestation, soil erosion, desertification, and wetland degradation. This has resulted in animals and humans having to move into unfamiliar areas and to share those spaces. The origins of zoonotic diseases are often historical – a result of decisions made decades ago – allowing conditions to develop that predispose certain populations to transmission. In this book, the impact of politics and socio-economic factors on vulnerability to disease comes up again and again. It is particularly evident with zoonotic diseases.

Going back to the Ebola outbreaks, it is worth considering how this zoonotic disease is suspected to have been transmitted to humans in the first place, and to link this process back to the book's various themes. This focus holds important lessons for the containment, if not prevention or eradication, of epidemics.

Ebola is likely to have emanated from human interface with wild animals (Edwards et al., 2018). The outbreak in West Africa is believed to have come from the hunting and handling of fruit bats (Leroy et al., 2009; Hogenboom, 2014; Rewar & Mirdha, 2014). Bats have been reported to host more viruses than any other mammal (Kupferschmidt, 2017). Transmission occurs from bites, scratches, bodily fluids, tissue, and excrement. Moreover, bats can infect other animals like gorillas and chimpanzees through their faeces or fruit they have touched (Hogenboom, 2014) and these primates can in turn infect humans through touch. Bats are ideal hosts for the Ebola virus because it is not lethal to them, unlike for humans and non-human primates (Hogenboom, 2014).

The practice of hunting and eating bats is common in parts of certain African countries, as either a necessary source of food or, for some, a luxury (Osborne, 2014; Kamins et al., 2015). However, the methods of capturing bats expose hunters and vendors to infections. Hunters often do not wear protective gear such as gloves when capturing and handling live bats, thereby leaving themselves vulnerable to scratches or bites (Osborne, 2014). Sometimes hunters shoot bats, leaving their blood exposed, posing an increased risk of infection to themselves and vendors (Kamins et al., 2015). Further, consuming bat-bitten fruits, or palm sap that has been tasted by fruit bats, can have detrimental health implications (Rajasekaran, 2018).

The case study of Ebola in the Democratic Republic of Congo (DRC) points to directions for future containment. In the DRC, between May and November 2007, an Ebola outbreak affected more than 260 people and caused 186 deaths (Leroy et al., 2009). A study by Leroy et al (2009) identified a mammoth annual fruit bat migration up the Lulua River (a tributary of the Kasai River, near the city of Kananga) prior to the outbreak. Particularly large numbers of fruit bats had migrated into the outbreak area, nesting in the fruit and palm trees of a deserted plantation. These bats were hunted in their numbers by villagers, likely causing the Ebola outbreak (Leroy et al., 2009). The outbreak raises issues of how humans have come to inhabit the same space and consume the same foodstuff as virus-infested creatures.

Bats are driven closer to human habitats by increased biological activity resulting from changes in ecological networks, including in deep forests (Rajasekaran, 2018). Field (2009) reported that deforestation, which is one of the consequences of oil palm planting, changes the feeding behaviour of bats. It causes them to focus on cultivated crops – thus bringing the interface between bats, humans, and livestock closer. As a case in point, fruit bats in Bangladesh were the most likely transmitters of the Nipah virus to human hosts via urine on the date fruit of planted palm trees (Luby et al., 2009). As the erosion of their habitats and food resources continues and they are forced to settle in unnatural habitats as a result (Rajasekaran, 2018), bats become increasingly malnourished – resulting in an increased viral load – Nipah virus, rabies, and other infectious viruses are then transmitted by these animals.

A similar phenomenon can be witnessed in the spread of Lassa fever in West Africa, this time with rodents as virus reservoirs. The socio-economic dynamics and civil wars in Liberia and Sierra Leone changed housing and agricultural patterns. This led to population displacement to dreadful, overcrowded living conditions, including in urban areas, and to refugee migrations, resulting in expanded human interface with rodents (Dzingirai et al., 2017). These are but a few examples of the impact of demographic, economic, political, and environmental changes on the way in which humans and animals interact and the resultant spread of zoonotic pathogens.

DIAGNOSIS AND CONTROL OF ZOONOTIC DISEASES

Despite the fact that zoonotic diseases are rife across tropical regions, particularly in Africa, they are seldom recognised, studied, and incorporated into plans for managing epidemic outbreaks (Halliday et al., 2015).

Zoonotic diseases present with general symptoms such as fever, headache, fatigue, and joint or muscle aches. Because these are common in a wide range of infectious diseases in tropical regions, it is difficult to differentiate them clinically (Halliday et al., 2015). Clinicians are more likely to diagnose patients with malaria or typhoid fever, which have similar symptoms to zoonotic diseases. Patient Zero in the 2014 Ebola outbreak in Nigeria was initially misdiagnosed with malaria, but thanks to Dr Ameyo Stella Adadevoh, who subsequently correctly diagnosed the patient with Ebola, the outbreak was contained (DRASA, 2018).

Apart from the difficulty in differentiating zoonoses from other common diseases, the inability of various health system infrastructures to contain disease becomes apparent (Kock et al., n.d). The lack, in some African countries, of laboratories in which to conduct diagnostics adds to the challenge of detecting zoonotic diseases (Kock et al., n.d). Furthermore, in these areas it is often not common practice to seek urgent medical care; people tend to seek out health care only in the late stages of the infection (Halliday et al., 2015), which is when the detection of pathogens is more difficult. Thus, seeking health care once the infection is advanced decreases the chances of accurate diagnosis (Halliday et al., 2015).

These diagnosis issues are mostly found in low-income countries with adverse socio-economic conditions. Whereas globally various zoonoses have been contained, in many African countries they remain prevalent and disproportionately affect people who are not only at high risk of pathogen exposure, but also have little access to adequate primary health care (Kock et al., n.d). This perpetuates misdiagnosis and underdiagnosis of zoonotic (and other) diseases in Africa, leaving poor communities, which most likely were forced into the areas they occupy, with the burden of these diseases.

A MULTI-LAYERED APPROACH TO ADDRESSING EPIDEMICS

If one is truly to address epidemic diseases, one needs to go beyond interventions that are made during an outbreak. Rather, a more complex approach linked to the roots of the epidemic needs to be taken. Epidemics are more than just a problem of public health. Ultimately, they are a political and social problem and, as such, they require political solutions from both the international community and national governments. Moreover, because epidemics can result from a multitude of influences, addressing them requires a dynamic approach from diverse sectors of society. Stakeholders who should be included would be drawn from those involved in public health, medicine, environmental science, animal health, food safety, economics, and public policy.

This book takes a multidisciplinary and transdisciplinary research approach, and the experts contributing to the research project reflect this. They are medical doctors, community health specialists, public health specialists, health science researchers, pharmaceutical scientists, policy analysts, sociologists, and historians. The chapters are divided into four sections, exploring (1) epidemics and syndemics: disease in context; (2) contending with epidemics and health systems in Africa; (3) contending with chronic conditions in African health systems; and (4) the future of health systems in Africa.

The overall aim of the book is to enhance understanding of the intricacies of epidemiological issues such as the reasons why epidemics occur and the underlying structural drivers that allow them to reoccur. Some of the reasons lie in political actions and the effect of public funds being redirected away from essential services. The insights in this volume can thus be used as a basis for improved planning and implementation of national and international strategies. The epidemical diseases discussed and the locations of the outbreaks examined were selected for the lessons that can be drawn from them. In putting forward these case studies, the book aims to assist with developing policies that will provide an enabling environment for the development of strong health systems.

Chapter 2 presents the conceptual framework of syndemics, which is an alternative to more conventional, mainstream epidemic frameworks. The concept of syndemics offers a nuanced approach to understanding the social and economic conditions in which diseases occur and the factors which exacerbate their impact. The author uses chronic undernutrition (stunting) in Zimbabwe – the extent and gravity of this syndrome are not duly appreciated – to highlight how specific local environmental conditions encourage stunting. The chapter highlights the importance of putting diseases and medicine in context in order to understand their subtleties, including that they do not occur in isolation. This also applies to epidemic outbreaks and their containment. An understanding of the underlying structural drivers that make certain populations vulnerable to diseases will inform strategies to contain such diseases.

Cholera is a preventable and treatable disease yet outbreaks still occur periodically. Chapter 3 uses the 2008–2009 outbreak of cholera in Zimbabwe (and references the 2018 outbreak) to demonstrate the crucial role political factors play in creating conditions for an epidemic outbreak. The economic crisis in Zimbabwe and the collapse of the health system and water and sanitation facilities there – and these factors being undergirded by political agendas – made conditions ripe for a prolonged outbreak and the deaths of thousands of people. This example illustrates how resources in a country can be politicised to gain power, with disregard for the well-being of citizens.

A lack of preparedness for outbreaks is common across various African countries. Many have weak health systems, which means that avoidable diseases are not being contained timeously. When regions suffer extreme floods or experience unusually high temperatures, the risk of a malaria outbreak is omnipresent, yet many health systems have not been strengthened sufficiently to anticipate or contain an outbreak. However, over the years actions have been taken in southern Africa to control outbreaks (and these attempts are continuously strengthened). Cross-border and regional collaborative efforts have led to the implementation of interventions to advance southern Africa's transition to malaria elimination. Chapter 4 describes successful strategies applied within the SADC region and emphasises the importance of networks in successful campaigns.

Creating strong health systems includes improving surveillance systems to help with the early detection of disease. There has been solid progress in this regard, albeit with occasional relapses. Nigeria's successful containment of the Ebola virus can be attributed to the meticulous diagnosis of the index patient by Dr Adadevoh, followed by a quick response and action and deployment of a health care workforce. There is a stark contrast between Nigeria's response strategies and those of the three other West African countries that experienced Ebola in the same period. Nigeria's response reveals the importance of good and decisive leadership when faced with an outbreak. This success story is analysed and systematically presented in Chapter 5.

Increasing chronicity on the continent places a different type of burden on national health systems to that which comes with epidemic outbreaks. NCDs, which are on the rise in sub-Saharan Africa, require long-term treatment and monitoring. Given the predicted increase in NCDs, and given health systems that are under-resourced, an evaluation of long-term care within the African setting is required. Health systems are now required to manage these chronic conditions and at the same time be prepared to contain any possible epidemic outbreaks. With HIV gradually becoming a chronic illness with similar implications to those of NCDs, health systems need to encompass long-term care. Lessons on addressing chronic illnesses can be drawn from examining care practices in health facilities, communities, and homes in response to long-term HIV. Health workers play a big role in rolling out disease-specific programmes such as the distribution of ART; thus they are central to the efficiency of health systems. Health care workers and nurses, who are at the frontline of both epidemic outbreaks and chronic care, are also expected to carry out administrative duties and these duties can outweigh their health care responsibilities. Chapters 6, 7 and 8 address these issues in depth.

Some of the building blocks of a strong health system are addressed in the last three chapters and in the book's conclusion. One of the building blocks is ensuring equitable access to medical products, vaccines, and technologies of assured quality, safety, efficacy, and cost-effectiveness, and their scientifically sound and cost-effective use. Nanotechnology has been shown to provide cost-effective, safe, and efficient treatment of certain diseases. Chapter 9 explores the potential of this technology to provide solutions to the need for accessible and efficient treatment. Contaminated water, which causes diarrhoeal diseases, can be treated using nanotechnology. Nanotechnology can therefore be used for both treatment and prevention.

Another important building block is financing the health system. The national health insurance (NHI) schemes in Rwanda and Ghana, which are reviewed in Chapter 10, serve as case studies of the implementation of national health insurance in Africa. Chapter 11 explores South Africa's health system, and assesses proposals for the anticipated NHI against current health needs. The chapter also explores South Africa's readiness to deal with known epidemics and those of the future. With all the common diseases the South African health system has to contend with, there are other conditions, like listeriosis, for example, which occur less frequently, and mental health, which is a neglected area. Both have exposed cracks in the SA health system. While the NHI is a ray of hope for people who anticipate that it will be a solution to equitable access to health care, there is also fear that it will worsen a health system that might be described, as the author of Chapter 11 demonstrates, as dysfunctional. The state of the South African health system and also what is required to enhance its capabilities is outlined in this chapter.

In shining a light on some of the structural and political drivers of disease in Africa, the authors of this compilation go some way to demystifying the notion that the continent must always bear an inevitable burden of sickness, manifesting from time to time in a well-publicised epidemic. The argument is made that a syndemic, multifaceted approach to disease is required in order to expose these drivers and to suggest how solutions might be developed. Through varied case studies, the authors demonstrate that Africa can only combat the epidemics that plague it by developing a different narrative about sickness, one that offers a wider, deeper understanding of the context for disease. Multiple lessons are drawn for the effective control and elimination of epidemics on the continent, and so are the limitations of the panicked, short-term responses that diseases in Africa so often evoke. The contributors, who are drawn from across sub-Saharan Africa, make a convincing case for the fact that we already have the knowledge and capacity to save the many lives lost to epidemics in Africa.

REFERENCES

André, A. M., Lopez, A., Perkins, S., Lambert, S., Chace, L., Noudeke, N., Fall, A. & Pedalino, B. 2017. 'Frontline field epidemiology training programs as a strategy to improve disease surveillance and response'. *Emerging Infectious Diseases*, 23, Supplement.

Banks, L. M., Zuurmond, M., Ferrand, R. & Kuper, H. 2017. 'Knowledge of HIV-related disabilities and challenges in accessing care: Qualitative research from Zimbabwe'. PLOSONE, 12 (8), DOI: E0181144.

Bardosh, K. L., Scoones, J. C., Grace, D., Kalema-Zikusoka, G., Jones, K. E., De Balogh, K., Waltner-Toews, D., Bett, B., Welburn, S. C., Mumford, E. & Dzingirai, V. 2017. 'Engaging research with policy and action: What are the challenges of responding to zoonotic disease in Africa?'. *Philosophical*

Transactions of the Royal Society of London, Series B, Biological Sciences, 372 (1725), 20160172.

Barnett, T. & Blaikie, P. 1991. AIDS in Africa: It's Present and Future Impact. London: Belhaven and London: John Wiley & Sons.

Barnett, B. & Whiteside, A. 2006. *AIDS in the Twenty-First Century: Disease and Globalization*. New York: Palgrave Macmillan.

Brown, C. 2004. 'Emerging zoonoses and pathogens of public health significance – an overview'. *Revue Scientifique et Technique (International Office of Epizootics)*, 23 (2), 435–442.

Canning, D., Raja, S. & Yazbeck, A. S. 2015. Africa's Demographic Transition: Dividend or Disaster? Washington, DC: World Bank.

Center for Disease Control and Prevention (CDC). 2017. 'Zoonotic diseases'. CDC, https://www.cdc.gov/onehealth/basics/zoonotic-diseases.html, accessed 16 January 2019.

Chersich, M. F., Scorgie, F., Rees, H. & Wright, C. Y. 2018. 'How climate change can fuel listeriosis outbreaks in South Africa'. *South African Medical Journal*, 108 (6), 453–454.

Child, K. 2018. 'Polony can come back into your diet: Listeria outbreak declared over'. *Timeslive*, https://www.timeslive.co.za/news/south-africa/2018-09-03-polony-can-come-back-into-your-diet-listeria-outbreak-declared-over/, accessed 20 November 2018.

Cleaveland, S., Laurenson, M. K. & Taylor, L. H. 2001. 'Diseases of humans and their domestic mammals: Pathogen characteristics, host range and the risk of emergence'. *Philosophical Transactions of the Royal Society of London, Series B, Biological Sciences*, 356, 991–999.

Corbett, E. L., Watt, C. J., Walker, N., Maher, D., Williams, B. G., Raviglione, M. C. & Dye, C. 2003. 'The growing burden of tuberculosis: Global trends and interactions with the HIV epidemic'. *American Medical Association Archives of Internal Medicine*, 163 (9), 1009–1021.

Courage, K., H. 2014. 'How did Nigeria quash its Ebola outbreak so quickly?'. *Scientific American*, https://www.scientificamerican.com/article/how-did-nigeria-quash-its-ebola-outbreak-so-quickly/, accessed 26 October 2018.

Cox, F. E. G. 2010. 'History of the discovery of the malaria parasites and their vectors'. *Parasites & Vectors*, 3 (1), 5 DOI: 10.1186/1756-3305-3-5.

Crouth, G. 2018. 'New food-safety regulations imminent'. IOL. https://www.iol.co.za/pretoria-news/new-food-safety-regulations-imminent-13904842, accessed 20 November 2018.

De Waal, A. 2017. 'Famine and Epidemic Disease in Africa', in Schiffrin, A.

& Lugalambi, G. (eds.) *African Muckraking*. Johannesburg: Jacana Media.

Department of Health, Republic of South Africa. 2018. 'Listeriosis outbreak situation report 11 June 2018'. Pretoria.

Dobson, A. P. & Carper, E. R. 1996. 'Infectious diseases and human population history'. *BioScience*, 46 (2), 115–126.

Doherty, T., Jackson, D., Zarowsky, C. & Sanders, D. n.d. 'HIV and health systems in Southern Africa'. *UWC HIV and AIDS Research Centre*, https://www.hivaids-uwc.org.za/docs/wrking_paper_no_1.pdf, accessed 9 December 2018.

Dramowski, A., Lloyd, L. G., Bekker, A., Holgate, S., Aucamp, M., Reddy, K. & Finlayson, H. 2018. 'Neonatal listeriosis during a countrywide epidemic in South Africa: A tertiary hospital's experience'. *South African Medical Journal*, 108 (10), 818–827.

DRASA Health Trust, 2018. 'Dr. Ameyo Stella Adadevoh'. DRASA, https://www.drasatrust.org/dr-adadevoh/, accessed 26 October 2018.

Duncan, C. J. & Scott, S. 2005. 'What caused the black death?'. *Postgraduate Medical Journal*, 81, 315–320.

Dzau, V. J. & Sands, P. 2016. 'Beyond the Ebola battle – winning the war against future epidemics'. *New England Journal of Medicine*, 375 (3), 203–204.

Dzingirai, V., Bukachi, S., Leach, M., Mangwanya, L., Scoones, I. & Wilkinson, A. 2017. 'Structural drivers of vulnerability to zoonotic disease in Africa'. *Philosophical Transactions of the Royal Society*, B 372: 20160169.

Edwards, S. J. L., Norell, C. H., Illari, P., Clarke, B. & Neuhaus, C. P. 2018. 'A radical approach to Ebola: Saving humans and other animals'. *The American Journal of Bioethics*, 18 (10), 35–42.

Ezzati, M., Pearson-Stuttard, J., Bennett, J. E. & Mathers, C. D. 2018. 'Acting on non-communicable diseases in low- and middle-income tropical countries'. *Nature*, 559, 507–516.

Farmer, P. 2004. 'On suffering and structural violence: Social and economic rights in the global era', in Farmer, (ed.) *Pathologies of Power: Health, Human Rights, and the New War on the Poor*. Los Angeles: University of California Press.

Fèvre, E. 2015. 'Zoonoses in Africa'. *Zoonotic & Emerging Disease Group*, http://www.zoonotic-diseases.org/zoonoses-in-africa/, accessed 15 January 2019.

Field, H. E. 2009. 'Bats and emerging zoonoses: Henipaviruses and SARS'. *Zoonoses and Public Health*, 56, 278–284.

Fonn, S. 2018. 'Want to solve complex health issues? Train scholars to think across disciplines'. *The Conversation*, https://theconversation.com/want-to-solve-complex-health-issues-train-scholars-to-think-across-disciplines-92188, accessed 26 October 2018.

Grace, D., Gilbert, J., Randolph, T. & Kang'ethe, E. 2012. 'The multiple burdens of zoonotic disease and an ecohealth approach to their assessment'. *Tropical Animal Health and Production*, 44 (1), S67–73.

Halliday, J. E. B., Allan, K. J., Ekwem, D., Cleaveland, S., Kazwala, R. R. & Crump, J. A. 2015. 'Endemic zoonoses in the tropics: A public health problem hiding in plain sight'. *Veterinary Record,* 176, 220– 225.

History.com. 2018. 'Cholera'. History, https://www.history.com/topics/inventions/history-of-cholera, accessed 22 January 2019.

Hoffman, S. J. & Silverberg, S. L. 2018. 'Delays in global disease outbreak responses: Lessons from H1N1, Ebola, and Zika'. *American Journal of Public Health*, 108 (3), 329–333.

Hogenboom, M. 2014. 'Ebola: Is bushmeat behind the outbreak?'. *BBC News*, https://www.bbc.com/news/health-29604204, accessed 15 January 2019.

Horgan, J. 2014. 'Justinian's Plague'. *Ancient History Encyclopedia,* https://www.ancient.eu/article/782/justinians-plague-541-542-ce/, accessed 22 January 2019.

Institute of Medicine (US) Committee on the Economics of Antimalarial Drugs. 2004. 'A brief history of malaria', in Arrow, K. J., Panosian, C. & Gelband, H. (eds.) *Saving Lives, Buying Time: Economics of Malaria Drugs in an Age of Resistance*. Washington DC: National Academies Press.

Kamins, A. O., Rowcliffe, J. M., Ntiamoa-Baidu, Y., Cunningham, A. A., Wood, J. L. N. & Restif, O. 2015. 'Characteristics and risk perceptions of Ghanaians potentially exposed to bat-borne zoonoses through bushmeat'. *EcoHealth,* 12, 104–120.

Kemunto, N., Mogoa, E., Osoro, E., Bitek, A., Njenga, M. K. & Thumbi, S. M. 2018. 'Zoonotic disease research in East Africa'. *BMC Infectious Disease*, 18, 545.

Kock, R., Croft, S., Dixon, M., Fletcher, C., Good, L., Guzman, J., Heymann, D., Liyanage, R., Mckeever, D., McNerney, R., Peeling, R., Moran, M., Pfeiffer, D., Waage, J. & Wu, L. n.d. 'Prioritising the need for new diagnostics, medicine, vaccines and management practices of zoonoses which have significant impact in the developing world'. DFID Zoonoses Report 6.

Korsten, L. 2018. 'What led to world's worst listeriosis outbreak in South Africa'. *The Conversation,* https://theconversation.com/what-led-to-worlds-worst-listeriosis-outbreak-in-south-africa-92947, accessed 20 November 2018.

Krishnan, A. 2016. 'Sustainable surveillance systems for noncommunicable diseases in developing countries: A bridge too far or a realizable dream?'. *International Journal of Non-Communicable Diseases*, 1 (2), 53–54.

Kumar, S., & Preetha, G. 2012. 'Health promotion: an effective tool for global health.' *Indian Journal of Community Medicine: Official publication of Indian Association of Preventive & Social Medicine, 37* (1), 5–12.

Kupferschmidt, K. 2017. 'Bats really do harbor more dangerous viruses than other species'. *Science Mag*. https://www.sciencemag.org/news/2017/06/bats-really-do-harbor-more-dangerous-viruses-other-species?r3f_986=https://www.google.com/, accessed 15 January 2018.

Leroy, E. M., Epelboin, A., Mondonge, V., Pourrut, X., Gonzalez, J., Muyembe-Tamfum, J. & Forment, P. 2009. 'Human Ebola outbreak resulting from direct exposure to fruit bats in Luebo, Democratic Republic of Congo, 2007'. *Vector-Borne and Zoonotic Diseases*, 9 (6), 723–728.

Lessler, J., Moore, S. M., Luquero, F. J., McKay, H. S., Grais, R., Henkens, M., Mengel, M., Dunoyer, J., M'bangombe, M., Lee, E. C., Djingarey, M. H., Sudre, B., Bompangue, D., Fraser, R. S. M., Abubakar, A., Perea, W., Legros, D. & Azman, A. S. 2018. 'Mapping the burden of cholera in sub-Saharan Africa and implications for control: An analysis of data across geographical scales'. *The Lancet*, 391 (10133), 1908–1915.

Luby, S. P., Gurley, E. S. & Jahangir Hossain, M. 2009, 'Transmission of human infection with Nipah Virus'. *Clinical Infectious Diseases*, 49, 1743–1748.

Lund, C. 2018. 'Why Africa needs to start focusing on the neglected issue of mental health'. *The Conversation*. https://theconversation.com/why-africa-needs-to-start-focusing-on-the-neglected-issue-of-mental-health-91406, accessed 21 November 2018.

Mackey, T. K., Liang, B. A., Cuomo, R., Hafen, R., Brouwer, K. C. & Lee, D. E. 2014. 'Emerging and reemerging neglected tropical diseases: A review of key characteristics, risk factors, and the policy and innovation environment'. *Clinical Microbiology Reviews*, 27 (4), 949–979.

Malaria Consortium. 2016. 'Malaria prevention through insecticide treated nets'. Malaria Consortium Advocacy Brief, London, UK.

Marquez, P. V. & Farrington, J. L. 2013. 'The challenge of noncommunicable diseases and road traffic injuries in sub-Saharan Africa: An overview'. Washington, DC: The World Bank.

Mendenhall, E., Kohrt, B. A., Norris, S. A., Ndetei, D. & Prabhakaran, D. 2017. 'Noncommunicable disease syndemics: Poverty, depression, and diabetes among low-income populations'. *The Lancet*, 389, 951–963.

Meštrovi, T. 2018. 'Salmonella sources of infection'. News: Medical Life Sciences, https://www.news-medical.net/health/Salmonella-Sources-of-Infection.aspx, accessed 22 January 2019.

Moleko, N. 2018. '5 diseases we can get from animals'. *Health24*, https:// https://www.health24.com/News/Public-Health/5-diseases-we-can-get-from-animals-20171215, accessed 16 January 2019.

Morand, S. 2018. 'Biogeography and the ecology of emerging infectious diseases', in Morand, S. & Figuié, M. (eds.) *Emergence of Infectious Diseases: Risks and Issues for Societies.* Versailles: Quae, pp 13-33.

Morse, S. S. 1995. 'Factors in the emergence of infectious diseases'. *Emerging Infectious Diseases*, 1 (1), 7–15.

Moyo, S. & Rehle, T. 2017. 'Accelerating tuberculosis control: Addressing the structural drivers of the disease in South Africa'. *Human Sciences Research Council*, https://www.hsrc.ac.za, accessed 18 November 2018.

Musa, E., Nasidi, A., Shuaib, F., Nguku, P. M. & Vaz, R. G. 2016. 'Nigeria's Ebola outbreak response: Lessons for future epidemic preparedness'. *Archives of Medicine*, 8 (6), DOI: 10.21767/1989-5216.1000171.

Musemwa, M. 2008. 'The politics of water in post-colonial Zimbabwe, 1980-2007'. Seminar paper presented at the African Studies Centre, University of Leiden, The Netherlands, 19 June 2008.

Mutsaka, F. 2018. 'Zimbabwe declares cholera outbreak after 20 deaths'. *Medical Press.* https://medicalxpress.com/news/2018-09-zimbabwe-declares-cholera-outbreak-deaths.html, accessed 27 November 2018.

Muzondi, L. 2014. 'Urbanization and service delivery planning: Analysis of water and sanitation management systems in the city of Harare, Zimbabwe'. *Mediterranean Journal of Social Sciences*, 5 (20), DOI: 10.5901/mjss.2014.v5n20p2905.

Naik, R. & Kaneda, T. 2015. 'Noncommunicable diseases in Africa: Youth are key to curbing the epidemic and achieving sustainable development'. *Population Reference Bureau: Policy Brief*, https://www.medbox.org/sz-studies-reports/noncommunicable-diseases-in-africa-youth-are-key-to-curbing-the-epidemic-and-achieving-sustainable-development/preview?, accessed 21 November 2018.

Nandini, R. (ed.) 2010. *Current Conservation Special:* Wildlife-Human Conflict, 4 (4), https://www.currentconservation.org/, accessed 16 January 2019.

Newman, M. E. J. 2002. 'Spread of epidemic disease on networks'. *Physical Review*, E 66, 016128.

Nixon, S. A., Hanass-Hancock, J., Whiteside, A. & Barnett, T. 2011. 'The increasing chronicity of HIV in sub-Saharan Africa: Re-thinking "HIV as a long-wave event" in the era of widespread access to ART'. *Globalization and Health,* 7 (41), 1–5.

Nyoka, S. 2018. 'Zimbabwe's cholera emergency: "Stench of sewage" in Harare'. *BBC Africa,* https://www.bbc.com/news/world-africa-45546699, accessed 7 November 2018.

Obeng-Odoom, F. 2015. 'The social, spatial, and economic roots of urban inequality in Africa: Contextualizing Jane Jacobs and Henry George'. *American Journal of Economics and Sociology*, 74 (3), 550–586.

Olu, O. 2017. 'Resilient health system as conceptual framework for strengthening public health disaster risk management: An African viewpoint'. *Front Public Health*, 5, 263, DOI: 10.3389/fpubh.2017.00263

Osborne, H. 2014. 'Ebola outbreak: Why do people eat bat meat?'. *International Business Times*, https://www.ibtimes.co.uk/ebola-outbreak-why-do-people-eat-bat-meat-1469295, accessed 15 January 2018.

Pariona, A. 2018. 'The 10 worst epidemics in history'. *World Atlas*, https://www.worldatlas.com/articles/the-10-worst-epidemics-in-history.html, accessed 11 December 2018.

Polio Eradication Global Eradication Initiative. 2017. 'Could this little girl become Africa's last case of polio?'. http://polioeradication.org/news-post/could-this-little-girl-become-africas-last-case-of-polio/, accessed 11 December 2018.

Rajasekaran, G. 2018. 'Where bats are sacred and bat meat is eaten, health communication on Nipah is lacking'. *The News Minute*, https://www.thenewsminute.com/article/where-bats-are-sacred-and-bat-meat-eaten-health-communication-nipah-lacking-81931, accessed 15 January 2019.

Reidl, J. & Klose, K. E. 2002. 'Vibrio cholerae and cholera: Out of the water and into the host'. *FEMS Microbiology Reviews*, 26 (2), 125–139.

Rewar, S. & Mirdha, D. 2014. 'Transmission of Ebola virus disease: An overview'. *Annals of Global Health*, 80 (6), 444–451.

Rosenberg, C. E. 1992. 'Explaining Epidemics', in *Explaining Epidemics and Other Studies in the History of Medicine*. Cambridge: Cambridge University Press.

Sands, P. 2017. 'The first line of defense against outbreaks is to finance pandemic preparedness at a national level'. *The World Bank*, http://blogs.worldbank.org/health/first-line-defense-against-outbreaks-finance-pandemic-preparedness-national-level, accessed 28 November 2018.

Sands, P., Mundaca-Shah, C. & Dzau, V. J. 2016. 'The neglected dimension of global security – a framework for countering infectious-disease crises'. *New England Journal of Medicine*, 374, 1281–1287.

Save the Children. 2015. 'A wake-up call: Lessons from Ebola for the world's health systems', https://www.savethechildren.net/sites/default/files/libraries/WAKE%20UP%20CALL%20REPORT%20PDF.pdf, accessed 27 November 2018.

Sharma, A. 2017. 'Syndemics: health in context'. *The Lancet*, 389, 10072.

Sharp, P. M. & Hahn, B. H. 2011. 'Origins of HIV and the AIDS Pandemic', in Bushman, F. D., Nabel, G. J & Swanstrom, R. (eds.): *Cold Spring Harbor Perspective in Medicine,* New York, Cold Spring Harbor Laboratory Press.

Shoman, H., Karafillakis, E. & Rawaf, S. 2017. 'The link between the West African Ebola outbreak and health systems in Guinea, Liberia and Sierra Leone: A systematic review'. *Globalization and Health*, 13 (1), DOI: 10.1186/s12992-016-0224-2.

Singer, M., Bulled, N., Ostrach, B. & Mendenhall, E. 2017. 'Syndemics and the biosocial conception of health'. *The Lancet*, 389, 941–950.

Tapela, N. 2017. 'Africa must reboot its health systems to cope with non-communicable diseases'. *The Conversation,* http://theconversation.com/africa-must-reboot-its-health-systems-to-cope-with-non-communicable-diseases-77773, accessed 26 November 2018.

Tatem, A. J., Rogers, D. J. & Hay, S. I. 2006. 'Global Transport Networks and Infectious Disease Spread'. *Advances in Parasitology*, 62, 293–343.

Temu, F., Leonhardt, M., Carter, J., & Thiam, S. 2014. 'Integration of non-communicable diseases in health care: Tackling the double burden of disease in African settings'. The Pan African Medical Journal, 18, 202. DOI: 10.11604/pamj.2014.18.202.4086.

UNAIDS. 2017. 'Ending AIDS: Progress towards 90-90-90 targets'. UN AIDS.

UNAIDS. 2018. 'AIDS info'. UNAIDS, http://aidsinfo.unaids.org/, accessed 9 December 2018.

United Nations (UN). 2015. 'Population 2030: Demographic challenges and opportunities for sustainable development planning'. *UN Department of Economic and Social Affairs*, New York.

United Nations Development Programme (UNDP). 2014. 'Human Development Index. Report on human development 2014'. *United Nations Development Programme,* http://hdr.undp.org/en/content/table-1-human-development-index-and-its-components, accessed 26 November 2018.

UNESCO. 2015. 'EFA Global Monitoring Report'. www.unesco.org, accessed

11 December 2018.

UNESCO. 2017. 'Gender Equality in SSA. Innovative Programmes, visible results'. UNESCO, Paris France. www.unesco.org, accessed 11 December 2018.

Wassilak, S. G. F., Williams, C. L., Murrill, C. S., Dahl, B. A., Ohuabunwo, C. & Tangermann, R. H. 2017. 'Using acute flaccid paralysis surveillance as a platform for vaccine-preventable disease surveillance'. *The Journal of Infectious Diseases*, 216 (S1), S293–298.

Wilke, M. 2017. 'The 10 deadliest epidemics throughout history'. *News24*, https://www.health24.com/Medical/infectious-diseases/News/the-10-deadliest-epidemics-throughout-history-20170928, accessed 11 December 2018.

World Health Organization (WHO). 2000. *The World Health Report 2000 – Health Systems: Improving Performance*. Geneva: World Health Organization.

World Health Organization (WHO). 2007. 'Everybody's business: Strengthening health systems to improve health outcomes: WHO's framework for action'. WHO Press, World Health Organization, Geneva, Switzerland.

World Health Organization (WHO). 2010a. 'Equity, social determinants and public health programmes'. Geneva: World Health Organization.

World Health Organization (WHO). 2010b. The WHO Global status report on noncommunicable diseases (Chapter 2). https://www.who.int/nmh/publications/ncd_report2010/en/, accessed 9 December 2018.

World Health Organization (WHO). 2014. 'Atlas of African Health Statistics'. *WHO African Health Observatory and Knowledge Management*, 1, 1–181. DOI::10.1007/s13398-014-0173-7.2.

World Health Organization (WHO). 2015. 'WHO publishes list of top emerging diseases likely to cause major epidemics'. WHO, https://www.who.int/medicines/ebola-treatment/WHO-list-of-top-emerging-diseases/en/, accessed 22 January 2019.

World Health Organization (WHO). 2016a. 'Mapping the risk and distribution of epidemics in the WHO African region: a technical report'. *WHO/AFRO Library Cataloguing – in – Publication Data.* WHO Regional Office for Africa: Brazzaville, Congo.

World Health Organization (WHO). 2016b. 'Global health estimates 2015: Deaths by cause, age, sex, by country and by region, 2000–2015'. December. www.who.int/entity/healthinfo/global...disease/GHE2015_Deaths_

Global_2000_2015.xl, accessed 9 December 2018.
World Health Organization (WHO). 2016c. 'Health systems: key expected results'. WHO website: http://www.who.int/healthsystems/about/progress-challenges/en/, accessed 20 November 2018.
World Health Organization (WHO). 2018a. 'Ebola virus disease: Key facts'. WHO, https://www.who.int/news-room/fact-sheets/detail/ebola-virus-disease, accessed 22 January 2019.
World Health Organization (WHO). 2018b. 'List of blueprint priority diseases'. WHO, https://www.who.int/blueprint/priority-diseases/en/, accessed 22 January 2019.
Youde, J. 2010. 'Don't drink the water: Politics and cholera in Zimbabwe'. *International Journal*, 65 (3). *Democracy Assistance* (Summer), 687–704.

TWO

Syndemics, Food Security, Health, and Local Environments

Chronic Undernutrition in Zimbabwe

Bill H. Kinsey

Of the millions of children living in Africa, more than 38 per cent suffer from chronic undernutrition (stunting) (WHO, 2006). In 2011 stunting affected at least 165 million children worldwide (Black, 2012). One of the short-term consequences of this pattern is that more than one-fifth of all mortality for children aged under five is related to stunting. Among the longer-term consequences are that stunted children suffer lasting cognitive defects, go through fewer years of schooling and exhibit poorer performance while in school; they experience more severe consequences of common infections, and grow up to manifest lower economic productivity in their adult lives (Black, 2012).

Stunting presents a significant public health challenge due to increased morbidity and mortality over the life course. The scale of the stunting problem is global, and chronic undernutrition is frequently referred to as an epidemic. For reasons explored in this chapter, the common understanding of epidemics does not fit well with the near universal presence of undernutrition[i] in sub-Saharan Africa. First, there has been no outbreak; stunting is omnipresent and the casualties it claims far exceed those of conventional epidemics. Yet its presence has been under appreciated. Second, the conditions that favour undernutrition tend to be related to specific local environmental conditions; leaving such an environment reduces risks and the risks are not transmitted upon relocation. Third, current evidence suggests that stunting and its accompanying physiological changes cannot be considered a disease; rather it is a syndrome with multiple signs and conditions pointing to one or more medical abnormalities (Prendergast & Humphrey, 2014).

The syndemics model of health, as most recently elaborated by Singer et al. (2017), centres on the biosocial complex, comprising interacting diseases and the social/environmental factors that heighten the negative effects of disease interaction. This approach creates a new perspective on the conventional understanding of diseases as distinct entities, separate from other diseases and independent of the social contexts in which they occur. In the syndemics model multiple factors interact synergistically in important ways and have a significant impact on the health of individuals and entire populations. As Singer et al. emphasise, the syndemics approach specifically explores why some diseases cluster and investigates the pathways through which they interact biologically in individuals and within populations and thus increase their overall burden. An added focus is the ways in which socio-economic environments, particularly conditions of inequality and injustice, contribute to disease clustering and interaction, as well as to vulnerability.

This chapter explores the relationship between worsening child nutrition and underlying socio-economic indicators, using Zimbabwe as a primary case. Through a syndemics framework, the chapter highlights the correlates between nutritional status and the setting of rural households. It then spotlights environmental, demographic, and socio-economic factors and their challenges to health. It broadens the debate about food security and

---

i *Undernutrition* as used here refers to chronic undernutrition, or stunting, a much more narrowly delimited concept than malnutrition, which embraces both overnutrition and the dual burden of a spectrum extending from starvation to obesity.

improving nutritional status through an encounter between conventional wisdom on food supply and broader biomedical understandings. In Zimbabwe, the mean prevalence of stunting over decades is high. The deterioration in a child's nutritional status begins very soon after birth (and perhaps before) and continues at least until its second birthday. This pattern, which is common across Africa, is leading to a deepening recognition that the first 1,000 days of life – from conception to the second birthday – are absolutely vital in shaping a child's biosocial trajectory for the rest of its life. Limited evidence of catch-up growth, either physical or cognitive, reinforces the unique importance of this early period of life.

Recently there has been a growing shift away from identifying nutritional status exclusively with food intake and towards a developing recognition that with broader conceptual frameworks the policy implications might differ strikingly. The recognition that undernutrition is a multifactorial problem has also strengthened a trend towards convergence between biomedical and social science researchers. It is now widely accepted that nutritional status depends not only on the intake of nutrients, but also upon non-nutrient food attributes that affect nutrition (such as cleanliness and freshness of foodstuffs), publicly provided goods (sewage, potable water, electricity, nutritional and health services, education, and the like), and privately provided inputs (such as the time and care taken to prepare food and look after children). Although closely related, food security and nutritional status are not the same things. It is here that a syndemic perspective can assist to draw together what have previously been separate disciplinary strands.

The remainder of the chapter is structured in seven sections. The first sets out the scale of the chronic undernutrition problem in Africa and points out the challenges posed by its coexistence with food security. The next section serves to break the assumed link between food intake and nutritional status. Then the trajectories of child nutrition in Zimbabwe are detailed, at both macro- and micro-levels. In the following sections, attention turns to an examination of the relationship between nutritional status and indicators of welfare, at both household and at per-capita levels. The concluding section recaps the theme of a complex nutritional syndemic, and suggests policy dimensions that need to be addressed if nutritional interventions are to become more effective.

THE PARADOX OF CHRONIC UNDERNUTRITION WITH FOOD SECURITY IN AFRICA

The shorthand for chronic undernutrition is stunting, defined as a delay in linear growth due to a failure to thrive.[ii] While the determinants of stunting are complex, the factors most commonly associated with impaired linear growth include poverty – manifested in households' low socio-economic status, inadequate food supply, repeated episodes of infection in infants, poor domestic hygiene, and maternal health before, during and after pregnancy (WHO, 2014).

Stunting is associated not only with increased morbidity and mortality over the life course, but also with a lifetime of negative economic and social consequences. Globally stunting affects at least 165 million children annually (WHO, 2014). Nearly 40 per cent of children in Africa and Asia suffer from stunting. The scale of undernutrition in Africa is staggering – it has been estimated that some 58 million children aged under five years are stunted (UNICEF, WHO & World Bank, 2012). Research shows that poor nutritional outcomes in childhood are linked to a lifetime of negative economic and social consequences: impaired development, compromised immunity, reduced energy levels, infection and disease, diminished educational performance, reduced productivity, and decreased prospects of moving out of poverty (Alderman, 1990; Hoddinott & Kinsey, 2006). There are also suggestions that stunting may be a transgenerational phenomenon; children who were stunted in childhood grow up to have stunted children of their own. Indeed, the adversities consequent upon stunting – the multiple pathological changes marked by linear growth retardation, increased morbidity and mortality, and reduced physical, neurodevelopmental and economic capacity – have led to stunting being characterised as a syndrome (Prendergast & Humphrey, 2014). And these impacts at the individual level are multiplied many times over to create adverse national consequences. Hence, the complexities of stunting can best be understood through a syndemics framework.

ii The technical definition of stunting is having a height-for-age (HA) index score more than two standard deviations (z-scores) below the median of WHO's international child growth standards (UNICEF, 2013; WHO, 2007).

The prevalence of stunting among children aged fewer than five years in Africa ranges from a low of 10 per cent to some 60 per cent. Only nine of the 54 African countries are estimated to be on course to meet global targets on nutrition. Because of methodological controversies, however, even these prevalence figures may be too low. Recent work suggests, for example, that the number of children globally suffering from severe acute malnutrition, or wasting,[iii] may be as high as 110 million instead of the 17–19 million usually quoted. Table 1 compares the mean prevalence of stunting for rural and urban children across Africa with patterns elsewhere in the world.

Table 1: Stunting prevalence (%) in children under five years of age by area of residence, 2009–2015*

	Urban (%)	Rural (%)
Least-developed countries	29	41
Sub-Saharan Africa	26	41
Eastern & Southern Africa	29	40
West & Central Africa	25	41
South Asia	33	42
Latin America & the Caribbean	13	26
Global	21	35

Source: UNICEF Global Databases, Stunting Disparities, 2016.
*Based on the most recent year available.

The concept of food security has continuously evolved since the term was first used at the 1974 World Food Conference. The definition almost universally used today, however – 'Food security exists when all people, at all times, have physical and economic access to sufficient, safe and nutritious food that meets their dietary needs and food preferences for an active and healthy life' (FAO, 2002) – still focuses on supply issues and food quality. Interpretations vary, of course, but there is an implicit assumption that once access to food is assured the world's nutritional problem is solved.

iii Low weight-for-age, a form of undernutrition more directly linked to inadequate food supplies or quality than is stunting.

For decades, development practitioners believed that the key to improving nutritional status in Africa lay in boosting food security to provide a nutritionally adequate diet. Observations about the millions of undernourished people living in Africa usually became a call for increasing food supply through increasing agricultural productivity or supplying more food aid.

Development economists have tended to focus on undernutrition in one of two ways. In the first, they have sought statistical evidence to examine the relationship between nutrition and income. Over some 30 years, a growing body of literature has examined the interactions among nutritional status in low-income countries (LICs) and nutritional intake and household income. Recommendations on how to improve nutrition have been made based on empirical studies of food expenditure systems at the household level.[iv] The second focus has been to take nutritional status as a given – the outcome of behavioural decisions at the household level – and to examine the consequences of poor nutritional outcomes in childhood for the life trajectories of afflicted children.[v]

Over time, the perspectives adopted in empirical studies have broadened as it has been found that the policy recommendations derived from analyses depend both on the definition of nutrition and, more broadly, on the conceptual framework employed. For example, critical elements of the pathway from changes in income to their effect on nutritional status are still questioned. Moreover, by showing that nutrient intakes are unresponsive to changes in income even at very low-income levels, some studies have questioned whether nutrition in LICs will improve with income gains (for example, Behrman & Deolalikar, 1987). There has thus been a trend away from identifying nutritional status exclusively with nutrient intake and towards a wider recognition that the policy implications might differ strikingly with broader conceptual frameworks (Skoufias, 2016). Phrased differently, there is a growing awareness that a narrow focus on discipline-based indicators masks the fact that numerous single-channel interventions,

---

iv Surveys of such studies include Alderman (1990), Behrman & Deolalikar (1987), and Shah (1983), among many others.

v For examples see Alderman (1990), Behrman & Deolalikar (1987) and, for Zimbabwe, Alderman (1990) and Hoddinott & Kinsey (2006).

even if successfully implemented, have minimal or no impact on more-encompassing nutritional outcomes.

THE PHYSIOLOGY OF DEPRIVATION: AN OVERVIEW

Chronic undernutrition in Africa is persistent. It is relatively unaffected by agricultural output, household incomes, or food security. Stunting remains widespread in Africa's rural areas despite consumption of diets that are adequate according to nutritional standards (Prentice, 1993; Prendergast & Humphrey, 2015). This lack of association challenges conventional thinking. Current research suggests that unhygienic conditions at the household level, exposure to pathogens borne by domestic animals, and the consumption of mycotoxins lead to a condition – environmental enteric dysfunction (EED) – in which food consumed is unable to be fully utilised. This condition is widespread throughout the tropical world.

The evidence examined in this chapter suggests that nutritional status reflects things other than a straightforward causal chain linking agricultural production and economic wellbeing to food availability, and food availability to nutritional outcomes. Nutritional status is an outcome of not only the quantity and quality of food consumed, but is also determined by the body's ability to extract and utilise the nutrients contained in the food.

EED has been known for some 50 years, after recognition that most people in LICs had an abnormality of the small intestine (Prendergast & Kelly, 2012). This disorder was hypothesised to arise from unhygienic conditions, because among sufferers who relocated to high-income countries the condition slowly resolved. Essentially EED has two basic effects: it causes the villi to atrophy and creates cellular overgrowth, thus impeding absorption of nutrients; it also impairs the intestinal barrier function, allowing virulent organisms to stimulate an immune response and causing the body to waste nutrients in fighting the resulting inflammation. Thus EED impacts the ability of a child's body to absorb nutrients from the diet, facilitates infections, and may impair the efficacy of oral vaccines.

EED is normally asymptomatic: the sufferer does not experience any overt symptoms, and there are no pains to complain about. It is invisible to those experiencing it. Moreover, EED is also both socially and medically invisibilised. It falls into that category characterised as chronic illnesses that 'do not necessarily involve ... an evident change or physical deterioration that makes others think that somebody is sick' (Masana, 2011: 130). Since high proportions of the children in the Zimbabwe panel are stunted in any given year (see below), socially acceptable ideas about what constitutes a healthy body are strongly influenced by this pattern. If everyone is sick (stunted), then sick (stunted) is the normal. Thus neither the parents nor the community detects anything unusual when stunted, underweight children are observed. Further supporting this argument is that parents in the Zimbabwe panel feel more shame about whether their children wear decent clothes, have shoes and attend school than about whether they are visibly undernourished and stunted. EED is medically invisibilised because medical practitioners tend to interpret stunted status as a consequence of a dietary problem and because diagnosis requires sophisticated laboratory equipment and trained clinicians.

While much more still needs to be learned about the precise aetiology of EED, the redesignation of tropical enteropathy as environmental was a reflection of the growing awareness that it is largely a complex of factors related to diet, hygiene and sanitation, and mycotoxins that is the cause of the condition. Efforts to understand EED, therefore, fit well into a syndemics framework.[vi]

The characterisation of chronic undernutrition as a stunting syndrome, marked by a plethora of adverse pathological changes, with different consequences manifesting over the short, medium, and long term, helps to shift researchers' focus away from a preoccupation with food supply as a unidimensional solution. Stunting is also a transgenerational phenomenon because women who were themselves stunted in childhood tend to have stunted offspring, contributing to a cycle of poverty and reduced human capital that is difficult to break. Moreover, EED modifies the effects of oral medications and vaccines, alters the outcomes of trials in the treatment and prevention of stunting, and is associated with low-level immune responses – diverting resources away from child growth. For

---

vi EED is one of a number of conditions common in the tropics and characterised by malabsorption, a feature that has led to its also being known as leaky gut syndrome (Manson-Bahr & Apsted, 1982).

these reasons, using Singer's conceptualisation, the chapter characterises chronic undernutrition in sub-Saharan Africa as a syndemic, the aetiology of which is yet fully to be understood.

TRAJECTORIES OF CHILD NUTRITION OVER TIME IN ZIMBABWE

At the time when Millennium Development Goals (MDGs) became a focal concern for development practitioners, per-capita income in Zimbabwe was only fractionally higher than at independence 20 years earlier. The absence of changes in income was not, however, mirrored in other spheres. On the contrary, several developments initiated dramatic changes: a land redistribution programme launched only six months after independence; drought (in the 20 years following 1980 at least six droughts were experienced); economic reform (an economic adjustment programme began in 1991); and the arrival and rapid spread of HIV/AIDS.

In 1980 Zimbabwe began a programme of land reform that was generally well planned and implemented (in contrast to the experience since 2000). This original land reform was intended to do many things, among them increase agricultural productivity, enhance food security, and improve rural welfare. Since 1982, the author has conducted a panel study of some 500–700 households, including both beneficiaries and non-beneficiaries of land reform. A component of this study has been the use of multiple measures of the welfare of these rural households, among which are anthropometric measures of the nutritional wellbeing of both children and their parents.

An unexpected finding is that the nutritional status of children included in the study for nearly 20 years declined by an average of 1.4 per cent annually, so that children whose families benefited from land reform had nutritional levels two decades later that were worse, by 25 per cent, than when land reform began. These declines mirror secular worsening elsewhere in Zimbabwe and occurred despite generally rising farm productivity and incomes, a gradual accumulation of assets, and improvements in social welfare.

The investigation upon which this chapter is based was launched to answer a basic question: what are the effects of land redistribution on the welfare of rural families? Starting with a baseline data set established in the early 1980s, data have been collected over a 30-year period from 22 randomly selected communities in three of Zimbabwe's earliest resettlement schemes. These schemes were chosen to ensure representation of the three major agro-ecological zones in Zimbabwe suited to cropping. Beginning in 1997, coverage was extended to include households in villages in the communal areas (CAs) from which the resettled households originated in the early 1980s. This supplemental data permits explicit comparisons between the resettlement and communal experiences and between living conditions in the CAs and the resettlement areas (RAs).

The nutrition data from the panel study can be best understood if it is appreciated that they come from what is a moving cohort sampled across many years. In 1983 and 1984, all children aged between six months and five years and resident in the household were weighed and measured. The same procedure was followed in all subsequent years with two exceptions: the upper age cut-off point was moved initially to six years and subsequently to seven years in order to include as many children as possible from previous survey rounds, and children were included in the panel from birth instead of at age six months. Thus the pool of children included in any given year will contain neonates born since the previous round and will drop older children who are then above the age of seven years. To the extent that there are secular influences from incomes or poverty on long-term child nutrition, these will be manifested as each year's recruits to the cohort grow to the age of seven years and then exit the cohort.

With these comments, the chief anthropometric indicator of interest here is height for age (HA), the indicator normally used to assess chronic undernutrition. As noted, HA is assessed using z-scores – the difference above and below the expected median value (Dibley et al., 1987), with a z-score of -2 as the threshold of stunting. Rather than work directly with z-scores, Figure 1 plots over time the percentage of children falling below -2 standard deviations. The figure also plots comparable data from the periodic Zimbabwe Demographic and Health Survey (GoZ, 2012).

Two important differences between the data series in Figure 1 should be noted. ZRDHS (Zimbabwe Rural Demographic and Health Survey) is a panel study that involves the same households in three areas in every iteration, whereas for the ZDHS a new random sample is drawn nationally for every round. Thus the ZRHDS allows a true assessment of annual changes, or changes over short intervals, while the ZDHS presents a more representative national picture over longer intervals.[vii]

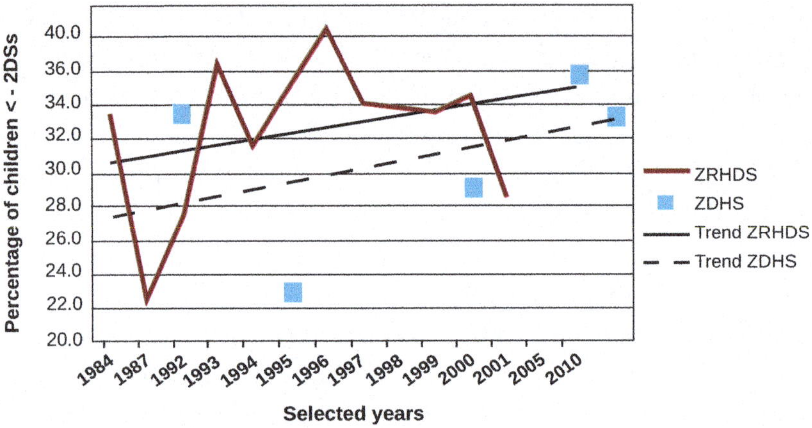

Figure 1: The evolution of nutritional outcomes for rural households, HAZ, 1984–2011

Sources: The annual rounds of the ZRHDS, the rural households from the ZDHS surveys at roughly five-year intervals, and the 2005–06 data are from Mbuya et al (2010). The ZDHS plot for 1994 represents only children aged less than three years, whereas the other years are results for children aged less than five years. The expected value for all years is 2.3 per cent.

The perspective in the plots represents the proportion of the children assessed lying below the threshold of stunting. HA exhibits dramatic changes. In 1983/84, nearly 34 per cent of children were stunted. In the following assessment period, 1987, the extent of stunting dropped by more than a third. This improvement was a consequence of several factors. Among them was a rapid expansion in social welfare expenditure, which supported cost-effective, community-based health interventions and improvements in child immunisation rates. And

vii In addition, the ZDHS (Zimbabwe Demographic and Health Survey) prevalence rates are based on the 2006 WHO standards (Victora et al., 2010) while the ZRHDS (Zimbabwe Rural Households Dynamics Study) rates use the NCHS standards (NCHS, 1977). Compared to the WHO standards, the NCHS reference tends to report lower height-for-age z-scores for children aged 12, 24 and 60 months and higher z-scores for ages 1, 36 and 48 months.

although the early 1980s experienced three consecutive years of drought, an effective drought-relief programme meant that crop failures were seldom experienced in the form of pronounced checks to child growth.

In the late 1980s or early 1990s, however, this improvement in HA was reversed. By 1992 stunting was close to the level of eight years earlier, while the following year, 1993, was the second worst ever recorded. The 1993 outcomes reflect the severe drought of the 1991–1992 season, but they may embody also the early signs of the cutbacks in public health services as part of Zimbabwe's structural adjustment programme. Following 1993, there was one year of marked improvement, but this was then succeeded by a continuation of poor outcomes. The linear trend is clearly for a growing proportion of children in resettlement areas to be stunted. In addition to the worsening of average nutritional status, 12 per cent more children were likely to be stunted at the end of the period than at the beginning.

The data plotted from the ZDHS represents only rural families from the national data set and thus provides a useful comparison with the panel data set. Looking at the two trend lines, Figure 1 strongly suggests that nutritional outcomes have worsened over time for all rural areas of Zimbabwe. Moreover, an assessment of progress toward the MDG targets for eradicating extreme poverty and hunger concludes that the targets are unlikely to be met (UNDP, 2012).

While it is far from obvious what is driving the changes observed, they are consistent with two possible but very different explanations. First, they match well the timing of the reversal of other health care indicators – infant, child, and maternal mortality – at the national level. This pattern is explained in part at least by the fact that real per capita health spending – which had increased more than 60 per cent between 1980 and 1990 – was in the late 1990s marginally lower than at independence (GoZ, 2006). A second factor that helps explain worsening nutritional outcomes during the 1990s is the fact that every growing season between 1988 and 1996 (seven consecutive years) experienced below long term average rainfall, including the two serious drought years of 1992 and 1995. When heavy rains came, as they did in 1996 and 1999, they brought with them national epidemics of malaria (see Chapter 4), which is particularly serious in the case of already undernourished children.

In summary, the ZRHDS data in Figure 1 shows a somewhat mixed picture, but the worsening of chronic undernutrition over time tells us that the resettlement experience has not led to general improvements – either in food security or in other underlying conditions – sufficient to reduce this dimension of undernutrition.

The analysis underlying the figure suggests that two related processes are unfolding together. Using median values for z-scores, we know half the children assessed will have better scores than the values used; and half will have worse scores. This latter group generates the consistently worsening results shown in Figure 1. What appears to be happening is that serious child undernutrition is becoming increasingly concentrated in one group of households and, moreover, that children in this particular group of households are becoming increasingly badly nourished. The focus to this point has been on aggregate indicators of nutritional status. But what underlies the patterns observed?

The first two years of life are a critical time for linear growth and particularly for brain growth and development of complex neural networks. Stunting develops during what has been termed the vital first 1,000 days – nine months of foetal life up to the second birthday – and its effects are thought to be largely irreversible.[viii] Figure 2, which plots the average z-scores for both height-for-age and weight-for-age (WA) over eight consecutive years, shows clearly the pattern of the onset of stunting in Zimbabwe. At the age of six months, children's HAZ begins a rapid decline that continues until just before the second birthday. At that point, some modest catch-up growth begins, but it never becomes complete.

Two features of Figure 2 are important. First, the fact that the youngest children have postpartum z-scores above expected values suggests that maternal nutrition and health may not be causes for major concern in rural Zimbabwe.[ix] Second, the very rapid decline in nutritional wellbeing from the age of six months to 18–25 months

viii The reversibility of stunting remains controversial, and divergent findings are reported depending upon whether studies address physical or cognitive stunting and the stage of life when assessments are done (for examples see Victora et al., 2010; Leroy et al., 2014 and 2015; Lundeen et al., 2014; Bhutta & Yackobovitch-Gavan, 2016; Georgiadis et al., 2017; Desmond & Casale, 2017; Prentice, 2017).

ix The major characteristic associated with low birth weights is the interval between the birth of the previous child and the child being assessed. Of multiple-birth children, 60 per cent had low birth weight (< 2500g), while 58 per cent were stunted at the time of the national survey (Mbuya et al., 2010).

(which is also reflected in national data (GoZ, 2014)) corresponds with two changes in infant-rearing practices: (1) the abandonment of exclusive breastfeeding and the introduction of supplementary foods and beverages, and (2) increasing exposure of infants to pathogens in their immediate environment. The latter arises because busy mothers or caregivers are likely to place infants and young children on the floor/ground while they do their chores or farm work. Anyone who has raised children knows that children explore their world by putting bits of it in their mouths; such exploratory ingestion creates direct pathways for bacterial infection (Ngure et al., 2013).[x]

In their study in Zimbabwe, Ngure et al (2013) observed caregiver-infant pairs to identify pathways of transmission of bacteria among infants. They tested the fingers, food, and drinking water of infants. Some infants actively ingested handfuls of soil and some also ingested chicken faeces. Hand-washing with soap was rare, and drinking water was contaminated with E. coli in more than half the households.

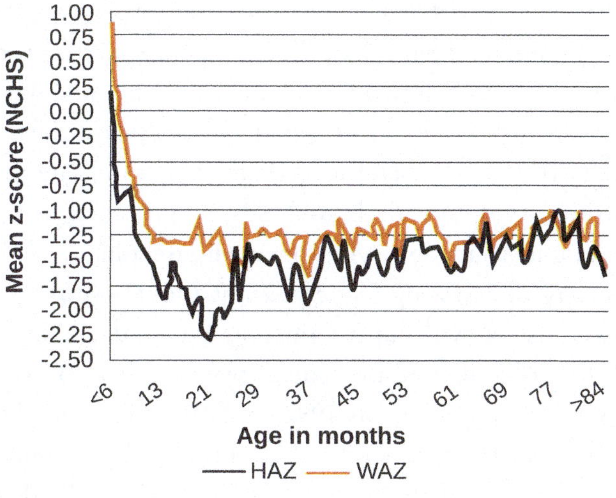

(n=7,235)

Figure 2: Timing of growth faltering among rural Zimbabwean children, 1993–2001

Source: Author's data. The expected value for all ages is 0.00.

x The compulsion in RAs to live in nucleated villages (in contrast to the dispersed pattern of dwellings in CAs) also almost certainly increases the risk of contamination.

NUTRITIONAL INDICATORS AND SOCIO-ECONOMIC MEASURES

In earlier work investigating nutritional status and socio-economic status (Kinsey, 2010b), anthropometric data (measurement of the size and proportions of the human body) were collected for both children and their parents, and households were identified where the phenomenon of undernutrition was present in adults, children, or both. Undernutrition exists among adults in a household if any one parent of young children has a body mass index (BMI) below 18.5.[xi] Similarly, undernutrition among children exists if any one of the three z-scores (HA, WA, and weight-for-height (WH)) for any young child in the household lies beneath two standard deviations below the median,[xii] the standard threshold for undernutrition.

Two new binary variables – BMI and Z – were created. The variable BMI is set to 0 in cases where no parent has a low BMI and to 1 where any parent has a BMI score below 18.5. An identical procedure was followed in creating the second variable: Z is assigned a value of 0 if *all* of the young children in the household have WA, HA and WH z-scores greater than two standard deviations below the median. If *any one* child has *any one* of the three z-scores below two standard deviations below the mean, Z is assigned a value of 1. Values of 0 for BMI and Z thus indicate an absence of undernutrition-symptomatic households, while values of 1 indicate the presence of undernutrition-symptomatic households.

A simple way of assessing *household* nutritional status is to create a two-by-two matrix with adults on one axis and children on the other. This cross-tabulation procedure was applied to the pooled data sets for the five years from 1997 to 2001.[xiii] The distribution of households obtained by applying this approach is summarised in Table 2. The four cells of the matrix contain: (1) households with no undernourished children or adults (the 0/0 households); (2) households with both undernourished children and undernourished adults (the 1/1

xi A threshold for the diagnosis of chronic energy deficiency using BMI has been defined as less than 18.5 (Shetty & James, 1994).

xii Including all three anthropometric indicators along with BMI for adults means that both chronic and acute undernutrition are being considered.

xiii None of these years was affected by drought.

households); (3) households with one or more undernourished adults but no undernourished children (1/0 households); and (4) households with one or more undernourished children, but no undernourished adults (0/1 households).

A third of households exhibited no sign of undernutrition on the basis of the z-scores of the children, while nearly 80 per cent of resident parents had BMIs above the cut-off.[xiv] The significance level for the cross-tabulation indicates that the hypothesis that intra-household child and adult nutrition levels are independent can be rejected. Examining the cross-tabulations, the most common outcome is a household with at least one undernourished child, but no parent below the cut-off point. The rarest outcome is a household with an undernourished adult, but no undernourished child; there are only 89 such cases across the five years in this category.

Looking only at the outcomes where neither adults nor children are undernourished or both are, in 14.4 per cent of households undernourishment exists in both groups, while it exists in neither group in about a third of all cases. Each cell of the matrix thus represents households that differ in significant ways. The 0/0 households exhibit no adverse nutritional phenomena and are therefore not regarded as impoverished or vulnerable. If both adults and children from the same household are undernourished, the 1/1 households, this suggests the same pathways may be affecting nutrition among the young and the old and that poverty, health, food availability and/or EED may be major contributing factors. The mixed cases present greater challenges to interpretation. If adults are well-nourished and children poorly nourished (the 0/1 households) – which is the case for nearly half the households – the primary cause is not likely to be so much a lack of food as poor intra-household distribution of food, poor child-feeding practices, child neglect, or complications of nutritional status caused by child-specific, health-related, and hygienic factors, such as EED.

---

xiv Many instances exist where children were assessed but no parent was present. These cases are excluded here. This exclusion may, however, bias the results since children who are being fostered, as the result of the death of parents, because of a broken marriage, or as a family coping mechanism, may be particularly prone to failure to thrive.

Table 2: Distribution of rural households by nutritional category, 1997–2001

	Children's z-scores		
	Symptomatic (1)	Asymptomatic (0)	Totals
Adults' BMIs	*(per cent (n))*		
Symptomatic (1)	14.4 (225)	5.7 (89)	20.1 (323)
Asymptomatic (0)	46.2 (722)	33.7 (526)	79.9 (1251)
Totals	60.6 (960)	39.4 (614)	100.0 (1562)

Pearson $X^2 = 20.0252$ Pr = 0.000.

In the other mixed case, where adults are undernourished and children well-nourished (the small number of 1/0 households), the intra-household allocation of food is likely to be satisfactory but adults are perhaps experiencing a situation in which physical activity levels are high relative to the supply of food; or the time available to prepare and eat nutritionally satisfactory meals is inadequate. An alternative, or additional, explanation is that adult-specific health-related factors, such as HIV/AIDS, are at work.

If the 14.4 per cent of symptomatic households (undernourishment in both parents and children) constitute the same group in each year, this would further implicate structural and social factors, such as poverty, hygiene, and sanitation. But it is not the same households that show up in each category over time. Indeed, on average, the doubly undernourished households appear somewhat less than twice over the five years.[xv] However, an assessment of 7,235 children across nine consecutive years from 1993 to 2001 reveals an average of one-third of children stunted (with a range of 28.1 per cent in 2001 to 38.1 in 1996), a pattern strongly suggesting that undernutrition is structural in nature and that environmental factors may be implicated.

Analysis of the nutritional data revealed that, contrary to all

xv There is, however, some indication of a neighbourhood effect because of the much greater frequency of appearance of doubly undernourished households in certain villages. This finding again suggests structural, social and environmental factors may be responsible.

expectations, children's nutritional levels in Zimbabwe's RAs are lower than virtually anywhere else in the country.[xvi] It was originally thought that this outcome might have been a consequence of the experience of relocating at a time of great environmental stress – the three-year drought of the early 1980s. Subsequent reporting suggests, however, that the relatively poor nutritional status of children in RAs appears to reflect persistent structural causes (Kinsey, 1998; GoZ, 1989; 1995; 1997; 2006).

Household-level outcomes

A syndemics approach dictates an examination of the proposition that undernutrition is structural in the RAs through scrutiny of underlying biosocial indicators. Accordingly, with households divided into the four groups shown in Table 2, a set of 90 variables was constructed comprising multiple indicators of socio-economic wellbeing. Although detailed explanation is impossible here, the significant outcomes serve to illustrate the frequent mismatch between nutritional status and presumed steps along a causal pathway linking food supply to nutrition. Because household size is such an important variable in assessing outcomes, this treatment merely highlights major findings from the aggregated analysis.[xvii]

A few results were anticipated. For example, households with no undernutrition have a significantly lower incidence of illness and a significantly higher income from the sale of livestock. Many more results, however, were seemingly perverse. Examples include the fact that the highest-income group in terms of revenue from cash crop sales has the worst nutrition and that neither total off-farm income nor total income is significantly associated with any nutritional category. Other findings were also counterintuitive.

The enigmatic association between nutritional status and the underlying measures suggests that the relationship between nutrition and traditional indicators is not as straightforward as intuition might suggest, certainly not as an indicator of household welfare.[xviii] Evidence for this contention can be found by correlating the entire set of indicators with

xvi Jenkins and Prinsloo (1995) report similar patterns.

xvii Full details of the calculations can be found in Kinsey (2010a; 2010b).

xviii See Behrman & Deolalikar (1987: 505) for an analysis of rural panel data which concludes that 'increases in income will not result in substantial improvements in nutrient intakes'.

the separate nutritional indicators for adults and children, a procedure that reveals some startling relationships. Of the four groups based on nutritional status, only the group of poorly nourished adults appears at all well differentiated according to the indicators used, and some of the differentiating factors are counterintuitive. Examples are households with a poorly nourished adult that possess cattle herds with lower market values and earn less from sales of livestock. Such households also receive more remittances in cash – 80 per cent more than the mean – and plant larger areas of cash crops (mainly tobacco and cotton) and have the highest ratio of cash crops to food crops. In comparison, households with only well-nourished children earn more from sales of livestock.

The presence of a poorly nourished adult is a good predictor that there will also be a poorly nourished child; just under 80 per cent of households with a poorly nourished adult will also contain a poorly nourished child. These households also have very low expenditure on staple grain and possess low-valued livestock holdings from which they earn relatively little in sales. They do, however, plant the largest area of cash crops, both in absolute terms and in relation to the area of food crops. These households also have mean total incomes more than 8 per cent above those of households with only well-nourished adults and have the lowest incidence of incapacitating illness.

Unambiguous results emerge from the correlations between crop- and livestock-related indicators and the nutritional outcomes of both adults and children. An increase in a crop-related indicator *always* worsens nutritional status, while an increase in a livestock-related indicator *always* enhances nutritional outcomes. Why should this pattern occur so clearly?

Answers to this question may come from a deeper appreciation of both the data and the farming systems from which they come. The data is collected annually at a period of peak labour stress and when food supplies are at their lowest point in the season. Collectively, an increase in the crop-related indicators can be interpreted as an increase in the seasonal demand for labour for field operations. This increase implies, in turn, two other associated shifts: an increase in the demand for caloric energy to sustain the labour inputs and a reduction in the amount of time available for women to care for children. Thus, greater commitments to cropping (and especially to cash-cropping) are associated with poorer nutritional outcomes. Nor do higher crop incomes from the previous harvest compensate during the current season.

Why do the livestock-related indicators have consistently the opposite effect? There are likely to be at least four effects at work. First, livestock are probably the best single indicator of wealth for rural households and of their ability to cope with cash shortfalls.[xix] Second, the labour demands for livestock keeping are non-seasonal and require little caloric expenditure; moreover, cheap, unskilled labour is often hired for herding during the busy cropping period, and cattle are often herded collectively, thereby saving labour. Third, the value of the herd is positively associated with possession of draft oxen, which can significantly substitute for human labour in the demanding tasks of land preparation and weeding. Finally, revenue from sales of livestock products is indicative that households have surpluses of milk and eggs, suggesting that the family is consuming all of these food sources.

A more simplified explanation is also possible. Households with large livestock holdings are the wealthy; they have made it, and they have decreased their vulnerability to the vicissitudes of rain-fed farming. Households with many positive crop-related indicators aspire to make it in a similar fashion and are working extremely hard to do so. Much of their income from crops may, therefore, be used to increase investment rather than improve consumption.

In contrast to the crop, livestock, and health indicators, however, the income and consumption indicators exhibit ambiguous outcomes. For example, in almost half the cases, the indicators exhibit opposite signs for adults and children, suggesting that the pathways to better household nutrition are more complex than is sometimes suspected. It feels intuitively correct that total household non-food consumption would be positively associated with child nutrition since there has to be a strong association with household income, but why should it be negatively associated with adult nutrition? And why should food purchases be negatively associated with nutrition for both children and adults, while grain purchases and the amount of grain in storage have positive effects for adults and negative ones for children? The income

xix See Kinsey, Gunning & Burger (1998).

variables are, if anything, even more paradoxical. Why should all sources of cash income (aside from crop income and income controlled by women) be positively correlated with child nutrition and yet only one (non-agricultural income) correlate positively with adult nutrition?

Per-capita outcomes

Examination of the relationship between nutritional indicators and associated measures at the household level revealed some puzzles and suggested that the ability of the combined indicators to point out pathways for nutritional improvement was generally weak. This section replicates the analysis reported above, but transforms the measures from a household to a per-capita basis. Table 3 presents a selected subset of measures defined in per-capita terms and adds a new variable representing household size. Households with no undernutrition are significantly smaller than the average, whereas those with undernutrition among both adults and children are significantly larger than the average.

Overall, the undernutrition-free and the all-undernourished groups differ significantly according to some 70 per cent of the indicators, and in the manner expected. Expenditure on food differentiates the all-undernourished group as expected, but its significance for the undernourished-adults group is hard to explain. Other variables that differentiate the worst-nourished group of households include grain storage, both consumption measures, the value of livestock and sales of livestock products, total income, and the area planted to cash crops. The only measures that successfully differentiate all four groups in Table 3 are the two non-food consumption measures.

With the transformation of the measures to per-capita terms, the two groups with undernourished children tend to drop below the population means of the selected measures, while the two with well-nourished children tend to rise above the mean. Thus the procedure of transforming the values is picking up the same thing that inclusion of the household size variable does: larger households are far more likely to contain poorly nourished children.

Table 3: Mean levels of socio-economic measures on a per-capita basis according to combined nutritional indicators for the household

	Nutritional group profile of the household				
Measure	All households	No under-nutrition	Only under-nourished children	Only under-nourished adults	Only under-nourished
	(mean values)				
Grain purchases $	1.18	0.93	1.68	0.63	*0.30
Food purchases $	43	46	43	*51	*38
Stored grain kg	65	*76	63	*55	*53
Stored legumes kg	0.27	0.45	0.03	0.02	*0.73
Consumption 1 $a	593	*729	*516	*698	*533
Consumption 2 $b	686	*842	*604	*764	*607
Crops value $c	1 272	*1 510	1 132	*1 488	1 173
Crops revenue $d	975	*1 146	859	*1 201	930
Livestock value $e	1 765	*1 994	1 715	1 732	*1 473
Livestock sales 1 $f	16	*20	14	*35	*11
Livestock sales 2 $g	112	*162	95	95	*71
Remittances $h	75	76	62	*169	86
Non-ag income $	349	*494	288	*204	288
Total income $	1 824	*2 261	*1 590	1 990	*1 629
Female income $	69	76	66	78	60
Area cropped ha	0.34	*0.37	0.33	0.33	*0.31
Cash crops ha	0.09	0.10	0.09	*0.12	0.10
Household size	10	*9	11	10	*12

Source: Author's data.
*Significantly different from the mean at P=0.05.
[a]Non-food consumption excluding educational expenditure. [b]Non-food consumption including educational expenditure. [c]Market value of all crops grown. [d]Market value of actual crop sales. [e]Market value of all livestock holdings. [f]Revenue from sale of livestock products. [g]Revenue from sale of livestock. [h]Excludes in-kind remittances.

While there are clearly fundamentally different socio-economic situations represented in the data set, these are not well delineated by the distribution of the nutritional indicators. Nor is there any consistent evidence that households with adults identified as being underweight are any worse off in terms of food security or health status than households without thin adults. Moreover, the combined measures lack discriminatory power when a group in which undernutrition exists is the norm, as is the case here, where households with undernourished children and well-nourished adults are the expected outcome.

Several factors help to explain this weakness in discriminatory power. First, much has been lost by converting the anthropometric scales to simple 0-1 dummy variables depending upon the position of an observation relative to a defined threshold. This procedure fails to differentiate among degrees of undernutrition, and it may be the severity of undernutrition – rather than merely its presence – that accords better with the socio-economic indicators. It could well be that the extent of within-household undernutrition is more significant.

A basic problem, however, is that because BMI for adults does not correlate well with the anthropometric indicators for children, many of the most promising cause-and-effect variables operate in opposite directions for children and for adults. This makes generalisations about the household unit extremely difficult. Nubé et al (1997) note a limitation to the use of BMI: seasonal fluctuations in food availability and/or labour demands may affect measures. The adults assessed here were all examined during periods of peak labour demands and at a time when food supplies from the previous harvest would normally have been running low. The outcomes suggest that, in this setting, BMIs may be better at identifying stress in terms of arduous farm labour than at differentiating households with poorly nourished adults from other rural households.

Finally, while structuring analysis on the basis of per-capita rather than household values yields results more indicative of underlying relationships, improvements can still be made since a per-capita approach weights adults and children equally and thus masks significant differences arising from household composition.

The analysis above illustrates well some of the difficulties that arise in attempting to apply a syndemics framework to the problem of child and household undernutrition. Analytically, a syndemics approach calls for the broadest possible perspective and inclusion of all relevant variables. Anthropologists will appreciate that this methodology can yield deep insights into the complexities that underlie observed nutritional outcomes, while economists will lament the presence of so many confounding variables and the challenge of assessing significance.

Given the poor record of so many past nutritional interventions, however, it becomes increasingly clear that a belief in simplistic solutions or unilateral causal pathways is misguided.

The influence of ecology and tenurial regime

In order to test further the proposition that the selected indicators themselves are valid measures, the data were restratified using two criteria for Zimbabwe which we know a good deal about: by land tenure regime (RAs and CAs) and by agro-ecological zone (natural regions or NRs).

If the indicators are valid, we would expect to find two strong patterns. First, since 84 per cent of households in CAs are poor in total consumption terms[xx] (GoZ, 1997) and RAs have been provided access to a superior resource base, we would expect to find systematically stronger indicators of wellbeing in RAs than in CAs. Second, rural households attempting to make a living from agriculture will achieve more positive results in areas physically better suited to farming. Thus, it would be expected that the agriculture-related indicators will generally indicate a progressive worsening as one moves from the better areas – NR 2 – to areas of lower inherent potential – NR 3 and NR 4. How well do the indicators fit with these expectations?

In the case of the RA-CA comparison, all indicators, with the exception of four, have the expected relationship. The first two exceptions show that the probability of a household containing either an undernourished child or adult is less in the CAs than in the RAs. The second two exceptions show the CAs to be healthier places to live – especially for children – despite the fact that all the RAs were provided with new health facilities in the early 1980s. Agriculture and livestock income variables, and consumption indicators, show the advantage of living in a resettlement area, while remittance and off-farm income variables indicate some of the disadvantages of living in CAs, with the difficulty of earning a living from smallholdings with a poor resource base. The different nutritional and health outcomes for RAs and CAs thus suggest sets of influences operating at different levels.

---

xx On the basis of the income required to purchase a basket of basic food needed by an average person per annum and meet non-food needs (clothing, housing, education, health, transport, etc.).

Why are nutritional and health status worse in RAs, where households have generous land-holdings and preferential access to health and agricultural services? One explanation may lie in settlement patterns and the time allocations of women. Villages in RAs have been laid out in a nucleated pattern so neighbours and their small livestock live in close proximity. Travel time to fields is long in RAs, as are the hours spent in the field. Busy mothers may leave young children at home in the care of siblings or take them to the fields; in neither case are the children likely to be well fed or cared for. In contrast, in the CAs, the fields surround the homestead, travel times are short, and midday meals can be managed easily.

A further explanation may be that official exhortations to be productive have propelled RA households in the direction of producing non-consumable commodities such as cotton and tobacco, leading to high ratios between the areas planted to cash crops and food crops and/or reductions in diversity in the mix of food crops grown. Because of their small land-holdings, CA households tend to market surplus food crops, if they have any, rather than grow crops for market that cannot be consumed. Incomes from agriculture and livestock are generally much higher in RAs than in CAs. Conventional wisdom on the effect of commercialisation of agriculture on nutrition of farm families holds that there should be minimal, if any, adverse effects on nutrition because of the compensating effects of higher cash incomes. This is not the case here.

The study sites span zones of agricultural potential, ranging from fairly high to quite low. In the area of best potential, farming appears dynamic and cash incomes are high because of widespread cultivation of cash crops such as cotton and tobacco and novel crops such as paprika and soya. Across all the years surveyed, however, this area has consistently displayed the lowest nutritional outcomes. In the area of lowest natural potential, agriculture appears stagnant; and no unirrigated farming system produces reliable incomes. Yet it is in this weakly commercialised area that the best nutritional outcomes for children have consistently been found.[xxi] Furthermore, the probability of finding an

xxi The higher potential areas have higher rainfall, which provides beneficial conditions for certain disease vectors.

undernourished adult in a household is three times higher in the best agro-ecological zone than in the intermediate and low-potential zones.

DISCUSSION: WE ARE NOT WHAT WE EAT

In the context of syndemics, this chapter has addressed three main themes: the prevalence of undernutrition and its causes, associations, and paradoxes; the physiology of deprivation and stunting; and the outcomes of an intervention aimed at improving links between agriculture and food systems.

An overview of the intervention reviewed here shows that stunting persists no matter what. In particular, agriculture and food-based approaches fail to reduce stunting significantly. The limited impact on the severity of stunting is insufficient to meet the UN's Sustainable Development Goals and eliminate the consequences of stunting. Similarly, the effects of nutrition interventions on growth of stunted children in low- and middle-income countries (LMICs) are disappointing. In summarising actions to accelerate progress on nutrition, Haddad et al. (2015) even question the efficacy of nutrition interventions on growth. Previously, Sguassero et al. (2012) meta-analysed community-based supplementary feeding of young children in LMICs and concluded that, despite a scarcity of relevant studies, supplementary feeding has a negligible impact on child growth. Kristjansson et al. (2015) show that socio-economically disadvantaged children, when supplemented, only grew an average of 0.27 cm more over six months than those who were not supplemented. In an analysis of before-and-after studies, they find no evidence of an effect on height. Overall, the data indicates that the net effect of nutrition on height is generally small and significantly smaller than that reported in historic studies (Hermanussen & Wit, 2017).

While multisectoral nutrition interventions in the right environment have potential to improve child health,[xxii] donor support for nutrition is less than 5 per cent of international health assistance. Global efforts have increased awareness of the need to improve the provision of nutrition

xxii Two recent evaluations (Nabwera et al., 2017; Barnett et al., 2018), however, call into question the ability of even expensive, long-term, multisectoral interventions to address effectively and sustainably the causal pathways for undernutrition or to eliminate stunting.

services yet, despite these efforts, progress in scaling up policy and programmes is still challenged by poor understanding of the burden of child malnutrition, insufficient scientific evidence, and by weak or non-existent political commitment. The costs of chronic undernutrition to individuals become more apparent with each new report of field research. Less obvious, however, are the costs to the economies of countries that do nothing about alleviating chronic undernutrition.

If children are to escape the life sentence of deprivation imposed by stunting, those involved with implementing nutritional interventions must base their work on sound scientific evidence and work at multiple levels across multiple sectors. Single-channel efforts – particularly those focused on food-related interventions – cannot succeed. Such multisectoral efforts will involve not only decisions about which specific measures to take, where, and in which combinations, but also supporting frameworks shaped by political choices leading to firm commitments. Governments and donor agencies will also have to reshape their thinking about the provision of resources and financing through more complex arrangements and within appropriate time frames.

This chapter takes some steps toward severing the generally assumed link between consumption of a nutritionally adequate diet and the positive outcome of improved nutritional status. Under the environmental conditions where EED (environmental enteric dysfunction, the condition in which food consumed is unable to be fully utilised) arises, the body of the child is simply unable to utilise much of whatever nutrients may be fed to it. This fact suggests that a major rethink is needed about ways to address chronic undernutrition among future generations.

This reconceptualisation demands cross-disciplinary and holistic approaches to formulating interventions to improve nutritional outcomes. Despite the wide prevalence of chronic undernutrition and attempts to address it, past experiences with nutritional interventions have had only marginal impacts (Prendergast & Kelly, 2012). Indeed, EED renders almost obsolete many of the buzzwords – such as *hunger* and *food security* – that have been used to motivate development assistance in the past.

Many previous interventions aimed at improving nutritional status have been designed or implemented in ways that precluded reliable evaluation of their effects. In assessing results, there has been a noticeable focus on indicators rather than outcomes. Synergies among different elements of interventions remain poorly understood. Reviews of complementary feeding programmes, for example, in combination with nutrition education showed mixed effects on HAZ and stunting, both in food-secure and food-insecure populations (Lassi et al., 2013). While some interventions showed significant effects on HAZ from food supplements and nutrition education, the effect on chronic undernutrition was not significant.

Although the potential benefits of strategies to improve the quality and micronutrient density of foods consumed by small children are well recognised, few LICs have clear policies in support of effective strategies to eliminate micronutrient deficiencies (Eilander et al., 2010). A review of multiple micronutrient supplementation efforts showed small benefits on linear growth but little evidence of effects on morbidity outcomes (Allen et al., 2009). Another review of the effect of micronutrient supplementations on cognitive performance concluded that such interventions might be associated with a marginal improvement in one area but not in others (Eilander et al., 2010). In her review of single-target interventions, supplementary feeding, hygiene/sanitation, or water supply, Humphrey (2009) shows that the best outcomes appear capable of addressing only about one-third of the magnitude of the stunting problem. Partial solutions are clearly inadequate.

Suggestively, Spears (2013) has shown that there is a quantitatively important gradient between child height and sanitation that can statistically explain a large fraction of international height differences. This association between sanitation and human capital is robustly stable and appears to possess more explanatory power than the relationship between GDP and child height. This connection clearly points to the significance of environmental factors influencing nutritional outcomes.

Recent work by Skoufias (2016) highlights the need for greater awareness at the operational level of the limitations of an exclusive focus on tackling single dimensions of undernutrition without considering the wider context. He examines the extent to which three key underlying determinants of nutritional status – food security; childcare at the maternal, household, and community levels; and access to health services and a safe, hygienic environment – on their own and interactively are associated with nutritional outcomes. Skoufias's analysis underlines the point that the success of sector-specific nutritional interventions may be constrained by a lack of momentum in leveraging the synergies among the three broad clusters of underlying determinants of undernutrition: food security, child care, and environment and health.

In his analysis, Skoufias uses data from Zimbabwe as one example. Although 22 per cent of Zimbabwean children are rated adequate in food, 39 per cent adequate in care, and 10 per cent adequate in environment and health combined, many children (47 per cent) are not adequate in any single component and only very few (17 per cent) are adequate in more than one component (Skoufias, 2016: 34). Thus, the beneficial synergies from multisectoral approaches are not being realised.

Evidence from Zimbabwe, as from most of Africa, shows that EED is a greater problem in rural areas, where small isolated communities must fend for themselves. While the most challenging development intervention – inducing behavioural change – must underlie the elimination of EED, there is great scope for integrated initiatives featuring improvements to sanitation, hygiene, water supply, and feeding and childcare practices. At the same time, training and education for medical and community workers could assist in reducing the burden of EED among children in LICs.

Stunting affects well over a third of all African children. The analysis here suggests that the prevalence of undernutrition in one form or another among rural Zimbabwean children may be as high as 60 per cent – far higher than the 33 per cent for stunting reported in the most recent DHS study (GoZ, 2012) and an incidence that *places undernutrition in the realm of a pandemic.* This difference is too great to be explained by the use of somewhat different nutritional reference standards and, moreover, the high prevalence rates are disturbingly persistent.

The reviews of wider experience display the same contradictory patterns as does this interrogation of the Zimbabwean experience. At present, we have few examples of success that could be scaled up; what may rather be needed is first to scale down to seek solutions that are effective at the community level, and then to understand exactly what makes them successful. The vast network of professional organisations that work to end hunger – the UN agencies, the government bodies and NGOs, the academics, and the rock concert organisers – all face a challenging learning curve to harmonise their individual prescriptions for ending undernutrition into effective multisectoral approaches. It is encouraging, however, to note an apparent growing recognition that a common middle ground must be sought between approaches addressing undernutrition incrementally, activity by activity, and those tackling the wider context in a syndemic framework, on the premise that fundamental social change is a prerequisite for any solution to the problem of chronic undernutrition.

**

The author expresses his grateful appreciation to the Netherlands Ministry for Development Cooperation and the Royal Netherlands Embassy in Harare and to the American Anthropological Association and the Wenner-Gren Foundation for support in preparing some of the background materials for this chapter and in soliciting critical comments.

REFERENCES

Alderman, H. 1990. 'Poverty and malnutrition: How closely linked?' Paper. Cuadernos de Economia, Agosto.

Allen, L. H. et al. 2009. 'Provision of multiple rather than two or fewer micronutrients more effectively improves growth and other outcomes in micronutrient-deficient children and adults'. *Journal of Nutrition*, 139, 1022–1030.

Barnett, C. E. et al. 2018. *Impact Evaluation of the Sada Millennium Villages Project in Northern Ghana: Endline summary report*. Hove: Itad Ltd.

Behrman, J. R. & Deolalikar, A. B. 1987. 'Will developing country nutrition improve with income: A case study for rural South India'. *Journal of Political Economy*, 95 (3), 452–507.

Bhutta, Z. & Yackobovitch-Gavan, M. 2016. 'Malnutrition and catch-up growth during childhood and puberty', in Koletzko, B., Shamir, R., Turck, D. & Phillip, M. (eds.) *Nutrition and Growth: Yearbook 2016. World Review of Nutrition and Dietetics*. Basel: Karger, 120–127.

Black, R. E. 2012. 'The vicious cycle of diarrhoea and malnutrition: Nutritional risk factors'. http://www.globalpaediatricresearch.org/. http://www.slideshare.net/

PGPR, accessed 22 February 2013.

Desmond, C. & Casale, D. 2017. 'Catch-up growth in stunted children: Definitions and predictors'. *PLoS ONE* 12, e0189135.

Dibley, M. J. et al. 1987. 'Interpretation of Z-score anthropometric indicators derived from the international growth reference'. *American Journal of Clinical Nutrition*, 46, 749–762.

Eilander, A. et al. 2010. 'Multiple micronutrient supplementation for improving cognitive performance in children: Systematic review of randomized controlled trials'. *American Journal of Clinical Nutrition*, 91, 115–130.

Food and Agriculture Organisation (FAO). 2002. *The State of Food Insecurity in the World 2001.* Rome. http://www.fao.org/docrep/005/y4671e/y4671e06.htm#fn31, accessed 1 December 2018.

Georgiadis, A. et al. 2017. 'Growth recovery and faltering through early adolescence in low- and middle-income countries: Determinants and implications for cognitive development'. *Social Science & Medicine*, 179, 81–90.

Government of Zimbabwe (GoZ). 1989. *Zimbabwe Demographic and Health Survey 1988.* Harare: Central Statistical Office.

Government of Zimbabwe (GoZ). 1995. *Zimbabwe Demographic and Health Survey Country Report.* Harare: Central Statistical Office.

Government of Zimbabwe (GoZ). 1997. *Poverty Assessment Study Survey (1995).* Harare: Ministry of Public Service, Labour and Social Welfare.

Government of Zimbabwe (GoZ). 1998. *Poverty in Zimbabwe.* Harare: Central Statistical Office.

Government of Zimbabwe (GoZ). 2006. *2003 Poverty Assessment Study Survey, Final Main Report.* Harare: Ministry of Public Service, Labour and Social Welfare.

Government of Zimbabwe (GoZ). 2007. *Zimbabwe Demographic and Health Survey 2005-06.* Calverton, Maryland: Central Statistical Office & Macro International, Inc.

Government of Zimbabwe (GoZ). 2012. *Zimbabwe Demographic and Health Survey 2010-11.* Calverton, Maryland: Zimbabwe National Statistics Agency & ICF International Inc.

Government of Zimbabwe (GoZ). 2012. *Zimbabwe Demographic and Health Survey 2012.* Harare: Central Statistical Office.

Government of Zimbabwe (GoZ). 2014. *Zimbabwe Multiple Indicator Cluster Survey 2014: Key Findings Report.* Harare: Zimbabwe National Statistics Agency.

Haddad, L. E. et al. 2015. 'The Global Nutrition Report 2014: Actions and accountability to accelerate the world's progress on nutrition'. *Journal of Nutrition*, 145, 663–671.

Hermanussen, M. & Wit, J. M. 2017. 'How much nutrition for how much growth?' *Hormone Research in Paediatrics*, 88, 38–45.

Hoddinott, J. & Kinsey, B. H. 2006. 'Long-term consequences of early childhood malnutrition'. *Oxford Economic Papers*, 58 (3), 450–474.

Humphrey, J. H. 2009. 'Child undernutrition, tropical enteropathy, toilets and handwashing'. *Lancet*, 374, 1032–1035.

Jenkins, C. & Prinsloo, E. 1995. *Inequality Among Households in Zimbabwe: an assessment using the 1990/91 ICES*. Harare: Central Statistical Office.

Kinsey, B. H. 1998. Determinants of rural household incomes and their impact on poverty and food security in Zimbabwe. Workshop on Rural Household Dynamics, Harare, 15–16 June.

Kinsey, B. H. 2010a. 'Who went where ... and why: Patterns and consequences of displacement in rural Zimbabwe after February 2000'. *Journal of Southern African Studies*, 36 (2), 339–360.

Kinsey, B. H. 2010b. 'Poverty dynamics in rural Zimbabwe: The 30 years (lost) "war against poverty"'. Ten Years of War against Poverty – What Have We Learned since 2000? University of Manchester, 8–10 September.

Kinsey, B. H. et al. 1998. 'Coping with drought in Zimbabwe: Survey evidence on responses of rural households to risk'. *World Development*, 26 (1), 89–110.

Kristjansson, E. et al. 2015. 'Food supplementation for improving the physical and psychosocial health of socio-economically disadvantaged children aged three months to five years.' *Cochrane Database Systematic Review*, 5 (3), CD009924.

Lassi, Z. S., et al. 2013. 'Impact of complementary food and education on growth and morbidity of children less than 2 years of age in developing countries: A systematic review'. *BMC Public Health*, 13, Suppl 3-S13, 1–10.

Leroy, J. L. et al. 2014. 'Linear growth deficit continues to accumulate beyond the first 1000 days in low- and middle-income countries: Global evidence from 51 national surveys'. *Journal of Nutrition*, 144, 1460–1466.

Leroy, J. L. et al. 2015. 'Using height-for-age differences (HAD) instead of height-for-age z-scores (HAZ) for the meaningful measurement of population-level catch-up in linear growth in children less than 5 years of age'. *BMC Pediatrics*, 15, 145.

Lundeen, E. A. et al. 2014. 'Height-for-age z scores increase despite increasing height deficits among children in 5 developing countries'. *American Journal of Clinical Nutrition*, 100, 821–825.

Manson-Bahr, P. E. C. & Apsted, F. I. C. (eds.) 1982. *Manson's Tropical Diseases.* Eastbourne: Baillière Tindall.

Masana, L. 2011. 'Invisible chronic illnesses inside apparently healthy bodies,' in Fainzang, S. & Haxaire, C. (eds.) *Of Bodies and Symptoms: Anthropological Perspectives on Their Social and Medical Treatment.* Tarragona: URV Publications, 127–149.

Mbuya, M. N. N. et al. 2010. 'Biological, social, and environmental determinants of low birth weight and stunting among infants and young children in Zimbabwe'. *Zimbabwe Working Papers*, 7. Calverton: ICF Macro.

Nabwera, H. M. et al. 2017. 'Growth faltering in rural Gambian children after four decades of interventions: A retrospective cohort study'. *Lancet Global Health*, 5, 208–216.

National Center for Health Statistics. 1977. *NCHS Growth Curves For Children, Birth to 18 Years*. PHS publication No. 78-1650. Washington, DC: National Center for Health Statistics, Department of Health, Education and Welfare.

Ngure, F. M. et al. 2013. 'Formative research on hygiene behaviors and geophagy among infants and young children and implications of exposure to fecal bacteria'. *American Journal of Tropical Medicine and Hygiene*, 89 (4), 709–716.

Nubé, M. et al. 1997. 'Body mass index: Indicator of health and wealth', *Centre for World Food Studies.* Amsterdam: Free University. Staff Working Paper WP-97-01.

Prendergast, A. & Kelly, P. 2012. 'Review: Enteropathies in the developing world: Neglected effects on global health'. *American Journal of Tropical Medicine and Hygiene*, 86 (5), 756–763.

Prendergast, A. J. & Humphrey, J. H. 2014. 'The stunting syndrome in developing countries'. *Paediatrics and International Child Health*, 34 (4), 250–265.

Prendergast, A. J. & Humphrey, J. H. 2015. 'Stunting persists despite optimal feeding – Are toilets part of the solution?', in Embleton, N. D., Katz, J. & Ziegler, E. E. (eds.) *Low-birthweight Baby: Born Too Soon or Too Small.* Nestlé Nutrition Institute Workshop Series, 81. Basel: Nestec Ltd., Vevey/S. Karger AG, 99–110.

Prentice, A. 1993. 'Nutrient requirements for growth, pregnancy and lactation: The Keneba experience'. *South African Journal of Clinical Nutrition*, 6, 33–38.

Prentice, A. 2017. 'Stunting in developing countries', in Koletzko, B., Shamir, R., Turck, D. & Phillip, M. (eds.) *Nutrition and Growth: Yearbook 2017. World Review of Nutrition and Dietetics*, 116, 165–174. Basel: Karger.

Sguassero, Y. M. et al. 2012. 'Community-based supplementary feeding for promoting the growth of children under five years of age in low and middle-income countries'. *Cochrane Database Systematic Review*, CD005039.

Shah, C. H. 1983. 'Food preference, poverty, and the nutrition gap'. *Economic Development and Cultural Change*, 32 (1), 121–148.

Shetty, P. S. & James, W. P. T. 1994. 'Body mass index: A measure of chronic energy deficiency in adults'. *FAO Food and Nutrition* Paper 56. Rome: Food and Agriculture Organisation.

Singer, M. N. et al. 2017. 'Syndemics and the biosocial conception of health'. *Lancet*, 389, 941–950.

Skoufias, E. 2016. 'Synergies in child nutrition: Interactions of food security, health and environment, and child care'. *Policy Research Working Paper*

7794. Washington DC: The World Bank.

Spears, D. 2013. 'How much international variation in child height can sanitation explain?' *World Bank Policy Research Working Paper*, WPS 6351. World Bank. http://go.worldbank.org/ SZE5WUJBI0, accessed 6 June 2013.

United Nations Children's Fund (UNICEF), World Health Organization (WHO) & World Bank. 2012. *Levels and Trends in Child Malnutrition. Joint Child Malnutrition Estimates.* New York, NY: United Nations Children's Fund; Geneva: World Health Organization; Washington, DC: World Bank.

United Nations Children's Fund (UNICEF). 2013. *Improving Child Nutrition: The achievable imperative for global progress.* New York: Division of Communication, United Nations Children's Fund. www.unicef.org/publications/index_68661.html, accessed 10 May 2017.

United Nations Children's Fund (UNICEF). 2016. UNICEF Global Databases, Stunting Disparities. New York: United Nations Children's Fund.

United Nations Development Programme (UNDP). 2012. *Zimbabwe 2012: Millennium Development Goals Progress Report.* Harare: Ministry of Economic Planning and Investment Promotion & United Nations Development Programme.

Victora, C. G. et al. 2010. 'Worldwide timing of growth faltering: Revisiting implications for interventions'. *Pediatrics*, 125, 473–480.

Victora, C. G. et al. 2013. 'Maternal and child undernutrition and overweight in low-income and middle-income countries'. *Lancet*, 382, 427–451.

World Health Organization (WHO). 2006. *World Health Statistics.* Geneva: World Health Organization.

World Health Organization (WHO). 2007. *WHO Child Growth Standards: Methods and Development.* Geneva: Department of Nutrition for Health and Development, World Health Organization.

World Health Organization (WHO). 2014. *Global Nutrition targets 2025: Stunting Policy Brief* (WHO/NMH/NHD/14.3). Geneva: World Health Organization.

Section Two

Contending with Epidemics and Health Systems in South Africa

THIS SECTION ANALYSES THE LESSONS that can be drawn from specific epidemical diseases that have struck, to variable degrees, in sub-Saharan Africa. At the core of this section is the importance of the state of a health system when disaster strikes, and how this determines the extent to which an outbreak will be contained. Multiple countries in sub-Saharan Africa have weak health systems. This is often as a result of social, economic, environmental, and political factors. It links to the notion of syndemics and the impact that the coexistence of a range of adverse socio-economic factors have on health outcomes.

Sunanda Ray, Farai Madzimbamuto and David Sanders present a chapter on the state of cholera in sub-Saharan Africa, which is endemic in 47 sub-Saharan African countries. The authors cite the 2008–2009 and 2018 cholera outbreaks in Zimbabwe to draw lessons on the social, economic, and political determinants of outbreaks of such a preventable disease. Corruption and mismanagement of resources by local and central government led to water and sanitation infrastructure and delivery being neglected and medications and essential supplies in city clinics being in short supply. Ray and co-authors typify the issues faced by several African countries in addressing the weaknesses in their public health systems that lead to calamities. Despite a significant cholera outbreak occurring in 2017/2018 in Lusaka, in neighbouring country Zambia, public health authorities in Zimbabwe did not enhance surveillance nor carry out health education in preparation for a possible outbreak. The importance of surveillance systems in containing outbreaks is aptly explored in the next chapter by Kaka Mudambo. Mudambo offers an assessment of malaria in the SADC region and examines the factors that lead to an outbreak: environment and climate, politics, governance and demographics, and health systems. Mudambo shows that although malaria is still rampant in the region, multiple interventions implemented, including good surveillance systems, have helped SADC progress in containing malaria. The chapter also surveys the constraints on these interventions.

Finally, Nathaniel Umukoro's chapter explores the successful containment of the Ebola outbreak in Nigeria. The efficient deployments of health care workers, as well as decisive and fast-acting leadership by political and medical authorities, are shown to have made the difference in containing the outbreak. Compared to Guinea, Sierra Leone, and Liberia, which suffered devastating outbreaks, Nigeria's Ebola outbreak story is one that accentuates how an equipped health system and a timely response can limit the spread of an epidemic.

THREE

Cholera in Africa in the 21st Century

Questions of Justice and Human Rights

SUNANDA RAY, FARAI D. MADZIMBAMUTO,
AND DAVID SANDERS

INTRODUCTION

SUB-SAHARAN AFRICA HAS REPORTED more than 90 per cent of the total global cholera cases since 2001, despite having only 12 per cent of the world's population (Gaffga et al., 2007). Cholera is endemic in 47 countries of sub-Saharan Africa. There are an estimated 200 million people living in areas with some reported incidence (new cases) of cholera, ranging from those where cholera is endemic, to areas where high numbers of cases are reported every year or where there are large outbreaks, followed by periods of low activity (Lessler et al., 2018). Endemicity is defined as where confirmed cholera cases, resulting from local transmission, have been detected over the previous three years (GTFCC, 2017: 30). Between 2000 and 2015, 83 per cent of 63,658 cholera deaths reported to the World Health Organization (WHO) occurred in sub-Saharan Africa (Lessler et al., 2018).

This chapter provides an overview of the cholera situation in sub-Saharan Africa, the barriers to adequately addressing the pandemic, and some thoughts on innovative ways to move forward. The experiences from the outbreaks of 2008–2009 and 2018 in Zimbabwe are explored to exemplify the problems many countries in Africa face in addressing the failures in their public health systems that lead to such emergencies.

Cholera is transmitted through water or food contaminated with faecal material harbouring the causative bacteria Vibrio cholerae (V. cholerae), which, when ingested in a sufficient dose, infects the bowel and causes profuse watery diarrhoea with loss of water and salt. One in 20 infected persons suffers severe disease, while for others the infection can be mild or asymptomatic, with 70 per cent of infected persons continuing as carriers of the bacteria. Children are often worse affected in outbreaks because they have not been exposed to infection in the past and do not have immunity. Individuals with immune suppression, such as through HIV and some cancers, may also be at higher risk of becoming infected with cholera (Mushayabasa & Bhunu, 2012). In severe infections, dehydration is the main cause of rapid decline, with death occurring within hours. With appropriate treatment a case fatality rate (CFR)[i] of less than 1 per cent is expected (Yates et al., 2017). Vigorous oral rehydration or intravenous fluid and electrolyte replacement are the main therapies, with recovery within days. The dose required to cause infection is high, so direct person-to-person transmission through shaking hands and so on is not common (Leibovici-Weissman et al., 2014). Outbreaks die down when individuals no longer come in contact with contaminated water or when they have developed immunity to the strain of bacteria.

Cholera is a disease said to symbolise inequity because people who live in poverty are disproportionately affected, despite this being a disease that is easy to prevent and treat. Ninety-two million people in Africa still drink water from unsafe sources (WHO, 2018a). Outbreaks occur when water and sanitation infrastructure is non-existent, inequitably distributed, or breaks down as a result of political or economic neglect, or during humanitarian crises. Nation states

i The case fatality rate (CFR) measures the proportion of deaths of all those diagnosed with the disease, and is an indicator of the quality of treatment and care.

in Africa have failed spectacularly to provide basic facilities, despite worsening outbreaks over the last 50 years, with accompanying mortalities and disruption to health systems, and despite signing up to the UN Sustainable Development Goals (SDGs) and various human rights declarations. The crisis of cholera and other water-borne diseases in Africa has generated a huge literature on the biomedical aspects of the infection, but little that overtly challenges the underlying socio-economic and political determinants of outbreaks. Some have argued that neglecting to address the political determinants of complex epidemics limits the integrity of these scientific publications (Cuneo et al., 2017).

SOCIAL, ECONOMIC, AND POLITICAL DETERMINANTS OF CHOLERA

Cholera is increasingly an urban problem in sub-Saharan Africa. In many large cities, migration from rural to urban areas and natural population growth have contributed to large peri-urban informal settlements, with overcrowding and increased demand on fragile water, sanitation, and hygiene (WASH) infrastructure. The proportion of people living in urban areas of Africa is predicted to increase from 36 per cent in 2010 to 50 per cent by 2030, with a corresponding increase in slum dwellers, who already make up 60 per cent of the urban population (GTFCC, 2017). Conflict and humanitarian crises also encourage migration to peri-urban and slum areas. Increasing affluence in other parts of cities and industrial development where there is economic growth increase private and public demand for water services, which also puts pressure on infrastructure. Despite exposing tremendous inequalities in access to safe drinking water and sanitation facilities, these injustices continue. Minimal opportunities for formal employment force young people into informal economic activities, such as vending in urban areas. Slum dwellings around unregulated mining sites without proper WASH facilities have been identified as hotspots for cholera transmission, especially since the crude gold ore may be washed in contaminated water (Hilson, 2002). Informal gold mining has historically been associated with the spread of cholera and has been associated with outbreaks in Zimbabwe, Tanzania, Ghana, South Africa, and Sudan (APA, 2018; Isaäcson et al., 1974; Opare et al., 2012).

The year 2018 experienced a spike in cholera cases in sub-Saharan Africa, with eight countries reporting and struggling with outbreaks. In 2017, more than 150,000 cholera cases and more than 3,000 deaths were reported in 17 countries in Africa. Countries in sub-Saharan Africa are struggling with other humanitarian and public health crises. Civil conflict, displaced peoples, refugee camps, climate change, unmanaged urbanisation, and overcrowding in peri-urban areas that are poorly serviced by local government (WHO, 2018a) all contribute to cholera outbreaks. In Zambia, an outbreak of cholera began in October 2017 and resulted in 5,905 cases and 114 deaths, with a CFR of 1.9 per cent;[ii] 92 per cent of cases and 98 deaths were in Lusaka, the capital city (Sinyange et al., 2018). The highest risk of contagion was in the city's high-density informal peri-urban settlements, where 70 per cent of the population live, which still rely on shallow wells and pit latrines (Bahadur, 2018).

The case of Zimbabwe

In 2008–2009, following the worst cholera outbreak in Zimbabwe's history, with nearly 100,000 suspected cases, 4,282 deaths, and a CFR of five per cent (Ahmed et al., 2011), several commentators wrote critical analyses of the epidemic and the humanitarian crisis that precipitated it (Nyandoro, 2011; HRW, 2013; Sollom et al., 2009). A damning Human Rights Watch (HRW) report titled 'Troubled Water: Burst Pipes, Contaminated Wells, and Open Defecation in Zimbabwe's Capital', released in November 2013, described how limited access to potable water and sanitation services was forcing citizens to resort to using water from unprotected sources and to other unhygienic practices, such as open defecation (HRW, 2013).

Amnesty International reported that the Zimbabwe government's failure in 2008 to provide safe drinking water and to repair broken-down sanitation systems left residents surrounded by flowing raw

ii A CFR value of more than one per cent demonstrates the lack of access to basic health care facilities with shortages of oral rehydration therapy, oral zinc, antibiotics, and intravenous fluids.

sewage, which contaminated water supplies and resulted in the worst cholera outbreak in memory.

A decade later, the same failures caused a repeat outbreak, in 2018: broken-down sanitation infrastructure and poor sewerage management, worsened by shortages of drugs, intravenous fluids, and medical supplies (Amnesty International, 2018). As of April 2018, 107 cases and four deaths (CFR 3.8 per cent) had been notified in Zimbabwe, with 9 per cent of cases aged less than five years (McAteer et al., 2018). From September to November 2018, in the recent outbreak, 10,086 cumulative cases, including 163 laboratory-confirmed cases, and 61 deaths were reported (CFR 0.6 per cent) (Reliefweb, 2018). Ninety-eight per cent of these cases were reported from Harare, with the most affected suburbs being Glen View and Budiriro, which were similarly affected in 2008.

History shows that the massive investment by European cities in construction of safe water supplies and efficient sewerage systems as part of 'sanitary reforms' in the mid to late 19th century paved the way for the elimination of cholera and other water-borne diseases. Improved knowledge of bacteriology and the discovery of the causative agent of cholera in 1884 influenced public health legislation of the time, allowing for the quarantine and isolation of affected persons, the disinfection of premises, and mass public education on hygiene and prevention (Evans, 1992). Similarly, major investments in the 1990s in safe drinking water supplies and sanitation facilities, as well as local production and promotion of bleach for household treatment of water, hygienic water storage, and the implementation of oral rehydration led to the successful control of cholera outbreaks in Latin American countries (Gaffga et al., 2007).

Prior to Zimbabwe's independence in 1980, urban population growth was tightly controlled by the colonial state through the regulation of where Africans could reside and own property. Concerns about hygiene among white ratepayers in Harare led to the introduction of new technologies in water and sanitation infrastructure in white residential areas. These were developed to the same standard as the cities of Europe. Meanwhile poorer and cheaper water and sanitation solutions were implemented in the segregated high-density areas reserved for the black population. At independence in 1980 the new government diverted resources from the cities to rural water development. The rural areas had been the backbone of the liberation struggle and were to be maintained as the main political base of the ruling party. Young people from the rural areas migrated into the cities searching for work, often living in informal shanty dwelling settlements which were not serviced by either water or sewerage facilities. Harare's sewerage system, designed for a small population, discharged its treated effluent into the very water source it drew from, creating a need for more intensive water treatment as increasingly poorly treated effluent was discharged (Musemwa, 2010).

At the political level, the relationship between central and local government changed when urban councils came under opposition party control after 2002 but were still dependent on central government funding. By 2005 the media were commenting on the increasing state of decay in some parts of the capital city of Harare, of litter dumping in open spaces, the mushrooming of squatter shacks, and raw sewage flowing in the streets (Musemwa, 2010). Water supplies became erratic in Harare's northern more affluent suburbs. Foreign currency shortages were blamed for the lack of chemicals to treat the water supply and for the failure to repair water pipes that were leaking.

Shortly after the national general elections in 2005, the government launched Operation Murambatsvina (Move the Rubbish), although it was officially known as Operation Restore Order. This was a large-scale operation forcibly to clear slum areas across the country, thereby displacing more than 700,000 people. It was believed that the displaced were mainly opposition supporters who, having been rendered homeless, would now have to move back to the rural areas, where they would be under control of the ruling party political structures. Management of urban water supplies and sanitation was removed from local authorities and transferred to the Zimbabwe National Water Authority (ZINWA). This spiral of failure continued to worsen as the financial and technical problems mounted, and residents found their own solutions in sinking boreholes in the affluent areas and shallow wells in the poorer parts. At the same time, during the land occupations where farmers were forcibly displaced from their farms, people were encouraged to settle anywhere, including on peri-urban land. The urban authorities expected that this would be temporary, so they neglected to extend urban infrastructure to these settlements (which would make them permanent). The result was what people called a 'cholera time-bomb'. During March 2006, 26 cholera deaths occurred, presaging what was to come two years later (Cuneo et al., 2017).

The functions of ZINWA included advising the government on policy, standards, and the conservation of national water supplies, as well as promoting the equitable, efficient, and sustainable allocation and distribution of water resources. ZINWA was also meant to assist local authorities in the discharge of their functions with regard to the development and management of the water resources under their jurisdiction and, in particular, the provision of potable water. Commentators on the lead-up to the 2008 cholera crisis believe that the government nationalised municipal water authorities to provide additional revenue streams to fill its coffers and to deprive the opposition-run municipal councils of an important source of revenue (Musemwa, 2010; Sollom et al., 2009). The government was also credited with purposely using the water shortages to take back control of the cities from the opposition. The Bulawayo City Council resisted a ZINWA takeover and did not experience the same water shortages as Harare – and Bulawayo had very few cases of cholera both in 2008 and in 2018, with most cases that were reported there having been imported from elsewhere. They also managed to source chemicals with the help of local business communities. ZINWA received significant funding from the Reserve Bank to rehabilitate Harare's waterworks, but had little to show for it (Musemwa, 2010). The government allowed outdated and damaged water systems to go unrepaired and water supplies to go untreated. A water systems engineer in Harare stated that ZINWA had not improved water service delivery; instead the parastatal agency had caused its ruin (Sollom et al., 2009).

Corruption and mismanagement were features of both local and central government. During 2014, through audits carried out by the Auditor General's office on state enterprises and parastatals, it came to light that senior management in many of Zimbabwe's parastatal organisations (the Public Service Medical Aid Society, the Zimbabwe Broadcasting Corporation, the national airline, the revenue authority, the electricity supply authority, and others) were being paid hundreds of thousands of US dollars (USD) a month (Simpson & Hawkins, 2018: 350–351). Seven Harare City Council senior executives were paid monthly salaries and allowances in excess of USD 30,000 a month. With allowances for school fees, holidays, travel, on-call, and so on, their monthly pay was in the hundreds of thousands of USD. The seven executives included the Director of Water Services, the Director of Health Services, and the Director of Works in the City of Harare (Davies, 2016; Rusvingo, 2014). These salaries were being paid while general workers were stranded for over five months without being paid. It was in this context that repair work of facilities was left undone. When it came to health care infrastructure, city clinics were struggling with shortages of medications and essential supplies. Funding for water and sanitation infrastructure was not made available and fulfilling organisational obligations to ratepayers was not prioritised.

Many would wonder how senior civil servants would justify to themselves their entitlement to such huge sums of public money, clearly to the detriment of local services, to the extent that, in 2008, it directly caused the deaths of more than 4,000 people in Zimbabwe. Magaisa argues that Zimbabwe was and still is in the hands of a powerful clique of oligarchs, a small influential network of political, military, and business elites who control and run the country for their own benefit and without any concern for the welfare of its people (Magaisa, 2018). These elites are only interested in accumulation of private wealth. They do not pay taxes or utility bills, although they extract these payments from others. They use their economic power and military allegiances to never be held accountable for their misdeeds and to maintain political control. They also create a façade of democracy to keep international agencies still patching up the humanitarian consequences of their disastrous policies. A similar situation is likely to exist in other countries of Africa, to varying degrees, depending on the level of accountability governments have to their electorate.

Sustainable Development Goals

Most African countries did not meet the UN Millennium Development Goals' safe water target, which was to reduce by half the proportion of the population without sustainable access to safe drinking water from 1990 to 2015. Based on current trends, sub-Saharan Africa will not reach this target until 2040 (UNEP, 2010). As part of the UN Sustainable Development Goals (SDGs) adopted by the UN General Assembly in 2015 (UN, 2016), Goal Six states that by 2030 countries should aim to achieve universal and equitable access to safe and affordable drinking water for all and achieve access to adequate and equitable sanitation and hygiene. Performance against these targets will be measured by the proportion of the population using safely managed drinking water services, the proportion of the population using safely managed sanitation services (including a hand-washing facility with soap and water), and the amount of water- and sanitation-related official development assistance that is part of a government-coordinated spending plan. Despite supporting these ambitious targets, most African governments have not prioritised funding for their achievement, so progress is slow. The report on progress in line with the SDGs shows that 68 per cent of the population in sub-Saharan Africa had access to improved water sources in 2015, an increase from 55 per cent in 2000, but was still substantially lower than all four Asian regions (approximately 90 per cent) and Latin America (approximately 95 per cent). Some of these 'improved' water sources, such as borehole water, may still be contaminated with faecal matter. Only 30 per cent of Africans in sub-Saharan Africa had access to improved sanitation in 2015, having increased from 26 per cent in 2000, compared to over 70 per cent in most of Asia and Latin America (UN, 2016).

Human rights

Walsh and Johnson state that unless emergency responses include a recognition of what individuals are entitled to simply by virtue of being human, there is a risk of dehumanising them, of perceiving people as data to be analysed or as vectors of infection (Walsh & Johnson, 2018). These rights are embedded in several international declarations and charters. The United Nations General Assembly, through Resolution 64/292 in 2010, explicitly recognises the human right to water and sanitation and acknowledges that clean drinking water and sanitation are essential to the realisation of all human rights. The African Charter on Human and Peoples' Rights similarly includes the right to 'a general satisfactory environment' favourable to peoples' 'development', which is unattainable without access to water and sanitation. The Convention on the Elimination of All Forms of Discrimination against Women states that rural women have a right to 'adequate living conditions, particularly in relation to ... water supply'. The Convention on the Rights of the Child states that all children have a right to the highest attainable standard of health guaranteed, including 'through the provision of adequate ... clean drinking water'. The Convention on the Rights of Persons with Disabilities recognises 'the right of persons with disabilities to social protection ... including measures to ensure equal access by persons with disabilities to clean water' (HRW, 2013).

Although they voted for UN Resolution 64/292, most African countries do not have enshrined in their national constitutions any statement regarding the constitutional right to safe water and sanitation, although several mention the right to a healthy environment (Higuet, 2014). Some legislative frameworks are weaker than they might be, making it challenging for individuals and civil society to advocate for the realisation of their rights. The Ethiopian constitution states, '*To the extent the country's resources permit, policies shall aim to provide all Ethiopians access to public health and education, clean water, housing, food and social security.*' The Gambia, Egypt, Djibouti, Morocco, Niger, Somalia, South Africa, South Sudan, Uganda, and Zambia also have statements in their constitutions that citizens have a right to water or clean water. The Kenyan constitution states that '*Every person has the right to accessible and adequate housing, and to reasonable standards of sanitation and to clean and safe water in adequate quantities*' (Higuet, 2014).

In Zimbabwe, the new constitution adopted in 2013 clearly places an obligation on the state to guarantee the rights of persons to a clean environment (section 73), the right to health care (section 76), and the right to safe, clean, and potable water (section 77) (GoZ, 2013). In addition, the newly revised Public Health Act of 2018 directs every local authority '*to provide and maintain, or cause to be provided and maintained as far as may be reasonably possible, a sufficient supply of wholesome water for drinking and domestic purposes*' (GoZ, 2018).

AFRICAN AND GLOBAL INITIATIVES FOR CHOLERA PREVENTION AND CONTROL

African health ministers in August 2018 adopted the Regional Framework for Implementation of the Global Strategy for Cholera Prevention and Control, pledging to reduce by 90 per cent the magnitude of cholera outbreaks, particularly among vulnerable populations and in humanitarian crises. They agreed to take evidence-based actions to achieve this by 2030. These include increasing investments in clean water and sanitation infrastructure to avoid contamination of water supplies, enhancing epidemiological and laboratory surveillance, mapping cholera hotspots, improving access to timely treatment, strengthening cross-border surveillance, promoting community engagement, and the use of the oral cholera vaccine (OCV).

The Global Task Force on Cholera Control (GTFCC), set up in 2017 by the WHO and partners, has proposed a three-pronged strategic approach to eradicating cholera. The first axis is one of emergency preparedness, having a rapid targeted response to outbreaks using enhanced early warning surveillance, followed by rapid delivery of cholera control kits, OCV, and WASH supplies. A functioning health system that can anticipate outbreaks and respond rapidly to alerts is essential for this approach. The second axis involves a focus on hotspots of endemic cholera, using a multisectoral approach. Use of OCVs can reduce transmission in the short term during outbreaks (effective for three to five years), thereby reducing the disease burden and mortality while longer-term repairs to the WASH infrastructure are made. The third axis is the coordination of operational support, local and global resourcing, and technical expertise delivered by GTFCC. Strong community partnerships will be essential for all interventions to stop transmission. The plan is for the task force to support six to eight countries to develop cholera control plans, develop an investment case on cholera, and create operational guidance on integrated prevention strategies (GTFCC, 2017).

Emergency preparedness

To be effective, response to cholera outbreaks must be urgent and rapid, with active anticipatory public health and laboratory surveillance and leadership from key players in the health sector and related agencies. Governments in sub-Saharan Africa need to act on the lessons from past outbreaks. One problem is that these outbreaks are relatively uncommon in each country, so health agencies may not retain institutional memory of what actions to take. There were several warnings ahead of the 2018 Harare outbreak, but they did not trigger preparedness for another major outbreak in Harare. With substantial movement of people and trade across borders in southern Africa, there is always the potential for the spread of infections from one area to another. There is evidence that the strains that caused the 2008 outbreak in Zimbabwe were related to cross-border transmission from Zambia and Mozambique, and were originally from Bangladesh, suggesting that the same strain was spreading globally (Islam et al., 2011). There was a significant cholera outbreak in Lusaka which lasted from October 2017 to May 2018 (Sinyange et al., 2018) which should have alerted public health authorities in Zimbabwe to enhance surveillance and to carry out presumptive health education. Similarly, in January 2018 an outbreak of approximately 60 cases of cholera occurred in Chegutu, a small town 100 km from Harare, with a possible link to the Lusaka outbreak. Water quality monitoring at water points and boreholes in high-density areas of Harare revealed several water sources to be heavily contaminated with faecal bacteria, while sporadic cases of cholera and typhoid were notified all over the country (Machamire, 2017). Broken sewer pipes have been implicated repeatedly in outbreaks of typhoid and other water-borne diseases in Harare (Davis et al., 2018; Muti et al., 2014). The response to these red flags appears to have been limited to the mobilisation of volunteers to give hygiene education and to hand out disinfection tablets and buckets, mainly by non-governmental organisations (NGOs). Beyond this there has been little sustained activity from the relevant government ministries to prevent the escalation of another outbreak.

The emergency response to the cholera threat is often hampered by a lack of resources, inadequately staffed hospitals, limited health awareness activities, and unclean water. In the Zimbabwe outbreak of 2008–2009, two-thirds of the deaths were reported from communities with poor access to treatment facilities (Ahmed et al., 2011). Often international agencies take a leading role because they have more experience of emergency responses. They are geared to quickly organise medical supplies, protective clothing, raise funds and so on. At the request of the WHO Global Outbreak Alert and Response Network (GOARN), the International Centre for Diarrhoeal Disease Research (ICDDR) from Bangladesh sent a six-member team to Zimbabwe in 2008 to provide technical expertise to the Ministry of Health and Child Care. The review team reported that there was inadequate monitoring of patients, overuse of intravenous fluids on their own rather than combined with oral rehydration therapy, that antibiotic use did not follow guidelines, that laboratory facilities were limited, and staffing levels were low (Ahmed et al., 2011). Despite many warnings of persistent water contamination, especially of borehole water, preparedness was low and pre-emptive actions such as running drills for frontline health staff were not carried out. Many of the solutions implemented, such as training health professionals in case management, especially using computer-based interactive training, appeared not to endure to the next major outbreak ten years later.

The role of international partners

International partners have an important role in supporting communities in sub-Saharan Africa, especially when they are most vulnerable, such as during humanitarian crises and emergencies. However, their intervention often masks the inaction of governments. It is governments who are responsible for the long-term infrastructure requirements of communities. Funds become available to resolve the immediate crisis, rather than being made routinely available for investment in the medium- or long-term development of WASH infrastructure. As an example, the declaration of a state of emergency over the cholera outbreak in Harare on 11 September 2018 was followed by an appeal from the Zimbabwean government for USD 60 million to address life-saving, short- and medium-term needs in WASH infrastructure. The UN Resident Coordinator made an allocation of USD 3 million from the UN Central Emergency Response Fund (CERF) in response to the cholera outbreak, to be administered by UNICEF, WHO, and the World Food Programme (WFP). Ten hotspot areas in Harare, including Glen View, Budiriro, and Mbare, were identified: the funds were used to provide health care, WASH, and food aid interventions for 600,000 people at risk of infection. The fund allowed for the immediate rapid scale-up of cholera outbreak response activities while alternative resource mobilisation efforts continued. The UN strategic support to development in Zimbabwe is guided by the 2016–2020 Zimbabwe United Nations Development Assistance Framework (ZUNDAF), which aims to contribute to six result areas: Social Services and Protection; Food and Nutrition Security; HIV and AIDS; Gender Equality; Poverty Reduction and Value Addition; and Public Administration and Governance. As of 30 June 2018, the mid-point of the ZUNDAF implementation cycle, the UN delivered USD 1.1 billion in the form of various development projects, accounting for 70 per cent of the total USD 1.6 billion planned to be mobilised over a period of five years. A sustainable urban plan for medium- to long-term renovation and renewal of WASH infrastructure, as well as sustainable waste disposal management, is desperately needed. UN System also facilitated the deployment of an inter-agency Capacity for Disaster Reduction Initiative (CADRI) to assess the country's disaster preparedness. The actions taken up to that point, however, did not manage to prevent the 2018 cholera outbreak in Harare – despite numerous warnings.

Médecins Sans Frontières (MSF), also known as Doctors Without Borders, is an international humanitarian NGO of French origin. In 2017, MSF teams treated 143,100 people for cholera in 13 countries, compared with 20,600 people in 2016. MSF responded to cholera outbreaks in Nigeria, Chad, Kenya, and South Sudan. In Yemen, MSF treated more than 100,000 people in 37 treatment centres and at oral rehydration points. They similarly managed to treat half the reported cases in one of the worst cholera outbreaks in 20 years in the Democratic Republic of Congo (DRC), where around 55,000 people were reported as cases in 24 provinces, with more than 1,000 deaths (MSF, 2017). These are often people in crisis situations, in camps for displaced people, or in war or conflict zones. In Zimbabwe, MSF has brought safe, clean water to vulnerable communities in high-density suburbs in Harare, including drilling new boreholes and rehabilitating existing ones. They also provided logistical and technical support to the Ministry of Health and Child Care during the 2018 outbreak; they provided nurses, water and sanitation expertise, and logisticians to support the technical capacity of local authorities and government (MSF, 2018).

Treatment for cholera

With vigorous rehydration, mortality – expressed as the case fatality rate (CFR) – can be reduced to less than 1 per cent, even in makeshift tent treatment centres (Gaffga et al., 2007). Antibiotic treatment for cholera was introduced in 1964 and found to limit the duration of bacteria shedding and the diarrhoeal episode, as well as reducing diarrhoeal volume (CDC, 2015). Antibiotics were used for moderately to severely ill patients together with aggressive fluid therapy (Leibovici-Weissman et al., 2014). Antibiotic sensitivity is tested in each outbreak to guide treatment and to track the evolution of the organism for epidemiological purposes.

Resistance of *V. cholerae* to most antibiotics is increasing; this may have emerged from prophylaxis of household contacts of patients with severe cholera in past epidemics (Okeke et al., 2007). During the 2008–2009 outbreak in Zimbabwe, *V. cholerae* strains showed variable sensitivity to commonly used antibiotics. Specimens from the Zambia outbreak in 2017 similarly showed variable sensitivity to the main antibiotics recommended (Sinyange et al., 2018). The Bangladesh ICDDR team suggested that the limited availability of laboratory services led to uninformed antibiotic use, which may have contributed to poor treatment outcomes (Ahmed et al., 2011), and that experience from Bangladesh indicated that cholera caused by strains with reduced sensitivity to ciprofloxacin was associated with therapy failure (Islam et al., 2011). In the 2018 outbreak, however, the strain circulating showed multi-drug resistance (WHO, 2018b). Antibiotic stewardship to decrease irrational antibiotic prescribing generally, but especially in management of diarrhoeal diseases, requires more emphasis in the region. Alternative approaches to antibiotic treatment are being explored, including drugs that could counter the severe diarrhoeal effects of the V. cholerae. The use of bacteriophages, viruses that infect bacteria, in treatment and in environmental management of water sources, remains to be explored (Nelson et al., 2009). Originally studied in India from 1928–1934, they were found to be useful in cholera outbreaks, but were overtaken by the development and effectiveness of fluid-based therapies and antibiotics.

In resource-limited settings the outcome of therapy depends on the time it takes for patients to seek and receive care, as well as the response time of the emergency system to manage the outbreak. When patients begin therapy after a significant delay, their fluid losses have become severe and intravenous (IV) therapy is essential (Ahmed et al., 2011). Oral fluids are used in all patients, with IV fluids added in severe cases to achieve rapid rehydration, especially when patients are vomiting. Huge quantities of IV fluids are necessary to resuscitate patients with severe dehydration. All the IV fluids used for rehydration in the last ten years, including for the cholera outbreaks, were imported from South Africa and other manufacturing countries. Ghana is a major producer for the West African market. The market in Africa for IV fluids is expected to reach a billion dollars in value because of growth in medical care and epidemics, with South Africa as the largest producer (Srivastava & Jaiswal, 2018). Large volumes of IV fluids brought into the countries by donors have had a deleterious impact on local suppliers. The pharmaceutical manufacturing sector in Africa is very weak. Local markets are not big enough to sustain manufacture and they do not keep sufficient stockpiles for emergency situations. A local company in Zimbabwe (Datlabs) used to manufacture IV fluid packs but, having failed to secure investment, it has been non-functional for 15 years. In the wake of the 2018 cholera outbreak the government of Zimbabwe has now pledged to assist the company to rehabilitate its IV fluids manufacturing plant (Equity-axis, 2018).

Mapping of cholera hotspots in Africa

Cholera incidence is thought to be concentrated in high-burden hotspots. Mapping of incidence of cholera between 2000 and 2016 in Africa was used to identify high-risk populations that could be targeted for specific interventions, to prevent and control outbreaks (Lessler et al., 2018). Areas with previous outbreaks were divided into 20 km square grids and data about the incidence, location of outbreaks within the grid, population, and water and sanitation coverage were used to generate maps of cholera incidence throughout sub-Saharan Africa. Based on this model, almost 90 million people in 150 districts were identified as having high risk for cholera; they could be targeted with interventions such as oral cholera vaccine or water and sanitation measures to prevent or reduce infections. By targeting districts in order of their cholera incidence (from highest to lowest), an effective cholera intervention (e.g. vaccination campaigns combined with improved water and sanitation) could eliminate 50 per cent of reported cholera cases in the region by covering less than 4 per cent of the population (35 million people). More than 168 million doses of OCV would be needed to vaccinate all eligible individuals living in these high-risk districts, which is substantially more vaccine than has been stockpiled. However, by concentrating on a small proportion (< 5%) of districts, better value for resources can be gained.

Immunity to cholera has been known for over a hundred years, when survivors of cholera in India were observed to develop resistance to the disease that lasted several months. The first oral vaccine was tested in Bangladesh in 1980, the forerunner of vaccines in current use. The OCV, given as a single dose, confers protection for six months, while the two-dose vaccine gives 50–80 per cent protection at three years. Modelling results suggest that vaccinating twice the number of people with a single dose will save more lives than using the two-dose regimen in a smaller population during an outbreak, which may be necessary if vaccine supplies are limited (Azman et al., 2016). The single-dose vaccination was successfully implemented in an outbreak in South Sudan in 2015, and the two-dose vaccination was deployed during the Zambia outbreak in 2018 (Azman et al., 2016; Sinyange et al., 2018). Vaccines sourced from the global stockpile funded by Gavi, the Vaccine Alliance, were allocated and administered by the Ministry of Health and Child Care in Zimbabwe, with support from WHO and other partners, to protect over a million people in cholera hotspots (WHO, 2018c). The use of OCV is a temporary bridging strategy, however. It cannot be the mainstay of cholera prevention, since it relies on donor support and does not prevent the acquisition of other water-borne infections. There is agreement that provision and maintenance of WASH infrastructure (safe sustainable water, sanitation, and hygiene facilities) are essential for the long-term cessation of transmission of cholera, typhoid, and other diarrhoeal diseases (GTFCC, 2017; Ivers, 2017). Universal access to clean water and improved sanitation provision, apart from conferring dignity, encompasses far wider social and health benefits for communities than a single short-term intervention like the vaccine can provide.

Community engagement

A key lesson from the Ebola outbreak in West Africa in 2014 (see Chapter 5), which applies to any outbreak or emergency situation, was that community engagement is critical from the outset of the response and must be prioritised (Walsh & Johnson, 2018). Listening to communities that are affected is essential to understand the challenges they face and what they feel needs to be done to enable them to protect themselves. When interventions are potentially stigmatising, such as mandatory supervision of funerals, getting traditional and religious leaders and community organisers on board is crucial for success. NGOs can be mediators who assist communities to mobilise, to develop, and to implement and monitor their own action plans. Social, economic, and political relationships determine how epidemic diseases spread, what their impact on populations will be, and to what degree this impact will be manifested. The way communities cope and respond has been described as 'a test of social cohesion' where the interaction and cooperation between different layers of society may be stressed to their limits (Evans, 1992). In Zimbabwe, community engagement has taken two major forms: local action for prevention, and advocacy for protection of human rights.

MSF works with local communities to enable them to manage and maintain water points through trained community health clubs (MSF, 2018). Committee members oversee the provision of clean water to members who contribute a small monthly fee to pay for chlorine and maintenance of the points. Over 70 rehabilitated boreholes are now managed by more than 60 community health clubs in 13 high-density residential suburbs in Harare. Members trained in water and hygiene safety responded to the outbreak in September 2018 by conducting house-to-house awareness campaigns, especially those in the hardest hit areas (Glen View, Budiriro, Mbare). An initial survey conducted by MSF of 16 community health clubs covering more than 8,000 people in the four most affected suburbs found only four suspected cholera cases. As the outbreak progressed a significant number of new community members signed up to receive clean water, as they became convinced of the benefits of such clubs. Harare City relied heavily on volunteers to provide health and hygiene education (especially on treating water and hand-washing) to households in its high-density areas. More than a thousand Red Cross volunteers went door-to-door, handing out bleach, water purification tablets, and buckets for storing water.

Civil society organisations have campaigned for the government to be held accountable for the breakdown of WASH infrastructure yet again, and to be held accountable for the impact on families and people who became infected through contaminated water, notwithstanding a lower CFR because of a more rapid reaction to the numbers of people pouring into the Beatrice Road Infectious Diseases Hospital and into the cholera treatment centres in Glen View and Budiriro. In 2018 the Civil Society Health Emergency Response Coordinating Committee (CSHERCC) made a statement (Chibamu, 2018) that the government, and through it the local authorities and ZINWA, were accountable for the deaths of people, since they had failed to provide basic health services, medical treatment and services, clean running water, and a sanitary environment for people so as to contain the spread of the water-borne disease. CSHERCC reminded the government of the human right to health enshrined in the country's constitution and the human rights instruments to which the government was a signatory. It called on the relevant ministries to work collaboratively and swiftly together with communities and non-state actors, and to take corrective measures to prevent further deaths from cholera, contain the epidemic, and prevent further outbreaks, and to provide clean running water and sanitary environs to all affected communities. All local government (municipal) authorities were included in the call, as well as specifically relevant ministries: Health and Child Care; Lands, Agriculture, Water, Climate and Rural Resettlement; Environment, Tourism and Hospitality Industry; Local Government, Public Works and National Housing. CSHERCC also called on the Zimbabwe Human Rights Commission swiftly to investigate the violation of people's constitutional right to life, health, and clean water. The Ministry of Finance was called on to increase the budget allocation for water, sanitation, and hygiene, and to achieve the 15 per cent budgetary allocation to health as provided in the Abuja Declaration. Local authorities were reminded that they had a duty to account for funds raised from ratepayers for water and sewerage in order progressively to contribute towards the realisation of the right to health and water.

The CSHERCC statement was endorsed by several civil society organisations, including the Zimbabwe Association of Doctors for Human Rights, the Community Water Alliance, the Community Working Group on Health, Zimbabwe Lawyers for Human Rights, and the Vendors Initiative for Social and Economic Transformation (VISET) (Kubatana, 2018).

VISET is a group that advocates for the rights of vendors, who were particularly targeted and harassed by the municipality's police during the attempted clearing of the Harare Central Business District in the name of cholera prevention in 2018. In reality, there was no evidence that vending was a risk factor in cholera transmission, even when fruit was being sold.

The focus of much of the response to the alerts on other outbreaks and reports on water quality was to emphasise personal hygiene rather than allocating expenditure for repairs to the WASH infrastructure. Government officials tend to focus on individual responsibility and scold communities for not practising good hygiene, instead of paying attention to the sewage pouring through the gutters from broken sewer pipes, as was the case in Harare in 2018. This was despite good evidence that person-to-person contact was not the main source of transmission. Restrictions placed on public gatherings and banning vendors from the city centre is suspected of having a political basis, as vendors are often forced into informal occupation due to high levels of unemployment. In many countries vendors are vocal critics of government policies.

In the 2017–2018 cholera outbreak in Lusaka, Zambia, riots broke out, leading to arrests, following the clampdown on vendors. The Lusaka Water and Sewerage Company, wholly owned by the Lusaka City Council, was accused of prioritising water connections for formal households and business, while neglecting peri-urban areas where the majority of the poor resided. Water was sold as a commodity through kiosks (private intermediaries) as part of a World Bank-funded project (2007–2013) but the bank was unable to sustain the technical and commercial efficiency of operations. In 2015, 10 per cent of the kiosks were not functioning. As with the Harare situation, there was poor coordination between local government and central government structures and activities (Bahadur, 2018).

Financing the prevention and control of cholera

The UNDP Human Development Report (2006) advises that governments should be spending about 1 per cent of GDP on WASH provision, with funding from taxes and tariffs, but also with international aid assistance (UNEP, 2010). The finance minister of Zimbabwe sparked public outrage during the 2018 outbreak when he launched an online crowdfunding appeal for donations to pay for commodities required for the outbreak, especially IV fluids and antibiotics. The move was considered hypocritical in light of reports that the government was spending money on new vehicles for cabinet members, but not budgeting for funds to repair the ageing water infrastructure. The government subsequently pledged USD 1 million to enable Harare City authorities to contain the further spread of cholera.

Following its successful contribution to supporting the response to the Ebola outbreak in West Africa, mobile phone company Econet Zimbabwe donated USD 10 million towards resolving the cholera crisis in Harare. It pledged to repair the sewer systems in cholera-affected areas, including pipe replacement of sewerage and water infrastructure in Budiriro and Glen View. It agreed to complement Harare City Council's refuse collection efforts by removing dumpsites in Mufakose, Glen View, Budiriro, Glen Norah, and the city centre (Kadirire, 2018). By rescuing the local government in its failure to provide safe water and sanitation facilities, yet again Econet, along with other international agencies, was providing a short-term solution to a chronic problem. Other industries made contributions too. Zimplats, for example, donated to the ministries of Finance and Economic Development and Health and Child Care antibiotics for 1,000 patients, 1,350 litres of IV fluids, and water treatment chemicals for up to 4,000 households (Zimplats, 2018).

International structures are in place to address epidemic, pandemic, and humanitarian crises such as cholera and Ebola. The United Nations Inter-Agency Standing Committee (UN-IASC) was established in 1992 in response to UN General Assembly Resolution 46/182 on the strengthening of humanitarian assistance. The IASC is a unique inter-agency forum for coordination, policy development, and decision-making involving key UN and non-UN humanitarian partners. It has specified the immediate deployment of qualified personnel, supplies, and the automatic release of funds from the Central Emergencies Relief Fund to prevent outbreaks escalating out of control. The World Bank has also launched a Pandemic Emergency Financing Facility, an insurance facility that should enable a more rapid response in emergency situations (Walsh & Johnson, 2018). What is missing are structures and plans to raise funds for sufficient WASH infrastructure and technology, particularly in cholera hotspots, which have been demonstrated to be the most sustainable long-term solutions.

Sub-Saharan Africa is the region with the lowest per-capita expenditure on health (USD 199 purchasing power parity in 2015 compared to South Asia at USD 212 and the World at USD 1,300), with the highest under-five mortality (78 per 1,000 live births in 2016, compared to 48 in South Asia and 41 for the World), and lowest life expectancy at birth (60 years compared to 69 in South Asia and 72 for the World) (Darvas et al., 2018). The richer the country, the more it spends on health in both the public and private sectors, whereas out-of-pocket expenditures are highest in poorer countries, especially those in sub-Saharan Africa. Some have argued that investing in health significantly contributes to economic development, so high-income countries should be urged to contribute through financial aid to achieve this purpose (Sanders, 2004). According to this thinking, in the instance of cholera prevention and control, investment in WASH infrastructure to prevent diarrhoeal diseases such as cholera and others would in itself lead to healthier, more economically thriving communities.

This line of argument avoids scrutiny of currently dominant macroeconomic policies and structures that perpetuate financial disadvantage in medium- and low-income (MLI) countries. Poverty Reduction Strategy Papers are recommended as a mechanism to direct development assistance towards strengthening health systems and are an integral part of global economic governance regimes. However, often these international strategies result in reduced national public sector health expenditure. This leads to greater inequalities in income, and from this to inequities in access to health services and health outcomes (Sanders, 2004).

The regulation of trade and intellectual property, for example in relation to transnational pharmaceutical corporations, has been dominated by rich countries, and places many essential drugs beyond the economic reach of poor people in MLI countries. An example with the cholera outbreaks in Africa is where the mainstay of treatment is IV fluids with back-up use of antibiotics for severe cases. None of these is manufactured in the affected countries, so they have to be imported – the financial benefit remains in the manufacturing countries – which increases dependence on donors and reliance on international agencies to swoop in to rescue countries during outbreaks. The time delay between the start of the outbreak and importation of commodities is when most of the deaths occur. An alternative could be investment in regional manufacturing hubs for essential commodities, but this is slow in coming. Oral rehydration salts that are put into sachets and distributed through UN agencies are perceived as medicines, whereas the alternative of salt and sugar solutions are home remedies, but are not promoted or not available when families cannot afford to buy these basics.

CONCLUSIONS

Sub-Saharan Africa in 2018 carried the largest burden of cholera compared to other global regions. Progress towards the various WASH targets on the continent is slow, resulting from the very complex political and socio-economic context in which cholera thrives.

Squalid urbanisation is growing as a consequence of poverty, neglect by local and central government structures, poor leadership, rural underdevelopment, and inequitable distribution of resources. The growing population living in underserved and marginalised communities as a result of urban in-migration is not prioritised for basic services in most African countries. Poor economic growth and misgovernance have resulted in the failure to provide urban infrastructure, and have led to increased vulnerability to environmental threats. Corruption and the lack of accountability of central and local government structures, as well as dependency on international partners coming to the rescue during outbreaks, means that long-term solutions to the underlying causes of cholera outbreaks are hard to come by. Weakened health services, carrying the legacy of structural adjustment from the 1990s and the austerity policies that followed, are unable to respond adequately, resulting in high

CFRs. Biomedical and technical solutions include mapping of hotspot areas and providing cholera vaccination and intensive hygiene education to high-risk communities when alerts are raised of potential outbreaks, and for rapid response when an outbreak starts.

Repairing and upgrading water and sanitation infrastructure is the mainstay of prevention and must be prioritised. The impact of this investment was demonstrated in Latin America and historically in Europe in the 19th century as bringing to a halt outbreaks of this nature. However, resolving the major underlying causes of cholera outbreaks and preventable mortality will require radical changes in macroeconomic arrangements between rich countries and Africa, and within African countries. These changes are unlikely without broad social and political mobilisation at national and global levels.

REFERENCES

Ahmed, S., Bardhan, P. K., Iqbal, A., Mazumder, R. N., Khan, A. I., Islam, M. S., Siddique, A. K. & Cravioto, A. 2011. 'The 2008 cholera epidemic in Zimbabwe: Experience of the icddr, b team in the field'. *Journal of Health, Population and Nutrition*, 29 (5), 541–546. https://doi.org/10.3329/jhpn.

Amnesty International (AI), 2018. 'Zimbabwe: Cholera outbreak highlights failure to invest in infrastructure and health system.' www.amnesty.org/en/latest/news/2018/09/zimbabwe-cholera-outbreak-highlights-failure-to-invest-in-infrastructure-and-health-system/%0D, accessed 2 December 2018.

APA News. 2018. 'Resurgent cholera outbreak claims 2 lives in Zimbabwe's Mt Darwin'. Agence de Presse Africaine, English ed., Dakar, 28 November.

Azman, A. S., Parker, L. A., Rumunu, J., Tadesse, F., Grandesso, F., Deng, L. L., & Luquero, F. J. 2016. 'Effectiveness of one dose of oral cholera vaccine in response to an outbreak: a case-cohort study'. *The Lancet Global Health*, 4 (11), e856–e863. https://doi.org/10.1016/S2214-109X(16)30211-X.

Bahadur, A. 2018. 'Stench of state failure in Zambia's cholera outbreak'. www.pambazuka.org/human-security/stench-state-failure-zambia's-cholera-outbreak%0D, accessed 10 November 2018.

Center for Disease Control and Prevention (CD), 2015. 'Recommendations for the use of antibiotics for the treatment of cholera.' www.cdc.gov/cholera/treatment/antibiotic-treatment.html, accessed 20 November 2018.

Chibamu, A. 2018. 'Civic groups blame government for cholera outbreak'. *New Zimbabwe,* https://www.newzimbabwe.com/civic-groups-blame-government-for-cholera-outbreak/, accessed October 2018.

Cuneo, C., Sollom, R. & Beyrer, C. 2017. 'The Cholera Epidemic in Zimbabwe, 2008–2009: A Review and Critique of the Evidence'. *Health & Human Rights Journal*, 19 (2), 249–264.

Darvas, Z., Moes, N., Myachenkova, Y., & Pichler, D. 2018. 'The macroeconomic implications of health care'. *Policy Contribution*, 11, 1–22.

Davies, H. 2016. 'Leaked audit reveals massive council salary abuse'. *Harare News*, www.hararenews.co.zw/2016/11/leaked-audit-reveals-massive-council-salary-abuse/%0D, accessed 1 November 2018.

Davis, W., Chonzi, P., Masunda, K., Shields, L., Mukeredzi, I., Manangazira, P. & Al, E. 2018. 'Typhoid Fever Outbreak — Harare, Zimbabwe, October 2016–March 2017'. *Morbidity and Mortality Weekly Report*, 67 (11), 342–343.

Equity-axis. 2018. 'Datlabs upgrades plant.' equityaxis.net/2018/10/07/datlabs-upgrades-plant/%0D, accessed 1 December 2018.

Evans, R. 1992. 'Epidemics and revolutions: Cholera in nineteenth century Europe', in Ranger, T. & Slack, P. (eds.) *Epidemics and Ideas: Essays on the Historical Perception of Pestilence*. Cambridge: Cambridge University Press, pp. 149–173.

Gaffga N., Tauxe, R. V. & Mintz, E. D. 2007. 'Cholera: A new homeland in Africa'. *The American Journal of Tropical Medicine and Hygiene*, 77 (4), 705–713. https://doi.org/10.4269/ajtmh.2007.77.705.

Global Task Force on Cholera Control (GTFCC). 2017. *Ending cholera: A global roadmap to 2030. World Health Organization.* http://www.who.int/cholera/publications/global-roadmap.pdf?ua=1, accessed 20 November 2018.

Government of Zimbabwe (GoZ). 2013. *Constitution of Zimbabwe*. Harare: Government of Zimbabwe.

Government of Zimbabwe (GoZ). 2018. Public Health Act 2018, Pub. L. No. Ch 15, Part VIII, Section 86, Zimbabwe.

Higuet, F. 2014. 'The right to water and the African constitutions: Table of the African constitutions.' www.rampedre.net/implementation/territories/national/africa/constitutions%0D, accessed 20 November 2018.

Hilson, G. 2002. 'The future of small-scale mining: Environmental and socioeconomic perspectives'. *Futures*, 34 (9–10), 863–872.

Human Rights Watch (HRW). 2013. 'Troubled water: burst pipes, contaminated wells and open defecation in Zimbabwe's capital.'

Isaäcson, M., Clarke, K. & Ellacombe, G. 1974. 'The recent cholera outbreak in South African gold mining industry: a preliminary report'. *South African Medical Journal*, 48, 2557–2560.

Islam, M. S., Mahmud, Z. H., Ansaruzzaman, M., Faruque, S. M., Talukder, K. A., Qadri, F., Alam, M., Islam, S., Bardhan, P. K., Mazumder, R. N., Khan, A. I., Ahmed, S., Iqbal, A., Chitsatso, O., Mudzori, J., Patel, S., Midzi, S. M., Charimari, L., Endtz, H. P. & Cravioto, A. 2011. 'Phenotypic, genotypic, and antibiotic sensitivity patterns of strains isolated from the cholera epidemic in Zimbabwe'. *Journal of Clinical Microbiology*, 49 (6),

2325–2327. https://doi.org/10.1128/JCM.00432-11

Ivers, L. 2017. 'Vaccines plus water, sanitation, and hygiene interventions in the fight against cholera (authors' reply)'. *The Lancet Global Health*, 5 (4), e395. https://doi.org/10.1016/S2214-109X(17)30081-5.

Kadirire, H. 2018. 'Harare City Council will increase its water supply by 75 megalitres by this week as part of its drive to curb the spread of cholera'. http://nehandaradio.com/2018/09/26/harare-to-increase-water-supply/, accessed 26 September 2018.

Kubatana. 2018. 'CSOs hold government accountable for avoidable cholera deaths.' From kubatana.net/2018/09/14/csos-hold-government-accountable-avoidable-cholera-deaths/, accessed 14 September 2018.

Leibovici-Weissman, Y., Neuberger, A., Bitterman, R., Sinclair, D., Salam, M. & Paul, M. 2014. 'Antimicrobial drugs for treating cholera'. *Cochrane Database of Systematic Reviews*, 6, Art. No.: CD008625. https://doi.org/10.1002/14651858.CD008625.pub2.

Lessler, J., Moore, S. M., Luquero, F. J., McKay, H. S., Grais, R., Henkens, M., Mengel, M., Dunoyer, J., M'bangombe, M., Lee, E. C., Djingarey, M. H., Sudre, B., Bompangue, D., Fraser, R. S. M., Abubakar, A., Perea, W., Legros, D. & Azman, A. S. 2018. 'Mapping the burden of cholera in sub-Saharan Africa and implications for control: An analysis of data across geographical scales'. *The Lancet*, 391 (10133), 1908–1915. https://doi.org/10.1016/S0140-6736 (17) 33050-33057.

Machamire, F. 2017. 'More Harare boreholes contaminated'. *Daily News*, www.dailynews.co.zw/articles/2017/03/24/more-harare-boreholes-contaminated%0D, accessed 2 March 2018.

Magaisa, A. 2018. '"Our Thing" – Understanding Zimbabwe's Oligarchy'. www.bigsr.co.uk/single-post/2018/10/27/Big-Saturday-Read-Our-Thing---Understanding-Zimbabwe's-Oligarchy, accessed 2 December 2018.

McAteer, J., Danda, S., Nhende, T., Manamike, P., Parayiwa, T., Tarupihwa, A. & Al, E. 2018. 'Outbreak of Vibrio cholerae Associated with Attending a Funeral — Chegutu District, Zimbabwe'. *Morbidity and Mortality Weekly Report*, 67 (19), 560–561.

Médecins Sans Frontières (MSF). 2017. 'Easy to treat and prevent, yet cholera ravages communities in 2017'. https://www.msf.org/international-activity-report-2017/easy-treat-and-prevent-yet-cholera-ravages-communities-2017, accessed 2 March 2018.

Médecins Sans Frontières (MSF). 2018. 'A collective response to cholera in Harare'. www.msf.org/zimbabwe-collective-response-cholera-harare, accessed 2 December 2018.

Musemwa, M. 2010. 'From "Sunshine City" to a landscape of disaster: The politics of water, sanitation and disease in Harare, Zimbabwe, 1980-2009'. *Journal of Developing Societies*, 26 (2), 165–206. https://doi.org/10.1177/0169796X1002600202.

Mushayabasa, S. & Bhunu, C. P. 2012. 'Is HIV infection associated with an increased risk for cholera? Insights from a mathematical model'. *BioSystems*, 109 (2), 203–213. https://doi.org/10.1016/j.biosystems.2012.05.002.

Muti, M., Gombe, N., Tshimanga, M., Takundwa, L., Bangure, D., Mungofa, S., & Chonzi, P. 2014. 'Typhoid outbreak investigation in Dzivaresekwa, suburb of Harare City, Zimbabwe, 2011'. *Pan African Medical Journal*, 18 (18), 309.

Nelson, E., Harris, J., Morris Jr., J., Calderwood, S. & Camilli, A. 2009. 'Cholera transmission: The host, pathogen and bacteriophage dynamic'. *Nature Reviews Microbiology*, 7 (10), 693.

Nyandoro, M. 2011. 'Historical overview of the cholera outbreak in Zimbabwe (2008-2009)'. *Journal for Contemporary History*, 36 (1), 154–174.

Okeke, I. N., Aboderin, O. A., Byarugaba, D. K., Ojo, K. K. & Opintan, J. A. 2007. 'Growing problem of multidrug resistant enteric pathogens in Africa', *Emerging Infectious Diseases*, 13 (11). http://wwwnc.cdc.gov/eid/article/13/11/pdfs/07-0674.pdf.

Opare, J., Ohuabunwo, C., Afari, E., Wurapa, F., Sackey, S., Der, J., & Odei, E. 2012. 'Outbreak of cholera in the East Akim Municipality of Ghana following unhygienic practices by small-scale gold miners, November 2010'. *Ghana Medical Journal*, 46 (3), 116.

Reliefweb. 2018. 'Bulletin: Cholera and AWD Outbreaks in Eastern and Southern Africa, Regional Update for 2018'. https://reliefweb.int/report/zimbabwe/bulletin-cholera-and-awd-outbreaks-eastern-and-southern-africa-regional-update-2, accessed 4 November 2018.

Rusvingo, S. 2014. 'The Salarygate Scandal in the Zimbabwe Parastatals Sector: Another Darkside of the Nation (2013–2014)'. *Global Journal of Management and Business Research: Administration and Management*, 14 (10), 19–29.

Sanders, D. 2004. Macroeconomic reform is necessary to progress in the MDGs: Round Table Discussion.

Simpson, M. & Hawkins, T. 2018. *The Primacy of Regime Survival: State Fragility and Economic Destruction in Zimbabwe.* London: Palgrave Macmillan.

Sinyange, N., Brunkard, J. B., & Kapata, N. 2018. Cholera Epidemic — Lusaka, Zambia, October 2017–May 2018, 67 (October), 556–559.

Sollom, R., Beyrer, C., Sanders, D., Donaghue, A. F., Potts, H., Bradshaw, J., & Khalsa, G. 2009. *Health in Ruins: A Man-Made Disaster in Zimbabwe. An Emergency Report by Physicians for Human Rights.*

Srivastava, A., & Jaiswal, P. 2018. Africa large volume parenterals LVP market. https://www.alliedmarketresearch.com/africa-large-volume-parenterals-LVP-market.

United Nations (UN). 2016. *The Sustainable Development Goals Report 2016.*

United Nations Environment Programme (UNEP). 2010. 'Water challenges and opportunities', in *Africa Water Atlas* (pp. 123–173). United Nations

Environment Programme.

Walsh, S. & Johnson, O. 2018. *Getting to Zero: A Doctor and a Diplomat on the Ebola Frontline*. London: ZED Books.

World Health Organization (WHO). 2018a. 'African Health Ministers commit to ending cholera outbreaks by 2030'. https://afro.who.int/news/african-health-ministers-commit-ending-cholera-outbreaks-2030%0D

World Health Organization (WHO). 2018b. 'Emergency preparedness, cholera Zimbabwe'. www.who.int/csr/don/05-october-2018-cholera-zimbabwe/en/%0D, accessed 21 December 2018.

World Health Organization (WHO). 2018c. Zimbabwe to vaccinate 1.4 million people against cholera in Harare. https://afro.who.int/news/zimbabwe-vaccinate-14-million-people-against-cholera-harare, accessed 1 December 2018.

Yates, T., Allen, J., Joseph, M. & Lantagne, D. 2017. *WASH Interventions in Disease Outbreak Response: Humanitarian Evidence Programme*. Oxford.

Zimplats. 2018. 'Zimplats donates towards fighting cholera'. www.zimplats.com/5802-2/%0D, accessed 21 September 2018.

FOUR

Outbreaks and Epidemics of Malaria in SADC

Cycles of Frustration in Preventive Action

KAKA MUDAMBO

INTRODUCTION – THE ONGOING RISK OF MALARIA IN THE SADC REGION

The *World Malaria Report* (WHO, 2017a) revealed that while the rate of new cases of malaria had declined overall since 2014, the trend of reversals of malaria outbreaks and epidemics had been levelling off. In some world regions it had reversed. In 2017 around 216 million people contracted malaria (in 91 countries) compared with the 211 million in 2016. The estimated global number of deaths from malaria rose from 445,000 in 2016 to 446,000 in 2017. It was overwhelmingly Africa that was affected. Roughly 90 per cent of all malaria cases and deaths worldwide were in Africa (WHO, 2016). As WHO (2017a) pointed out, 15 countries (only one of them, India, not in sub-Saharan Africa) continued to bear 80 per cent globally of the malaria death burden.

These trends contrast with the objectives of the control and eradication, or elimination, of malaria. The words elimination, eradication, and control are often used loosely, which results in misunderstanding (Maharaj et al., 2016). Previously, eradication was used to describe what we now call elimination (Hemingway et al., 2016). Eradication is used with reference to the 'permanent reduction to zero of the worldwide incidence of infection caused by a specific agent as a result of deliberate efforts; interventions measures are no longer needed' (Dowdle, 1999).[i] As the bottom line, eradication means that follow-up measures are no longer required. For malaria, however, follow-up measures remain essential. WHO (2004) therefore defines malaria elimination with reference to 'interrupting local mosquito-borne malaria transmission in a defined geographical area'; there will be zero incidence of locally contracted cases (although imported cases will still occur), and continued intervention measures remain necessary. In Africa, estimates of the population at risk of malaria epidemics[ii] range from 52 million to 144 million (Delacollette, 2004). WHO estimates that 23 countries on the continent are known to be epidemic prone. This

---

i Control refers to the reduction of disease incidence, prevalence, morbidity, or mortality to a locally acceptable level as a result of deliberate efforts, and continued intervention measures are required to maintain the reduction (e.g. diarrhoeal diseases). Elimination of disease denotes the reduction to zero of the incidence of a specified disease in a defined geographical area as a result of deliberate efforts, and continued intervention measures are required (e.g. neonatal tetanus). Elimination of infections, in comparison, refers to reduction to zero of the incidence of infection caused by a specific agent in a defined geographical area as a result of deliberate efforts, and ongoing measures to prevent re-establishment of transmission are required (e.g. measles and poliomyelitis). Eradication, in contrast, has a bearing on the permanent reduction to zero of the worldwide incidence of infection caused by a specific agent as a result of deliberate efforts, and intervention measures are no longer needed (e.g. smallpox) (Dowdle, 1999).

ii Malaria epidemic is defined as a sharp increase in the incidence among populations in which the disease is rare or a seasonal increase in areas of low to moderate transmission beyond the normal pattern. However, the definition of 'normal' occurrence can only be defined for a particular population in a specific area and time. Therefore, malaria epidemics can generally be considered as a disturbance of a previously existing epidemiological equilibrium. The term 'true epidemics' refers to infrequent/cyclical outbreaks in relatively non-immune populations related to climatic anomalies. There can also be strongly seasonal outbreaks. This phrase, in turn, refers to variable but relatively predictable transmission influenced by variation in climate, e.g. southern region of Africa and highland fringe areas. Neglected control or the breakdown of control refers to the re-emergence of malaria in receptive areas, e.g. areas affected by civil unrest, internally displaced populations, refugees, population migration, complacence, insecticide/drug resistance, poor coverage/inappropriate intervention etc. A pandemic is an outbreak of a disease that occurs over a wide geographic area and affects an exceptionally high proportion of the population.

includes all the Southern African Development Community (SADC) countries, except malaria-free Lesotho and the islands of Mauritius and Seychelles. There have been marked improvements in the rate of malaria outbreaks and deaths since 2000, yet a range of factors continue to trigger new occurrences. Such trigger factors relate to environment and climate, politics, governance, and demographics; and health system factors both prompt outbreaks and affect the processes of countering, controlling, and eradicating these occurrences. Malaria epidemics usually affect populations that live in the highlands or in arid and semi-arid areas, where rainfall and/or higher temperatures play a big role in causing an epidemic, usually after an extended period of drought, thereby increasing general population vulnerability. Devastating epidemics[iii] have been recorded due to large-scale movements of non-immune populations to endemic regions as a result of the political displacement that accompanies civil wars or local conflicts. The regions or districts at risk are usually not sufficiently prepared to cope with the sudden increase of malaria transmission in which 30–50 per cent of at-risk people may develop the disease, with a mortality rate of 1–5 per cent, depending on the rapidity and the effectiveness of the response (WHO, 2009; 2012).

The 2017 WHO World Malaria Report highlighted that there has been recent stagnation in the progress towards reducing the global malaria burden: there was an unexpected upsurge in the number of cases and deaths, after significant gains in the preceding period. A situational analysis suggested that the resurgent outbreaks were caused by (Elimination 8, 2017: 6):

- weakening of the malaria control programme – caused by funding shortages, complacency, poor strategy execution and cessation of control activities;
- increases in the intrinsic potential for malaria transmission – due to movement of humans or mosquitoes, development and land-use changes, and changes in climate and weather patterns; and
- technical problems, including drug and insecticide resistance – as manifested in vector and drug resistance.

---

iii An epidemic is a widespread occurrence of an infectious disease in a community at a particular time; an outbreak carries the same definition as epidemic but is often used for a more limited geographic area.

Funding problems contributed adversely to the ability to get effective coverage with vector control interventions, such as indoor residual spraying (IRS), long-lasting insecticide-treated bed nets (LLINs), and larval source management (LSM). There were also delays in procurement of malaria commodities such as insecticides and rapid diagnostic test kits (RDTs), and artemisinin-based combination therapy (ACT) was constrained.

In SADC's 16 member states,[iv] as the SADC Malaria Report (2017) indicated, the burden of malaria was approximately 47 million cases in 2016, a rate therefore of 17 per cent in the SADC population of 277 million. Since 2014, several SADC countries have been affected by outbreaks. In 2016–2017 most SADC member states experienced malaria outbreaks. A comparison of the 2013 and 2016 levels of incidence and mortality (Table 1) reveals the variations among low- and high-transmission countries. The year 2017 proved to be the worst of these recent years in terms of malaria outbreaks in the SADC region (SADC, 2017). For example, Botswana had 9,478 cases and 76 deaths by March–April 2017, compared to 6,385 cases and 58 deaths for the same period in 2016. South Africa in comparison had 4,092 cases and 33 deaths in 2017, against the 1,543 cases and 18 deaths of 2016 (SADC, 2017). The SADC countries experienced significant increases in the numbers of malaria cases and deaths in the 2016–2017 season over those in the 2015–2016 season, when drought conditions had prevailed. In fact, there were peaks in March–April 2015, 2016, and 2017 in all high-transmission countries.

The trends in Table 1 demonstrate the heterogeneous nature of malaria transmission in SADC (WHO, 2017b; SADC, 2007a; SADC, 2017), making it difficult to mobilise a whole-region response. There is a risk in countries that no longer report local transmission (Lesotho, Mauritius, and Seychelles) that if this upsurge continues, they will be unprepared. In the high-transmission national areas (Angola, the Democratic Republic of Congo (DRC), Madagascar, Malawi, Mozambique, United Republic of Tanzania (Mainland), Zambia, and

iv Angola, Botswana, Comoros, Democratic Republic of Congo, Eswatini, Lesotho, Madagascar, Malawi, Mauritius, Mozambique, Namibia, Seychelles, South Africa, United Republic of Tanzania, Zambia, and Zimbabwe.

Table 1: Trends in malaria incidence and mortality in SADC, 2013–2016

Transmission rate – high/moderate or low	Trend	Malaria incidence	Malaria mortality
In countries with moderate to high transmission rates	Up	Malawi, Mozambique, DRC, Angola, Madagascar	Angola, DRC
	Stable	Zimbabwe, Zambia	Madagascar, Malawi, Mozambique
	Down	United Republic of Tanzania (Mainland)	United Republic of Tanzania (Mainland), Zambia
In countries with low transmission rates	Up	Namibia, Eswatini	Namibia
	Stable	Botswana	United Republic of Tanzania (Zanzibar)
	Down	United Republic of Tanzania (Zanzibar), South Africa	Botswana, South Africa, Eswatini

Source: Compiled from various data sets in SADC Malaria Report, 2017: 1–2

Note: In 2016 there were a total of 60,414 malaria-related deaths in SADC countries, which was 4 per cent higher than in 2013. Angola (27 per cent of total) and DRC (56 per cent of total) were the two SADC countries with the highest mortality rates. On incidence, DRC, Malawi, Mozambique, and Zambia are the four countries with the highest incidence by far.

Zimbabwe) the incidence in 2016 ranged from 11 to 381 malaria cases per 1,000 population, with corresponding mortality rates of 1.5–39 malaria deaths per 100,000 population. In the medium- and low-transmission areas (Botswana, Namibia, South Africa, and Eswatini), the incidence ranged from 0.3 to 9.7 cases per 1,000 population, with mortality rates of 0.1–2.4 per 100,000 population. In Mauritius, where there is no local malaria transmission, there were 25 malaria cases and no malaria-related deaths. Mozambique had increasing numbers of cases over the period, with a lower peak in 2015 than in 2017, while in Malawi and Zambia, the peak in 2016 was higher than those in 2015 and 2017. Thus, Angola, Malawi, and Zambia had lower peaks in 2017 than Mozambique. Angola recorded the largest number of cases to date (4.2 million) in 2016, with a peak in April of that year (583,000 cases), followed by a steady downward trend from May to September 2016.

Against this background of malaria incidence and mortality, the rest of this chapter reviews the overall levels of progress in the control and elimination of malaria in SADC. It draws on the observations by and participatory experiences of the author, as well as on research and reports generated by the WHO, structures of the SADC regions, and in particular on data and strategic programming generated by the SADC platform of Elimination 8 (E8). It also recognises and uses other scholarly contributions in the field. The chapter explores in depth the complexities, including constraints thereon, of the multiple interventions that have helped SADC progress in countering malaria in the region. In the final section it reviews the lessons learned from past actions and offers proposals for further strategic action.

PROGRESS IN FIGHTING THE ENCUMBRANCE OF MALARIA

Despite the high ongoing SADC burden of malaria, since 2000 the region has made remarkable progress in the fight to control malaria. This emanated from the SADC countries' scaling-up of interventions, which included surveillance, diagnosis and treatment, vector control, health promotion, and communication for behaviour change. This whole-system approach, rather than just a curative approach, has yielded positive results for the region.

These efforts have resulted in increased access to malaria prevention and treatment, associated with a 30 per cent increase in domestic financing for malaria between 2014 and 2015, as well as strong partnerships with other stakeholders. The 2017 SADC Malaria Report showed that in 2016 the case confirmation rate[v] was 85 per cent in 10 of the 11 countries in which this is measured, and in seven countries 95 per cent of uncomplicated cases received ACT, all contributing to constraining rates of incidence and mortality. All countries achieved a

v Confirmation of suspected malaria cases that had a parasitological test; see SADC, 2017: 4.

rate of reporting of cases by health facilities of 80 per cent (SADC, 2017: 9). However, the report highlighted that coverage with vector control did not meet the target of 80 per cent of the population – this was only achieved by six of the nine countries that reported IRS coverage and only three of the nine countries and areas that distribute LLINs (WHO, 2017b). Cross-border and regional initiatives have been established in the SADC region to address malaria transmission among mobile and migrant populations (Elimination 8, 2015; 2016). These include the:

- E8 SADC platform,[vi] an initiative for elimination of malaria in four countries (Botswana, Namibia, South Africa, and Eswatini) and pre-elimination in an additional four countries (Angola, Mozambique, Zambia, and Zimbabwe).
- Mozambique–South Africa–eswatini (MOSASWA) cross-border initiative for elimination in South Africa and Eswatini and pre-elimination in Mozambique (for details, see section on cross-border transmission and control).

These initiatives are complementary. It is anticipated that as those E8 countries with low transmission progress to eliminating malaria, the four second-line countries (Angola, Mozambique, Zambia, and Zimbabwe) as well as Madagascar, the DRC, and the United Republic of Tanzania (Mainland) will transition to elimination,[vii] which is anticipated to be achieved by 2030 (see also Delacollette & Rietveld, 2006).

To prevent outbreaks or epidemics, countries need to ensure that all communities receive health education aimed at behaviour change. This should go hand in hand with ensuring universal access to all interventions. Behaviour change should be mostly related to climatic conditions conducive to malaria transmission, to prepare the population

vi Key SADC frameworks form the foundation of the E8 Strategic Plan. They include the SADC Protocol for Health, the SADC Malaria Strategic Framework 2007–2015, the SADC Malaria Elimination Framework, the SADC Protocol on Health Implementation Plan, and the SADC Malaria Advocacy and Communication Framework. The E8 vision is to have a malaria-free Southern Africa, and its goal is to enable and accelerate zero local transmission in the four frontline countries by 2020 through the provision of a platform for collaboration and joint strategic programming.

vii For the comparative definitions of elimination and eradication see, for example, Cohen et al., 2010; Dowdle, 1999.

to take precautions. Countries also need to establish strong malaria surveillance systems because countering malaria depends on the accurate and complete identification of and reaction to outbreaks.

Malaria forms part of the United Nations Sustainable Development Goals (SDGs). The SDG are supported by the WHO Global Technical Strategy for Malaria 2016–2030 (GTS), WHO's Framework for Malaria Elimination and the Roll Back Malaria Partnership's Action and Investment to defeat Malaria 2016–2030 (AIM) (Roll Back Malaria Partnership, 2015). These activities are highly dependent on the availability of funding/resources through sustained domestic financing and innovative solutions to fill in gaps in countries receiving donor funding. Significantly, slow responses to outbreaks and epidemics have often been because of inadequate government funding, which in turn was due to over-reliance on international financing (Roll Back Malaria Partnership, 2015).

RISK FACTORS IN HEALTH SYSTEMS AND IMPLEMENTATION OF MALARIA INTERVENTIONS

In order to understand the forward momentum in the control and elimination of malaria, along with the setbacks and the conditions that need to prevail in order to avert relapses (see Feachem & Sabot, 2008, for example), it is essential to assess the quality and regularity of the initiatives to combat malaria. While the current section provides an overview of a selection of risk factors, much of the rest of the chapter presents detailed explorations of these risks, paired with deeper assessments of the success factors.

Important risk factors that are associated with malaria outbreaks and epidemics in the SADC region include (see also Figure 1):

Insufficient tracking and data recording:

The causes of malaria epidemics are multiple and may vary from one country to the next. There is general agreement that inadequate annual forecasting of the risks for malaria epidemics and emergencies at national level remains a challenge. This is compounded by inadequate flow of communication of the information to districts to allow for timely mitigation through targeted prevention. Information sources include:

- national surveillance systems (dealt with separately below)
- meteorological offices for climate updates
- population movements and displacements from local authorities
- development ministries
- the private sector
- humanitarian agencies

Weak surveillance systems:
Observation across country borders indicates that national malaria control/elimination programmes are not carrying out weekly tracking of malaria cases, which would enable the detection of abnormal rates of transmission, which would in turn lead to appropriate response measures (Elimination 8, 2015; 2016; Elimination 8 TWG, 2018; WHO, 2004). Some countries do not have updated thresholds for weekly reporting, and those that do may find that the given thresholds are no longer appropriate for the stratification zones (Elimination 8 TWG, 2018; Teklehaimanot et al., 2004; WHO, 2004).

Weak planning and preparedness:
During the rainy season, although programmes and associated staff may be aware that an unusually heavy rainy season is highly probable they often do not strengthen their epidemic and preparedness response at all levels, including the lowest level possible (Elimination 8, 2016; WHO, 2004; 2013; 2017b). Failure to put these systems in place may result in failure to detect and respond to outbreaks in a timely manner. Most countries have also failed to trigger an adequate response to malaria epidemics and emergencies due to lack of emergency stocks of the essential malaria commodities (insecticides, RDTs, ACTs, etc.) (Elimination 8 TWG, 2018; WHO, 2017a; 2013; 2004). This risk factor results from internal factors of planning by health system staff, and from environmental constraints of funding (see below), and 'natural' factors such as occasionally unpredictable weather change (Figure 1).

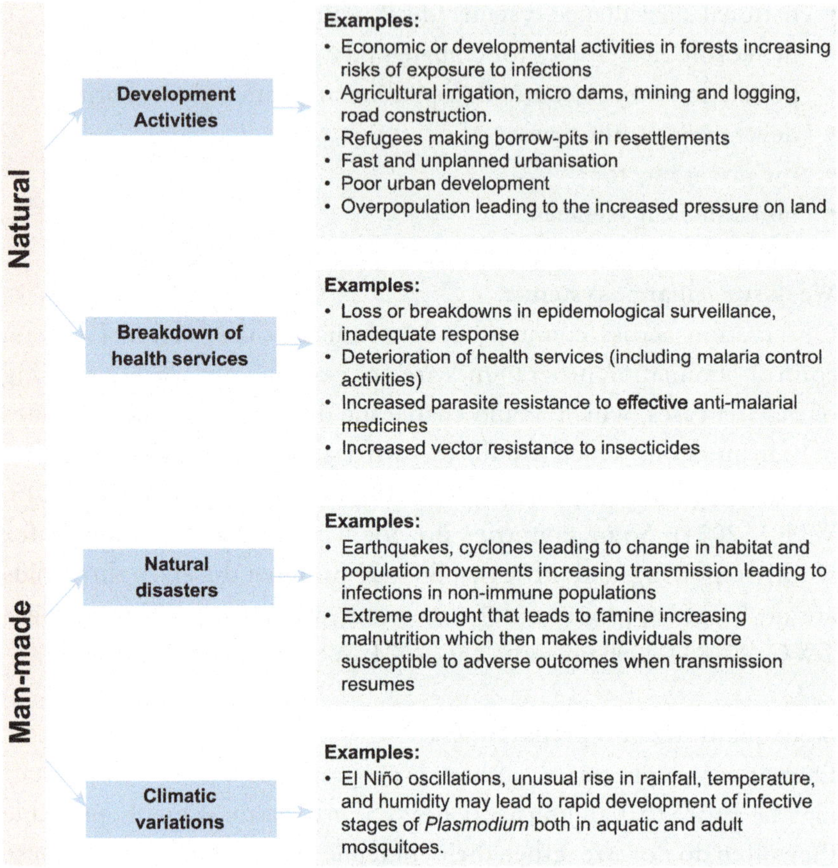

Figure 1: Human-made and natural factors that contribute to epidemics

Source: WHO, 2018a

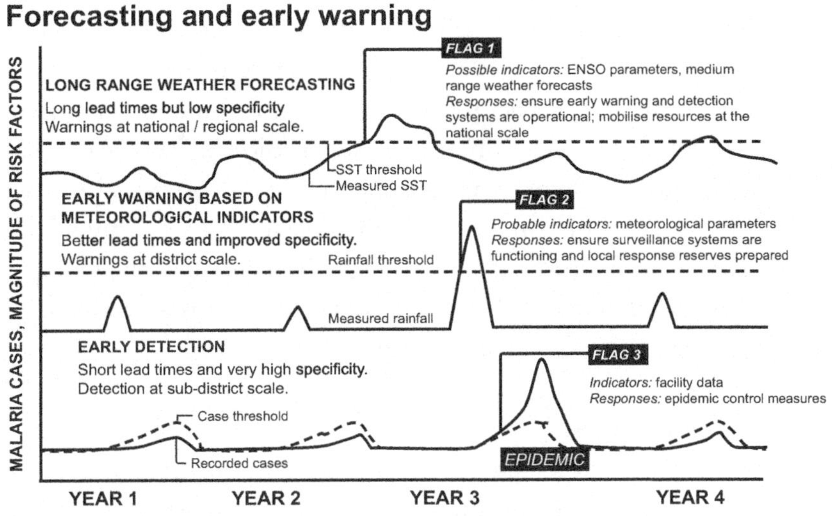

Figure 2: Surveillance system for epidemics

Source: WHO, 2018a

Delayed response and disbursement:

When a malaria epidemic is verified, early management of patients that report high fever cases by health workers and clinicians is the key to reducing the case fatality rate. As part of case management in non-immune people sick with malaria, it is particularly vital to use, and quickly make available, highly efficacious and safe drugs at village level through mobile clinics. Most countries rely on external resources to fund malaria efforts, and when disbursement is delayed, there is also delayed response to outbreaks (see also the risk factor of weak planning systems). Limited human, financial, and infrastructure capacity has been noted for impeding active case investigation in countries conducting elimination of malaria. There is no tool for assessing the efficacy of and responses to case investigations (WHO, 2018a).

Health system risk factors:

The countries often lack designated malaria and integrated disease outbreak and emergency teams at district level. Country data shown in the 2017 SADC *Malaria Report* showed that countries were failing to meet the 85+ per cent IRS target. The low IRS coverage reported in several countries has been attributed to factors such as delayed procurement of commodities such as insecticides, protective equipment, and spray pumps, along with insufficient recruitment of spraying teams, and inadequate capacity for supervision and microplanning of these operations. Poor or suboptimal supervision of IRS teams has affected the quality of spraying, which may be compromised further by late deployment of commodities, the delayed start of campaigns, and late payment of seasonal spray operators. Therefore, the strength of a health system outside of the malaria space also has a bearing on a country's ability to respond effectively.

Biological risk factors:

Epidemics are influenced, among other things, by emerging insecticide resistance and changing mosquito behaviour (issues that emerge in combination with favourable climatic and environmental factors). Resistance to pyrethroids, for example, is widespread in the SADC region, even though a large proportion of house structures are still sprayed with pyrethroids (Hemingway et al., 2016; Mpofu et al., 2016). In the past decade, use of pyrethroid insecticides in malaria vector control has increased dramatically through scale-up of the distribution of LLINs and IRS (see, for example, Ranson et al., 2011). In the process, major malaria vectors have developed resistance to pyrethroids, resulting in the decreased efficacy of the most commonly used insecticide class of pyrethroids. This decreased efficacy has increased mosquito survival, which signals the rising incidence of malaria morbidity and mortality. There is an urgent need for a key multisectoral approach to combat the threat of resistance, with research and development going into the creation of new and more effective pesticides.

Climate and environmental risk factors:

Unusually heavy rainfall leads to flooding, which creates favourable environmental conditions for malaria transmission (increased vector density and competence) and also leads to increased population displacement and limited delivery and access to health services. This requires countries to plan accordingly. Areas that are malaria prone display common characteristics of being in tropical and subtropical areas, relatively close to the equator, where it is warmer, with temperate climatic factors: temperature, humidity, and rainfall; also more frequently in areas where there are lapses in economic development and public health measures (CDC, 2017). All of these factors are important for outbreak anticipation and for taking timely preventive action.

In conditions where the natural ecology supports low levels of seasonal transmission, amidst limited immunity in the population, exceptions to this pattern (rebounds) may occur where (WHO, 2018a):

- Anomalous climatic or epidemiological conditions lead to increased transmission that extends beyond the typical pattern. This may be in highlands, arid, and semi-arid areas.
- Rates of parasite infections have been reduced over time due to interventions, but receptivity remains high. This is likely in conditions where coverage has reduced, the health system has suffered breakdown, efficacy of interventions has suffered, and importation levels have gone up.
- Sudden large-scale movements of infected populations happen due to conflicts or complex emergencies. They move into non-immune populations in receptive areas, or into areas of ongoing transmission.
- Areas undergoing rapid ecological (including human) changes in immunologically-naive populations start posing conditions receptive to malaria outbreaks. Deforestation, irrigation, construction of dams and roads, flooding, mining, and earthquakes may be some of the changing conditions.

The rest of the chapter explores in depth SADC country experiences and initiatives to counter risk factors through planning, action, and reaction on the ground.

STRATIFICATION FOR TARGETED INTERVENTIONS

Stratification in the context of malaria control refers to a dynamic and ongoing process involving research, diagnosis, analysis, and interpretation of the information, which serves as a basis for comprehensive and methodological classification of geo-ecological areas and population groups according to *malaria risk factors*, as was put forward by Castillo-

Salgado (2009). In the control of malaria outbreaks, stratification is a vital analytic step to determine epidemiological differences and socio-economic aspects such as conflict, population movement, human behaviour, poverty, and access to health services (see Figure 3). A stratum that will be identified for an intervention is a population or social group located in a well-defined geographical area that shares similar principal risk factors – consequently, the measures or interventions undertaken are to modify the risk factors.

In order to provide a tailored intervention, it is vital to determine epidemiological differences (such as spatial, vector, ecology, resistance) and socio-economic factors (including conflict, population movement, human behaviour, poverty, and access to health services). The purpose of stratification is therefore to be able to employ different and appropriate interventions in diverse geographical places or populations. The choices and actions to be determined could be, for example, IRS vs LLIN or LSM,[viii] or the choice to use mobile clinics in mobile populations.

The determinants for stratification and deployment of interventions against malaria are twofold, namely in epidemiology (with reference to receptivity, vulnerability, vector, and parasite species) and capacity (considering especially resources and health systems). When such interventions are undertaken one can foresee one of two scenarios: a rapid or a gradual decrease. A gradual decrease, the second scenario, entails protecting the same fraction of population in sub-regions with different baselines of receptivity to transmission. A rapid decrease, the first scenario, means achieving reductions to the same low level in all sub-regions – it requires protecting a greater fraction of the at-risk population in sub-regions that have a higher baseline.

Early detection remains the obvious basis on which the decisions of stratified interventions against malaria epidemics rest (see WHO, 2004). Epidemic threshold is a critical level at which the reported counts of cases or deaths, in a given space and time, are beyond what

viii Larval source management (LSM) refers to the targeted management of mosquito breeding sites. The goal is to reduce the number of mosquito larvae and pupae. LSM can help reduce the numbers of both indoor and outdoor biting mosquitoes, and in the malaria elimination phase it can be a useful addition to programme tools to reduce the mosquito population in remaining malaria hotspots (see WHO, 2013).

would be considered 'normal'. For operational purposes (see, for example, Teklehaimanot et al., 2004), four relatively simple statistical methods are recommended to determine thresholds.[ix]

MONITORING TRANSMISSIONS AND OUTBREAKS – SADC CONSTRUCTING SURVEILLANCE AND DATA SYSTEMS

Much of the ongoing challenge in moving from the control to elimination of malaria in Africa and SADC relates to surveillance, and specifically the recording and activation of information to counter transmission. In this respect we find that the main challenges experienced during the 2016–2017 SADC malaria season included (beside other factors, like insufficient emergency stocks and staff to give effect to operations):

- inadequate annual forecasting of the risks for malaria epidemics and emergencies at national level and communication of the information to districts to allow for timely, targeted prevention and mitigation; and
- insufficient weekly tracking of malaria cases in most programmes in the region to allow detection of abnormal rates in time for an appropriate response.

In its reflections on best practice (see also Figure 4), SADC refers to the case of Zimbabwe, noting that in 2016 Zimbabwe experienced a year free from outbreaks (ESARN, 2017; WHO, 2017b). It reflects specifically on aspects of surveillance and data systems. One of the strategic objectives of Zimbabwe's National Strategic Plan is to detect 100 per cent of epidemics within one week of onset and effectively to manage 100 per cent of malaria epidemics within two weeks of detection.

Although no epidemics were reported in Zimbabwe in 2016, epidemic preparedness was continued, including weekly monitoring of surveillance data. Training in integrated disease surveillance and response was given in some epidemic-prone districts, and alert and epidemic thresholds were updated based on recent data. In keeping

ix These four methods are constant case count thresholds; mean + 2SD; medium + upper 3rd quartile; and the cumulative sum (C-SUM).

with epidemic preparedness and response protocols, rapid response teams were given updated information, epidemic preparedness and response in provinces and districts were assessed, and partnerships and epidemic control funds were mobilised to support logistics for early outbreak response (SADC, 2017: 16). Although Zimbabwe experienced malaria epidemics in 2017, it was able to identify epidemic districts and health facilities through its weekly surveillance system and mounted a strong response with its preparedness and response plan (WHO, 2017a; ESARN, 2017). Consequently, their incidence occurrence per 100,000 population was at a low peak of 2 per cent in 2016 (compared with 9 per cent in 2015 and 7 per cent in 2017) (SADC, 2017: 14, 15).

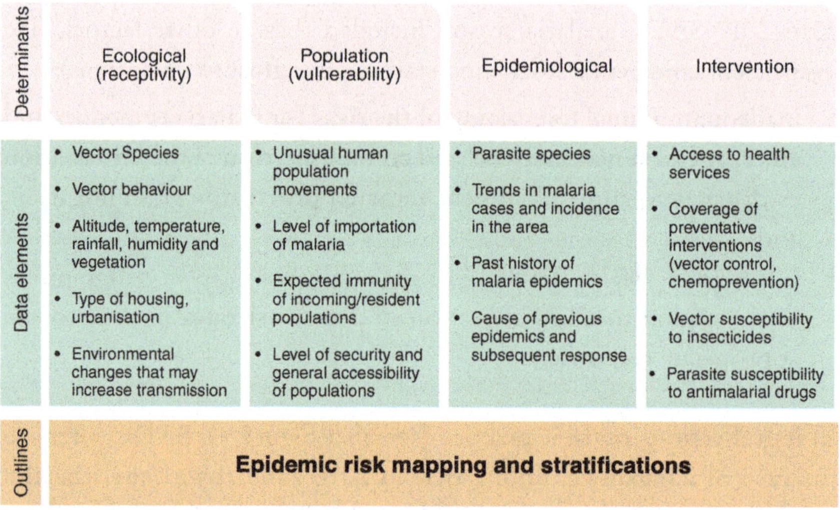

Figure 3: Defining areas that are prone to epidemics – the role of stratification

Source: WHO, 2018a

In addition, the African Leaders Malaria Alliance (ALMA) – a coalition of 49 African heads of government – adopted a malaria elimination agenda and the ALMA 2030 scorecard towards malaria elimination to monitor and encourage progress (ALMA, 2016; SADC, 2014). The scorecard has a set of indicators on which each country's achievements are scored.

EPIDEMIC PREPAREDNESS AND RESPONSE PLANNED CHECKLIST									
KEY ACTIVITY	SUB-ACTIVITY	COUNTRY							
		South Africa	Swaziland	Zambia	Zimbabwe	Angola	Botswana	Mozam-bique	Namibia
MONITORING SURVEILLANCE AND EARLY WARNING	Weekly data are generated accurate-ly at all reporting levels	UNDER-WAY	YES		YES		UNDER YES	YES	YES
	A reporting rate of 100% on a weekly basis from all health facilities	N/A	NO		YES		YES	YES	YES
	Routine (weekly) analysis of sur-veillance data for decision making	UNDER-WAY	YES		YES		YES	YES	YES
	Health facilities plot trend lines of the number of cases and deaths of malaria	NO	NO		YES		YES	YES	YES

EPIDEMIC PREPAREDNESS AND RESPONSE PLANNED CHECKLIST									
KEY ACTIVITY	SUB-ACTIVITY	COUNTRY							
		South Africa	Swaziland	Zambia	Zimbabwe	Angola	Botswana	Mozam-bique	Namibia
MONITORING SURVEILLANCE AND EARLY WARNING	National level notifies district health facilities of possible increases	YES	YES		YES		YES	UNDER-WAY	YES
	Private health facilities are included in national malaria surveillance system	YES	YES		UNDER-WAY		YES	NO	UNDER-WAY
	Annual health worker training on malaria surveillance and outbreak	YES	YES		YES		YES	NO	YES
	Early malaria outbreak detection system (alert threshold) predefined	NO	YES		YES		YES	UNDER-WAY	YES
	Key drivers of malaria epidemics identified in different areas	UNDER-WAY	YES		YES		UNDER-WAY	UNDER-WAY	UNDER-WAY

MONITORING SURVEILLANCE AND EARLY WARNING	Health facility or district data reported on monthly/ weekly basis	YES	YES		YES		YES	YES	YES
	Malaria risk map for transmission areas generated routinely	NO	YES		YES		UNDER-WAY	YES	YES
	Team regularly reviews data and provides evidence of malaria events	YES			YES		YES	YES	YES
	Team regularly reviews data and provides evidence of malaria events	YES	YES					YES	

Figure 4: Development of a checklist for epidemic preparedness – a means to identify priority areas for funding and/or partner support

Source: SADC, 2014

Critical questions on the checklist by Member States:

User guide for checklist?

List of tracked indicators for EPR and their relevance?

Frequency of updating E8 Situation Rwoom checklist?

Time taken for situation to change in countries and the region?

COMPLICATING FACTORS OF HUMAN RESOURCES AND FUNDING IN NATIONAL MALARIA CONTROL PROGRAMMES

SADC countries face multiple challenges in their fight against malaria. The main challenges relate to inadequate human resources, inadequate funding, and insufficient resources to accelerate interventions.

Most national malaria control programmes (NMCPs) encounter a combination of limiting factors. NMCPs are often understaffed, due to poor remuneration and working conditions, and the attrition rates in the NMCPs are high (Elimination 8, 2015; 2016; Maharaj et al., 2016; WHO, 2017a). The main beneficiaries of the drainage of malaria workers from the control programmes are the private sector, NGOs, foundations, universities, and UN agents, who are constantly on the lookout for high-calibre experts, a situation that is probably comparable across a range of epidemics.

NMCPs also face challenges in the procurement supply management (PSM) chain as a result of bureaucracy within the government system where approvals take a long time, leading to delayed procurement and slow arrival/supply of malaria commodities (Elimination 8, 2015; 2016; Maharaj et al., 2016; WHO, 2017a). This is compounded by a lack of transport – much needed to deliver commodities to targeted communities and also for rapid response to outbreaks. This leads to poor delivery and stockouts of essential malaria commodities, especially at health facility and community levels.

Funding shortages also delay the launch of operations, especially of spraying campaigns (Elimination 8, 2015; 2016; Maharaj et al., 2016; WHO, 2017a). Spraying campaigns require precise timing and include the training of spray operators and the start of the actual spraying. Very often programmes have no funds to hire spray operators. At times they also do not have the requisite protective clothing, spray pumps, and insecticide (due to delays in procurement and delivery). The structure of some NMCPs is not well defined – for example, when it comes to the malaria posts and where the programme manager is below the level of director, these persons do not have the authority to carry out certain functions and have to go through several stages to reach the permanent secretary (PS) or director general (DG) (Elimination 8, 2015; 2016; Maharaj et al., 2016).

EPIDEMIC RESPONSE – ACCESS TO EARLY DIAGNOSIS AND EFFECTIVE TREATMENT

Access to early diagnosis and effective treatment are essential in reducing the forward transmission of malaria (see Figure 5). The factors crucial to this enablement are, foremost, the use of a drug that has gametocytocidal effect, mass drug administration (MDA) (see, for example, Kobylinski et al., 2011) where feasible, and radical cure in the case of epidemics of P. vivax. In addition, and to reduce mortality, it is essential to have mass fever treatment if access is an issue and MDA is not feasible. In remote areas with low access to health care, temporary or mobile clinics are essential. Dealing with drug resistance is among the complicating factors. Other factors that affect effective treatment include the management of complex emergency situations, and the management of malnutrition and other comorbidities that increase susceptibility to malaria.

Dealing with insecticide resistance is an added complicating factor in preventing or countering malaria epidemics. There have in recent times been challenges with regard to the type of insecticide to deploy. Problems related to the manufacturers have been compounding these issues: manufacturers at times do not have adequate stocks of malaria commodities, which situation results in delayed supply. The high costs of the commodities, especially insecticides, also makes it difficult for countries to withstand the financial impact of prevention and early diagnosis, even though it is cheaper than dealing with an epidemic. High costs lead to the programmes reducing the quantities that are needed to attain the geographical coverage targets that will meet WHO standards. As indicated before, failure to attain high spraying rates leads to malaria outbreaks and consequently a rebound and loss of the ground gained in the fight against malaria. This was one of the main causes of the 2016–2017 malaria outbreaks in the SADC region. The shortages also mean that the programmes have no buffer stock, which is much needed for mounting rapid response to outbreaks and preventing the spread of the cases to other districts or communities.

Implementation of intermittent preventative treatment in pregnancy (IPTp) (WHO, 2018b) – which is the chemoprophylaxis given to pregnant women[x] (usually at each antenatal care visit) – remains a challenge because of failure to achieve the 60 per cent target. Very few countries in the SADC have attained a level of above 65 per cent. The WHO proposes currently that each woman should get this treatment more than three times in the course of a pregnancy. Birth complications in cases of malaria infection include premature deliveries and low birth weight (also infants being born laden with parasites). The WHO (2018c) reports that recent progress in Africa in adherence to this policy has increased only marginally: among the 23 countries that reported in 2016, an estimated 19 per cent of eligible pregnant women received three or more doses of IPTp, compared with 18 per cent in 2015 (and 13 per cent in 2014). The WHO believes that uncertainty among health workers pertaining to the exact administration protocols played a role, and hence it advocates for simplified IPTp messages and health worker training.

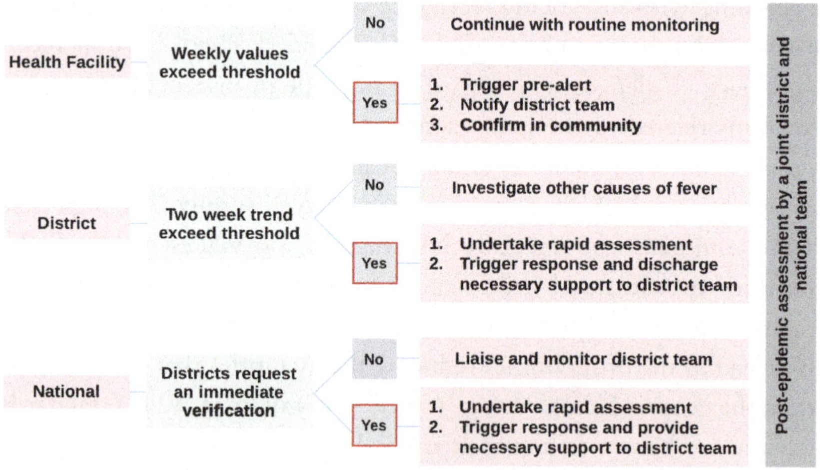

Figure 5: Early detection, verification, response and post-epidemic assessment process

Source: WHO, 2018a

x A full therapeutic course of anti-malarial medicine which is administered to pregnant women at their routine antenatal care visits, irrespective of whether they are infected with malaria or not.

CROSS-BORDER MOVEMENTS AND TRANSMISSION – AND INITIATIVES TO COUNTER MALARIA

Countries of the SADC region are also fighting to minimise both the importation of malaria from one district to another within the same country, and from one border district to another, including those coming from endemic regions such as East, Central, and West Africa (see Figure 6). The E8[xi] countries have recorded cases of transfer from as spread out as Ghana, Nigeria, Ivory Coast, Gambia, Somalia, South Sudan, Uganda, Burundi, Rwanda, Ethiopia, and Eritrea and, within SADC, from the DRC, Angola, Mozambique, Malawi, Zambia, and Tanzania. It is important to acknowledge that as long as there exist high endemic countries, importation will also always exist. Nevertheless it is important for the countries to eliminate at least the local transmission of malaria; by doing so this will decrease the risk of exportation.

One of the threats related to the importation of malaria concerns the military or uniformed forces involved in the SADC, African Union (AU), and UN Peacekeeping enforcement forces that operate within and outside the SADC region. The danger is that when returning from external deployment missions, soldiers often bring malaria parasites with them. Among them cases of *Plasmodium vivax* (Pv), *P. malariae* (Pm) and *P. ovale* (Po) (see Burrows et al., 2017) have been observed – these are either not found or exist on a very limited scale south of the Zambezi River (the northern boundary of Zimbabwe). Thus, there is the risk of spreading these in receptive areas. Because these strains are not common in some SADC countries, there is the added challenge of diagnosis and treatment. The malaria RDT used in countries like Botswana, Eswatini, Namibia, South Africa, and Zimbabwe is only sensitive to *Plasmodium falciparum* (Pf) and so Pv, Pm and Po are not detected. Therefore, there is the need for countries to have some RDTs that are able to detect these other forms as well, especially at border posts. There is no economic sense to provide them country-wide, where they will be under-utilised, as most cases are Pf.

---

xi The countries which constitute the E8 are Angola, Botswana, Mozambique, Namibia, South Africa, Eswatini, Zambia, and Zimbabwe.

Heavy and frequent population movement through several crossing points between the E8 countries (both formal and informal) for reasons of trade, migrant work, and education – combined with the fact that many borders in the region are artificial boundaries that cut across communities – further fuels the importation of malaria across countries. Work needs to be intensified, therefore, to optimise the containment and elimination of transmission across border regions. Preventing the importation of parasites from one country to another is central to the ability to achieve elimination (Elimination 8, 2015; 2016). Increasing avenues for surveillance through the establishment of border posts where testing and treatment can be carried out, and the availability of ongoing information for informed decision-making and planning are just two of the many important contributions that can be made.

Several initiatives to control and eliminate malaria unfold at regional level, given that nationally targeted efforts cannot address the interconnected nature of malaria transmission and importation across borders. The cross-border malaria control initiatives in the SADC region operate with varying levels of success. Within the E8, there are three operational cross-border malaria initiatives:

- MOSASWA: Malawi, Mozambique, and Zambia; and Mozambique, South Africa, and Eswatini (MOSASWA was formerly the Lubombo Spatial Development Initiative).
- the Trans-Kunene Malaria Initiative between Angola and Namibia.
- ZAM-ZIM (Zambia and Zimbabwe), a subset of the Trans-Zambezi Malaria Initiative.

Further cases are the Trans-Zambezi Malaria Initiative, comprising Angola, Botswana, Namibia, Zambia, and Zimbabwe, and the Botswana, Mozambique, South Africa, and Zimbabwe Malaria Initiative (formerly the Trans-Limpopo Malaria Initiative). These regional initiatives could advance malaria elimination through greater collaboration, the sharing of lessons to tackle common challenges, and direct cooperation with neighbouring countries on specific border issues. They are, however, limited by insufficient financial resources (Maharaj et al., 2016; WHO, 2017b). The Lubombo Spatial Development Initiative was reckoned to have been an example of success in cross-border malaria control.

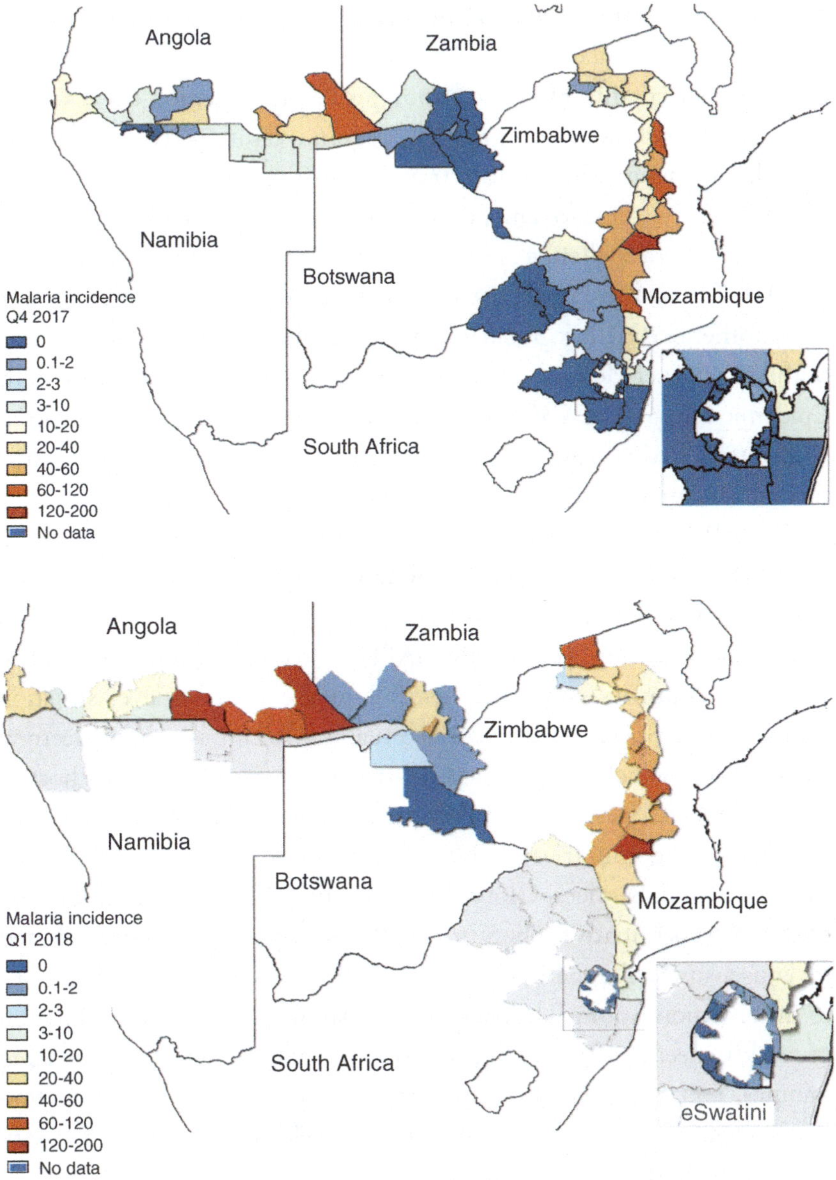

Figure 6: Informed decision-making through the use of data – 2017/18 Border District updated by month and during weekly calls

Source: Elimination 8 TWG, 2018

The goal of the malaria component of the project (to decrease the transmission of malaria in the region) was met and it was deemed to have been successful. However, upon project termination there was an upsurge of malaria cases in the sub-region, resulting from migration from high transmission to low transmission areas (see Maharaj et al., 2016). Clearly, the movement of people across borders in Southern Africa remains a challenge in sustaining malaria control and elimination.

The establishment of the E8 Regional Situation Room (Figures 7 and 8) is another pertinent regional initiative. It enables attempts at countering outbreaks of epidemics to focus on cross-country measures. The Epidemic Preparedness and Response (EPR) teams and situation rooms were established at regional and country levels to be able to monitor and track the occurrence of malaria epidemics and guide the responses.

The EPR body is required to be endorsed by the Minister of Health at country level, and the ministerial committee at regional level. These bodies work within the framework of what is known as a situation room. The situation room becomes the SADC body for regional outbreaks, while the countries concerned also adopt the national-level situation room model. Specifically, the E8 Situation Room is a multisectoral partner body which, at regional level (the E8 level), comprises a host of partners: SADC Secretariat, E8 Secretariat, Country M/E focal points (for all participating countries), WHO, RBM-SARN, Africa CDC, SADC Military Health Services, Global Public Health, ALMA, and the Clinton Health Access Initiative. The Situation Room is headed by a chair selected by consensus, while the E8 Secretariat EPR Focal Point is the Secretary to the Situation Room. The Secretary is responsible for the coordination of weekly meetings, the writing, distribution and publication of meeting minutes, and any other business that may be required. The Situation Room meets via teleconference once every week to deliberate on a variety of matters: updates of the current malaria situation in each country; status of malaria commodities (insecticides, spray pumps, protective materials, ACTs, RDTs, LLINs); status of preparedness, especially at the start of the season, with regard to launching spraying campaigns, LLIN distribution and buffer stocks and support needs (whether the country needs additional insecticides, ACTs, RDTs, etc.).

At country level it is made up of the NMCP M/E focal points, partners and EPR focal points from provinces and districts. The country level Situation Room feeds into the regional body and, in this way, both the country and regional bodies are able to access real-time weekly information that is much needed for informed decision-making and planning, in particular for immediate response in situations where increases are being observed.[xii] Figure 7 illustrates the E8 Situation Room and how it was established, approved, endorsed, and funded.

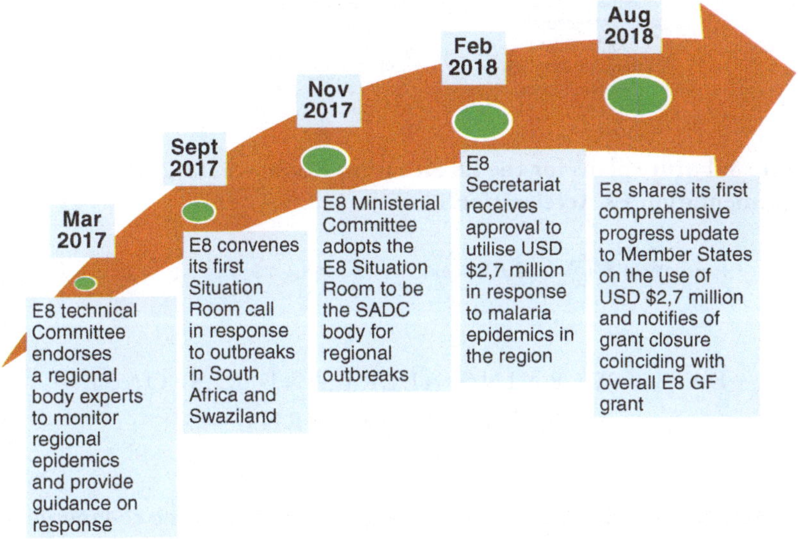

Figure 7:[xiii] Establishing the E8 Regional Situation Room – milestones and successes

Source: Elimination 8 TWG, 2018

xii Further background information to situation rooms, which indicate the high level of planning and coordination that is required, includes:

- Terms of Reference (ToR): The Situation Room should develop ToRs that are approved by the Technical Committee and it operates within the parameters of the ToRs.
- EPR planning checklist: The Situation Room should develop an EPR planning checklist which has components of monitoring, surveillance, and early warning activities, along with sub-activities, a user guide for the checklist, a list of tracked indicators and frequency of updating the checklist.
- Budget/resource allocation: For the Situation Room to be operational and have the capacity to organise responses to malaria epidemics in the region, it should have an approved budget allocated at regional and country level.

xiii Figure constructed prior to the former Kingdom of Swaziland's name being changed to Eswatini.

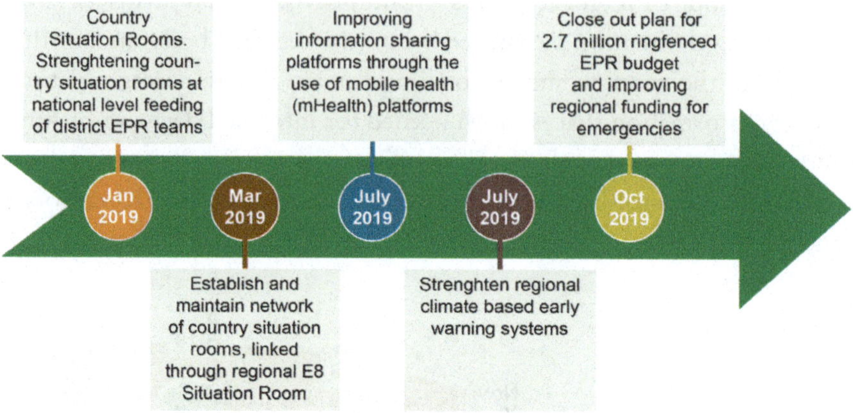

Figure 8: Future plans for the E8 Situation Room – 2018–2019 Implementation E8 Acceleration Plan

Source: Elimination 8 TWG, 2018

EARLY WARNING ALERT AND RESPONSE NETWORK (EWARN)

The figures on malaria outbreaks and epidemics reveal the re-emergence of malaria in areas where zero status had been achieved previously (where elimination targets appeared to have been met). This places immunologically naive populations at a very high risk (WHO, 2012; 2018a). In such humanitarian emergencies or disasters, national malaria control or elimination programmes should ensure availability of appropriate rapid diagnostic tests (RDTs). Here the Early Warning Alert and Response Network (EWARN) plays a central role in the early detection of outbreaks that require action (see WHO, 2009). The main condition for including malaria in EWARN is that it has been confirmed by RDT or microscopy. EWARN therefore is an adjunct, not a substitute, for the national disease surveillance system. Once the acute emergency phase is over, it should be reintegrated into the national surveillance system.

It is well known that humanitarian emergencies increase the risk of transmission of communicable diseases and conditions that have the potential of becoming epidemic (epidemic-prone diseases), thereby increasing morbidity (disease) and mortality (deaths) (WHO, 2012; 2018a). Conditions that result from such emergencies often involve the displacement of large numbers of people, mostly of those settled in temporary, highly crowded locations (WHO, 2012). Due to high population density there is usually inadequate food and shelter, unsafe water, poor sanitation, and lack of infrastructure. Because of the breakdown of the health systems, surveillance systems will be underperforming, disrupted, or non-existent, or they may quickly become overwhelmed.

Because the surveillance systems are unable to provide the required surveillance information associated with humanitarian emergency (including timeliness and high data quality), setting up an EWARN will temporarily fill this gap. This will be the case especially during the acute phase of an emergency and will also allow time for the routine systems to recover from the effects of the disaster.

To ensure functionality, an EWARN structure is to be made up of a network of people who collect information that will be fed into the next reporting level so that the set control measures will be implemented.

The EWARN setup has two main components: an immediate alert component (which signals the early stages of an outbreak), and a weekly reporting component (which reports weekly data aggregated by health facilities) needed for timely detection and verification of outbreaks, and effective monitoring of morbidity patterns.

The following aspects of the structure and operations need to be functional:

- To be effective, the EWARN should have management coordinated by a public health specialist or epidemiologist who has wide experience in disease surveillance, disease control in emergencies in particular, and knowledge of surveillance systems. The coordinator will ensure the operation of provincial and district focal points (one per province/district/health facility level).
- If well coordinated, this surveillance network takes over the assessment of the occurrence of epidemic-prone diseases. This network of people is responsible for collection, investigation, reporting, analysis, and dissemination of information from the

facilities/field through the reporting chain to the central level. The whole package should include adequate training and resources to ensure complete, reliable, and regular reporting. Based on information collected, alerts can be generated using alert thresholds.

- Thus, data collection and alerts should be reported in the quickest way possible, using weekly aggregated data. The data should include case definition, universal coverage, links with existing vertical surveillance programmes, and minimal data requirements.
- Data reporting and transmission methods and alert information, irrespective of their source, should be reported through the quickest means possible for verification and outbreak investigation. The coordinator and focal points should monitor the frequency of reporting (immediate, daily, or weekly) and reporting of mortality data.
- Another important function is the establishment of an outbreak preparedness system made up of a multisectoral outbreak control team (OCT) that is capable of responding effectively to outbreaks. It is essential to be prepared by arranging items such as an outbreak response plan, standard line-list forms for data collection, and standard treatment protocols for key diseases.
- Once an alert has been received by the EWARN district focal point or higher levels, a systematic alert verification process, starting at the field level, should be initiated within 24 hours. A standardised process should be used to verify the alert and, if an outbreak is confirmed, an on-site investigation should be started.
- An outbreak investigation involves determining the cause of an outbreak and who is at risk so that control measures can be implemented, thus reducing morbidity and mortality. It should begin as soon as an alert detected by surveillance has been verified. In the initial stage of an outbreak, the causative agent may not be known, and general control measures must be taken, based on the best available data. Once the cause has been confirmed, specific measures to control the disease can be undertaken.
- It is important, therefore, to get laboratory support (WHO, 2008a). Although normal routine reporting of EWARN syndromes does not require laboratory confirmation, diseases such as malaria require confirmation through RDTs or microscopy. Such confirmation is

mandatory before treatment can be started. Complex tests such as antimicrobial sensitivity validation or RDT validation need to be referred to a regional or international reference laboratory. This process is important because malaria at its onset has symptoms similar to other diseases such as chikungunya, dengue, and others. Hence the need for a proper case definition and confirmation through data analysis and interpretation.

SADC TAKING FORWARD THE LESSONS LEARNED

The lessons learned from preceding and ongoing engagement with countering malaria outbreaks and epidemics in the SADC region range in scope from specific medical diagnosis and treatment to procurement and delivery of malaria commodities, specifically targeted and capacitated systems on the ground, and management of cross-border movements – and many interventions in between. As the bottom line, the challenges are ongoing and the conditions and capacitation of the anti-malaria fight remain sub-optimal. There have been breakthroughs and improvements, but simultaneously relapses and recurrent problems are observed. This section provides an overview, summarising and interpreting the lessons highlighted in the preceding analysis. The lessons concern, in the main, joint regional surveillance and action on the occurrence of outbreaks or epidemics by developing coordinated plans of action and sharing best practices. These include innovative cross-border strategies, diagnostic methods and tools, community case management, vector control, entomological surveillance, and mass drug administration.

The Elimination 8 (2015) initiative is central to Southern Africa's endeavours to advance from control to elimination of malaria, and multiple lessons learned from past experiences have been, and continue to be, taken on board. The E8 countries recognise the need to plan pre-emptively. Sustainability of financing is a key component in driving the region's elimination agenda. It is essential to help ensure the switch from reorientation and control to the labour-intensive project of elimination. It requires, for example, sophisticated and comprehensive case detection and investigation (see Elimination 8, 2015). There is a need for stable and sustained flows of financing to prevent breaks in the chain of prevention and elimination. One of the key challenges facing the E8 is therefore the attainment of resources to achieve elimination in the medium to short term, and to sustain the gains in the long term. Innovative, donor-independent financing is critical to the long-term sustainability of the E8's malaria programming, helping to ensure that once elimination is achieved, it will also be sustained.

To sustain momentum towards achieving the vision of a malaria-free SADC, regional and multi-country funding mechanisms, mainly from governments and their public or private partners, need to be developed. According to Elimination 8 (2015), a regional public fund could contribute to accelerating progress to elimination throughout the region and help to reduce the importation of malaria into malaria-free zones. It is also stated as one of the Elimination 8 programme goals to see public-private partnerships playing a central role in malaria elimination, especially with a view to leveraging short-term financing, financial sustainability planning, usage of information and communication technology applications, laboratory services, and commodity availability.

On the ground, SADC countries continue to face challenges in malaria case management due to ongoing stockouts of essential malaria diagnostics (RDTs shortages) and treatment for both uncomplicated and complicated or severe malaria. Delays and challenges in the procurement and supply management (PSM) systems result in the delayed supply of anti-malaria medicines (and stockouts on the ground). The stockouts in anti-malaria commodities (medicines, RDTs, insecticides) have contributed to the failure to achieve targets: deaths due to malaria increased by 4 per cent in the SADC region between 2013 and 2016. An essential part of recommended best practice moving forward, SADC noted, is the need to define and establish minimum stockpiles of malaria commodities at SADC level. In collaboration with member states, it is necessary to pursue pooled procurement and warehousing of insecticides, RDTs, malaria medicines, and other relevant commodities in order to reduce prices and secure supplies for malaria outbreaks in the region.

Vector control using IRS is the main intervention in countries that are moving towards elimination of malaria, mainly Botswana, Eswatini, Namibia, South Africa, Zambia, United Republic of

Tanzania-Zanzibar, Mozambique, and Zimbabwe. However, a host of issues contribute to ongoing malaria outbreaks in the region. The problems include issues of environmental compliance, insecticide resistance, inadequate funding to procure insecticide, and delays in the PSM chain (including delayed delivery by the manufacturers). It is recommended, therefore, that the SADC communicable diseases centre should include malaria outbreaks in their mandate. Countries are encouraged to strengthen vector control, especially in areas of entomological surveillance. They should also strengthen malaria surveillance, when possible in integrated systems, and rigorously investigate potential drivers of transmission to ensure the completeness and timeliness of data.

Quality-assured diagnosis is a crucial component of malaria control and elimination programmes moving forward, and further advances build on this capacity. Every national malaria control/elimination programme has to ensure, therefore, its functional capacity for quality-assured diagnosis. WHO has trained certified microscopists (level one) to help ensure harmonisation of policies, standardisation of practices, and inter-operability in the SADC region. WHO countries have benefited from the regional programme for improving diagnosis, which includes capacity building, specialised testing, and a microscope slide bank (see, for example WHO, 2008b).

Other government and regulatory measures and factors contribute to the initiatives to eliminate malaria from Southern Africa by 2030, but difficulties remain. The movement of malaria commodities across borders is an example, as these materials are governed by regulatory restrictions. The impact of procurement and supply management challenges is that countries often lack buffer stocks and, consequently, cannot respond effectively or timeously to malaria outbreaks or epidemics. Delays in some countries in the registration of some medicines (primaquine, for example, which is a transmission-blocking medicine) have adverse implications for achieving the planned malaria elimination targets.

Only joint and concerted efforts can help the SADC countries reach the goal of ending cross-border transmissions. To facilitate the reduction of cross-border malaria transmission, the E8 provide technical support and operational guidance to control and end cross-border transmission.

They recognise that a regionally coordinated approach is critical. It is recognised that 72 per cent, 79 per cent, and 48 per cent of cases in Eswatini, South Africa, and Botswana, respectively, are imported from the countries' more endemic neighbours. To aid joint surveillance and monitoring of the cross-border movement of people with malaria parasites, the E8 has facilitated the establishment of border posts, which extend access to diagnosis and treatment of malaria to mobile and migrant populations and the under-served border communities (see Elimination 8 Strategic Plan 2015). Furthermore, the E8 advocates for the strengthening of communication for behaviour change in cross-border areas through the use of targeted messages and by empowering and engaging local communities to support the initiatives. This includes the use of data, information, and predictions provided by meteorological institutions to strengthen public communication appropriate for specific risk groups and for health workers (see Elimination 8, 2015).

Due to the ongoing instability of malaria in the SADC region it is crucial, in terms of climatic monitoring and associated planning, to be part of a network of systems that link the health sector to weather bureaus. The SADC Secretariat's SADC Climate Services Centre (see SADC, undated) provides regional operational services for monitoring and predicting extreme climate conditions. Every year it hosts a meeting of the Southern Africa Regional Climate Outlook Forum where a weather outlook for the coming season is analysed. This SADC centre collaborates with the United States National Oceanic and Atmospheric Administration to help get accurate forecasts as to pending malaria-conducive conditions. The weather forecasting infrastructure needs to link closely with health institutional infrastructure in the region. Hence, as proposed by SADC (WHO, 2004), malaria programme managers and directors should also work closely with the SADC Regional Communicable Diseases Centre in Lusaka, Zambia, to establish a thematic group on malaria outbreaks and emergencies, initiate a proactive approach to malaria surveillance, and strengthen the development and use of alert and epidemic thresholds for weekly reporting of malaria cases and deaths and surveillance of active foci (Elimination 8 TWG, 2018; SADC, 2007a; Teklehaimanot et al., 2004; WHO, 2004).

While there has been much progress in the SADC and E8 initiatives to control and advance towards the elimination of malaria in the region, further advances are required. These depend on systematic coordination and cooperation (see Elimination 8, 2016: 2). As stressed in SADC's Elimination 8 (2015) initiative, for E8 member states to move towards elimination, they need concertedly to deliberate on policies and the strategic and operational issues that affect their malaria elimination programmes. A collective effort is needed in order to eliminate malaria (Elimination 8, 2015). Such efforts to harmonise policies will support national programmes and regional actors to design and execute strategies that complement and reinforce one another. It is crucial equally for malaria control and elimination policies (see Feachem, 2009; Feachem et al., 2009) to be renewed suitably and be aligned across the SADC region. For example, the five-year Malaria Strategic Plan (SADC, 2007a; SADC, 2014) needs to undergo a mid-term review and end-term review. The Malaria Elimination Strategic Plan (SADC, 2007b; SADC, 2014), which is aimed at accelerating 'Zero Local Transmission' in all districts leading to country-wide Local Zero Transmission through the provision of a mechanism for collaboration and joint strategic programming needs to be evaluated. These documents should be aligned with the SADC Malaria Strategic Framework (2015, to be updated) and the SADC Malaria Elimination Framework. The document should also be aligned with the SDGs, GTS, and AIM.

CONCLUSION

Certain and important strides forward have been made in the campaign to consolidate Southern Africa's transition from malaria control to malaria elimination. The campaign has been carried powerfully by a set of international and regional organisations and platforms to these organisations. The analysis showed the important impact that was leveraged by the network in which the WHO, SADC, and its platform Elimination 8 have been powerful players. The E8 Technical Committee is an illustration of the already-existing network operations that will help sustain SADC programmes in future.

The analysis also articulated these organisations' goals and advocacy programmes moving towards elimination. It emphasised that multiple obstacles remain before elimination will be achieved. The battle against malaria in SADC continues, but the benchmarks achieved to date offer significant pointers to actors countering Africa's epidemics, particularly malaria. At the heart of these lessons is evidence of holistic approaches, multi-, inter- and trans-disciplinary, coming together to record the levels of success we continue to witness.

REFERENCES

African Leaders Malaria Alliance (ALMA). 2016. 'ALMA 2030 scorecard towards Malaria elimination'. http://alma2030.org/sites/default/files/elimination-sc/english_december_2016_malaria_elimination_scorecard.pdf, accessed 2 October 2018.

Burrows, J. N., Duparc, S., Gutteridge, W. E., Van Huijsduijnen, R. H., Kaszubska, W., Macintyre, F., Mazzuri, S., Möhrle, J. J. & Wells, T. N. C. 2017. 'New developments in anti-malarial target candidate and product profiles'. *Malaria Journal*, 16 (1), 26.

Castillo-Salgado, C. 2009. 'Concept Paper-Elimination 8'. Concept Note, Malaria Elimination Ministerial Meeting, Windhoek, Namibia.

Centers for Disease Control and Prevention (CDC). 17 March 2017. 'Where Malaria Occurs'. *Centers for Disease Control and Prevention*, https://www.cdc.gov/malaria/about/distribution.html, accessed 2 December 2018.

Cohen, J. M., Moonen, B., Snow, R. W. & Smith, D. L. 2010. 'How absolute is zero? An evaluation of historical and current definitions of malaria elimination'. *Malaria Journal*, 9 (1), 213.

Delacollette, C. & Rietveld, A. 2006. 'WHO GMP-Informal consultation on malaria elimination: Setting up the WHO agenda'. *World Health Organization, Fecha de consulta: 5 de abril de 2011,* Tunis. http://whqlibdoc.who.int/hq/2006/WHO_HTM_MAL_2006.1114_eng.pdf, accessed 3 March 2010.

Delacollette, C. 2004. 'Malaria Epidemic Response: What the clinician needs to know'. *Roll Back Malaria.*

Dowdle, W. R. 1999. 'The principles of disease elimination and eradication'. *Morbidity and Mortality Weekly Report*, 76 (supplement SU01), 23–27.

Eastern and Southern Africa Sub-Regional Network (ESARN). 2017. Zimbabwe Malaria re-stratification experience – evidence based programming presentation: ESARN Meeting, 8–12 October, Addis Ababa, Ethiopia.

Elimination 8. 2015. *Elimination 8 Strategic Plan, 2015-2020: Working Towards a Malaria-free Southern Africa*. Windhoek, Namibia.

Elimination 8. 2016. 'Reaching beyond borders to achieve a malaria-free southern Africa'. https://malariaelimination8.org/wp-content/uploads/2017/.../E8-Work-Two-Pager.pdf, accessed 2 November 2018.

Elimination 8. 2017. Concept note. https://malariaelimination8.org/wp.../2017/.../Malaria-Elimination-Concept-Note-2016, accessed 8 December 2018.

Elimination 8 EPR Technical Work Group (TWG). 2018: Establishment of E8 Regional Situation Room – milestones and successes. Addis Ababa, Ethiopia.

Feachem, R. G. A. The Malaria Elimination Group, 2009. *Shrinking the Malaria Map: A Guide on Malaria Elimination for Policy Makers.* The Global Health Group, Global Health Sciences, University of California, San Francisco.

Feachem, R. G. A., Phillips, A. A. & Targett, G. A. (eds.) 2009. *Shrinking the Malaria Map: A Prospectus on Malaria Elimination.* The Global Health Group, Global Health Sciences, University of California, San Francisco.

Feachem, R. G. A. & Sabot, O. 2008. 'A new global malaria eradication strategy'. *The Lancet*, 371 (9624), 1633–1635.

Hemingway, J., Ranson, H., Magill, A., Kolaczinski, J., Fornadel, C., Gimnig, J., Coetzee, M., Simard, F., Roch, D.K., Hinzoumbe, C. K. & Pickett, J. 2016. 'Averting a malaria disaster: Will insecticide resistance derail malaria control?' *The Lancet*, 387 (10029), 1785–1788.

Kobylinski, K. C., Massamba, S., Chapman, P. L., Moussa, D., Sarr, M. D. & Foy, B. D. 2011. 'Ivermectin mass drug administration to humans disrupts malaria parasite transmission in Senegalese villages'. *American Journal of Tropical Medicine and Hygiene*, 85 (1), 3–5.

Maharaj, R., Moonasar, D., Baltazar, C., Kunene, S. & Morris, N. 2016. 'Sustaining control: Lessons from the Lubombo spatial development initiative in southern Africa'. *Malaria Journal*, 15 (1), 409.

Mpofu M., Becker, P., Mudambo, K. & De Jager, C. 2016. 'Field effectiveness of microbial larvicides on mosquito larvae in malaria areas of Botswana and Zimbabwe'. *Malaria Journal*, 15 (1), 586.

Ranson, H., N'guessan, R., Lines, J., Moiroux, N., Nkuni, Z. J. & Corbel, V. 2011. 'Pyrethroid resistance in African anopheline mosquitoes: What are the implications for malaria control?' *Trends in Parasitology*, 27 (2), 91–98, DOI: 10.1016/j.pt.2010.08.004.

Roll Back Malaria Partnership. 2015. *Action and Investment to defeat Malaria 2016–2030. For a Malaria-Free World* (WHO). http://www. Action and investment to defeat malaria 2016–2030: https://www.mmv.org/sites/default/files/uploads/docs/publications/RBM_AIM_Report.pdf. Report, accessed 15 November 2018.

Southern African Development Community (SADC). nd. 'Climate Services Centre'. https://www.sadc.int/sadc-secretariat/services-centres/climate-services-centre/, accessed 1 November 2018.

Southern African Development Community (SADC). 2007a. *Malaria Strategic Framework, 2007–2015*. SADC. November.

Southern African Development Community (SADC). November 2007b. SADC *Malaria Elimination Framework, 2007–2015*. SADC.

Southern African Development Community (SADC). 2014. *E8 Malaria*

Elimination Scorecard. SADC. May.
Southern African Development Community (SADC). 2017. *Malaria Report*. SADC.
Teklehaimanot, H. D., Schwartz, J., Teklehaimanot, A. & Lipsitch, M. 2004. 'Alert threshold algorithms and malaria epidemic detection'. *Emerging Infectious Diseases*. 10 (7), 1220–1226.
World Health Organization (WHO). 2003. *Malaria epidemics: Forecasting, prevention, early detection and control: From policy to practice, report of an informal consultation*. Leysin, Switzerland, 8–10 December 2003.
World Health Organization (WHO). 2004. Malaria Epidemics: Forecasting, prevention, early detection and control – from policy to practice: report of an informal consultation: Leysin, Switzerland, 8–10. December 2003.
World Health Organization (WHO). 2008a. National Strategic Plan for Laboratories 2008–2012, Version 2, February 2007 . www.who.int/hiv/amds/amds_nat_strat_plan_lab_2008.pdf, accessed 2 October 2018.
World Health Organiszation (WHO). 2008b. Global malaria control and elimination: report of a technical review. Global Malaria Control and Elimination Meeting. http://malaria.who.int/docs/elimination/MalariaControlEliminationMeeting.pdf, accessed 4 March 2010.
World Health Organization (WHO). 2009. *Surveillance/EWARN in Emergencies*. www.who.int/diseasecontrol.../idhe_2009_london_surveillance_morbidity.pdf, accessed 2 December 2018.
World Health Organization (WHO). 2012. Outbreak surveillance and response in humanitarian emergencies – WHO guidelines for EWARN implementation: WHO/HSE/GAR/DCE/2012.1, accessed 20 October 2018.
World Health Organization (WHO). 2013. Global Malaria Programme. *World Malaria Report 2013*.
World Health Organization (WHO). 2016. *World Malaria Report 2016*. https://www.who.int/malaria/publications/world-malaria-report-2016/report/en/, accessed 2 December 2018.
World Health Organization (WHO). 2017a. *World Malaria Report 2017*. http://www.who.int/malaria/publications/world-malaria-report-2017/report/en/, accessed 3 December 2018.
World Health Organization (WHO). 2017b. *Southern African Development Community (SADC) Malaria Report 2017*. WHO Regional Office for Africa.
World Health Organization (WHO). 2018a. Outbreak surveillance and response in humanitarian emergencies Global Malaria Program (GMP): Malaria surveillance – surveillance, monitoring and evaluation presentation: ESARN Meeting 8–12 October, Addis Ababa, Ethiopia.
World Health Organization (WHO). 2018b. Intermittent preventive treatment in pregnancy (IPTp), http://www.who.int/malaria/areas/preventive_therapies/pregnancy/en/, 21 June, accessed 6 November 2018.
World Health Organization (WHO). 2018c. *World Malaria Report 2018*. Geneva Licence: CCBY_NC_SA: ISBN978-4-156565-3.

FIVE

Containing Ebola in Nigeria: *An African Success Story*

NATHANIEL UMUKORO

INTRODUCTION

EBOLA VIRUS DISEASE (EVD) IS recognised as one of the deadliest viral diseases in the world. The disease was called Ebola because the first outbreak occurred in a village close to the Ebola River in the Democratic Republic of Congo. Since 1976 most cases of EVD have occurred in Africa (Baseler et. al., 2017). The outbreak of the disease in Africa and other parts of the world from 2014–2016 recorded more casualties than in any prior outbreak (see Table 1).[i] In Sierra Leone, out of the 14,124

i According to WHO (2018), Ebola virus disease first appeared in 1976 in two simultaneous outbreaks, in South Sudan and the Democratic Republic of Congo (see Table 1). The 2014–2016 outbreak in West Africa was the largest since the virus was discovered in 1976. There were more cases and deaths in this outbreak than in all others combined. The virus family Filoviridae includes three genera: Cueva virus, Marburg virus, and Ebola virus. Within the genus Ebola virus, five species have been identified: Zaire, Bundibugyo, Sudan, Reston, and Taï Forest. The first three, the Bundibugyo, Zaire and Sudan viruses, have been associated with the large outbreaks in Africa. The virus causing the 2014–2016 West African outbreak belongs to the Zaire Ebola virus species cases recorded there were 3,956 deaths (28 per cent); 10,675 cases were recorded in Liberia, with 4,809 deaths (45 per cent); and Guinea recorded 3,811 cases, with 2,543 deaths (67 per cent) (WHO, 2018).

Nigeria was one of the African countries affected by the EVD epidemic of 2014,[ii] but because the outbreak was effectively contained there, Nigeria was able to paint a different picture to that of the other West African countries at that time. The outbreak caused anxiety in Nigerians and foreigners alike, most especially because of the huge size of the population in its capital city, Lagos – approximately 21 million – but also because of the challenges associated with health care services delivery. As United States consul general in Nigeria Jeffery Hawkins said: 'The last thing anyone in the world wants to hear is the two words, "Ebola" and "Lagos" in the same sentence.' That 'single juxtaposition', he noted, conjured up images of an 'apocalyptic urban outbreak' (Abubakar et al., 2014; Bureau of Public Services Reforms, 2015). Due to an early, accurate diagnosis, and appropriate action by medical practitioners, however, that image did not come to pass in Nigeria.

Nigeria's effective containment of the Ebola outbreak is a success story for two reasons. Firstly it prevented the transfer of the outbreak of the disease to other parts of Nigeria. Secondly it showed that the federal government could successfully, and effectively, manage health problems affecting the country's citizens if political leaders demonstrated the political will to do so.

Given the poor state of health services delivery in Nigeria, what lessons can be learned from the successful containment of the disease? This chapter investigates this question and extracts some lessons other

---

ii WHO (2018) provides details: Fruit bats of the Pteropodidae family are natural Ebola virus hosts. Ebola is introduced into the human population through close contact with the blood, secretions, organs, or other bodily fluids of infected animals such as chimpanzees, gorillas, fruit bats, monkeys, forest antelope and porcupines found ill or dead or in the rainforest. Ebola then spreads through human-to-human transmission via direct contact (through broken skin or mucous membranes) with the blood, secretions, organs or other bodily fluids of infected people, and with surfaces and materials (e.g. bedding, clothing) contaminated with these fluids. Health care workers have frequently been infected while treating patients with suspected or confirmed EVD. This has occurred through close contact with patients when infection control precautions are not strictly practised. Burial ceremonies that involve direct contact with the body of the deceased can also contribute in the transmission of Ebola. People remain infectious as long as their blood contains the virus.

countries in Africa might learn from the Nigerian experience. To do this the chapter is divided into five interrelated sections: a brief overview of Nigeria's health care system, a review of the introduction of EVD to Nigeria, analysis of the response of the federal government to the EVD epidemic, consideration of other factors that contributed to the successful containment of EVD in Nigeria, and lessons from the successful containment of EVD in Nigeria. The chapter draws on retrospective documentary analysis, the author's primary interview research conducted in 2016 in the aftermath of Nigeria's containment of EVD, and contemporary interpretations of data.

OVERVIEW OF NIGERIA'S PUBLIC HEALTH CARE SYSTEM

The public health care system in Nigeria reflects the country's federal structure of government. Nigeria has 36 states and 774 local government areas. This means that the federal, state, and local governments are all involved in the provision of public health care services (Umukoro, 2012). Additionally, private health care institutions exist to complement the role of the government. Health facilities in the private sector are not generally accessible to low-income earners, and private hospitals mainly provide services for higher income households. Poor health outcomes in public health care institutions can be attributed to the lack of appropriate targeting strategies for reaching the poor, the low levels of government funding of health institutions, and poor implementation of public health care policies (Osafo-Kwako & Apampa, 2009).

In Lagos, where the Nigerian outbreak of EVD started, there are 26 registered general hospitals, 256 public health care centres, 2,886 private hospitals or specialist clinics and laboratories or diagnostic centres, in addition to an estimated 160 tradomedical centres (see Musbau, 2017). In spite of the presence of these institutions, quality health care services remain a mirage in the city. Basically, this is because of inadequately qualified staff, overcrowded emergency wards, fake drugs, financial constraints, and, sometimes, lack of empathy from health workers. These were some of the things contributing to the high anxiety levels when news broke of the EVD outbreak in Lagos.

Table 1: Chronology of previous Ebola virus disease outbreaks

Year	Country	Ebola virus species	Cases	Deaths	Case fatality %
2015	Italy	Zaire	1	0	0
2014	DRC	Zaire	66	49	74
2014	Spain	Zaire	1	0	0
2014	UK	Zaire	1	0	0
2014	USA	Zaire	4	1	25
2014	Senegal	Zaire	1	0	0
2014	Mali	Zaire	8	6	75
2014	Nigeria	Zaire	20	8	40
2014–2016	Sierra Leone	Zaire	14,124*	3,9568	28
2014–2016	Liberia	Zaire	10,675*	4,809*	45
2014–2016	Guinea	Zaire	3,811*	2,543*	67
2012	Democratic Republic of Congo	Bundibugyo	57	29	51
2012	Uganda	Sudan	7	4	57
2012	Uganda	Sudan	24	17	71
2011	Uganda	Sudan	1	1	100
2008	Democratic Republic of Congo	Zaire	32	14	44
2007	Uganda	Bundibugyo	149	37	25
2007	Democratic Republic of Congo	Zaire	264	187	71
2005	Congo	Zaire	12	10	83
2004	Sudan	Sudan	17	7	41
2003 (Nov–Dec)	Congo	Zaire	35	29	83
2003 (Jan–Apr)	Congo	Zaire	143	128	90
2001–2002	Congo	Zaire	59	44	75
2001–2002	Gabon	Zaire	65	53	82

Year	Country	Ebola virus species	Cases	Deaths	Case fatality %
2000	Uganda	Sudan	425	224	53
1996	South Africa (ex-Gabon)	Zaire	1	1	100
1996 (Jul–Dec)	Gabon	Zaire	60	45	75
1996 (Jan–Apr)	Gabon	Zaire	31	21	68
1995	Democratic Republic of Congo	Zaire	315	254	81
1994	Côte d'Ivoire	Taï Forest	1	0	0
1994	Gabon	Zaire	52	31	60
1979	Sudan	Sudan	34	22	65
1977	Democratic Republic of Congo	Zaire	1	1	100
1976	Sudan	Sudan	284	151	53
1976	Democratic Republic of Congo	Zaire	318	280	88

Source: WHO, 2018
Note: Includes suspect, probable, and confirmed EVD cases.

Introduction of Ebola virus disease to Nigeria

Although several outbreaks of epidemics had occurred in Nigeria over the years, no case of Ebola was documented there until 2014. On 20 July 2014, a traveller from Liberia who was infected with Ebola landed at the Lagos Murtala Muhammed International Airport. He passed the disease to everyone who assisted him, from the officer who escorted him to the hospital to nine of the doctors and nurses who treated him there (Umukoro, 2016).

The Ebola outbreak created panic in Nigeria for a number of reasons: the known deadly impact it had had on some African countries, the poor state of public health care in the country, and the possibility of the disease spreading from Lagos to other areas. The estimated population of Lagos at the time was 21 million, which is almost the combined populations of Guinea, Sierra Leone, and Liberia (Bureau of Public Services Reforms, 2015). Following the confirmation of this first case, contact tracing in the densely populated urban environment became the government's primary concern.

Response of the government of Nigeria to the regional Ebola epidemic

The first action taken by the government was to announce that the EVD outbreak was a public health emergency and that a swift response was essential (Umukoro, 2016). Calling the outbreak a public health emergency ensured that the government and health workers would give priority attention to the management of the EVD problem. Financial resources were promptly made available to prevent the spread of the disease (Bureau of Public Services Reforms, 2015). The government also approved a special national intervention plan and released the sum of 1.9 billion (USD 11.5 million) to support the implementation of the plan at both national and sub-national levels (News Agency of Nigeria, 2014). The implementation of the intervention plan resulted in the deployment of additional health workers for contact tracing, screening at borders, establishment of additional isolation centres, and procurement of more health care facilities and safety equipment. In order to strengthen the efforts of the Lagos state government in curbing the spread of EVD, the federal government provided financial resources to the state government.

This approach to combating the Ebola crisis was based on a modification of the existing polio programme infrastructure. The government also used some of the experts in the polio programme for the management of the Ebola crisis (Fatiregun & Isere, 2017). For example, the Ebola Emergency Operations Centre (EEOC), which coordinated the response to the EVD outbreak in Nigeria, was led by the deputy incident manager of the National Polio Emergency Operations Centre. Generally, the support from the polio programme infrastructure, in particular the coordination mechanism adopted, the availability of skilled personnel from the polio programme, and lessons that had already been learned from managing the polio eradication programme, added significantly to the quick prevention of the spread of Ebola in Nigeria in 2014 (Vaz et al., 2016).

In personal research conducted in 2016, in order to obtain insights into the government's Ebola outbreak response, the author interviewed multiple actors (see Umukoro, 2016). One key informant (Joseph), who was a health worker in the Federal Ministry of Health (FMH), stated that 'the first priority of the government was to locate all who likely had contacts with anyone infested by Ebola'. This confirmed contact tracing as a key strategy in reacting to the Ebola crisis. It involved looking for people who had interacted with an Ebola patient and then keeping them under careful observation. It helped to ensure early detection of new cases and the prompt quarantining of those who were believed to be infected. During the period of EVD crisis, cases were identified rapidly and put under inspection for 21 days (the maximum incubation period of Ebola virus) from the last day of contact (WHO, 2014).

Another key informant (Femi), a member of the Nigerian Medical Association, gave the opinion that the response to the Ebola crisis of health workers in various health care institutions in Nigeria was nothing short of remarkable. Health workers played key roles in the disease's containment. When the first case of EVD was confirmed (in July 2014), some health workers in public health institutions were on strike. In order that all health workers could be available to participate fully in the fight against EVD, on 25 August the strike was suspended. In truth many health workers risked their lives to prevent the spread of the disease. Key health worker informants (Kemi, Johnson, Ihenacho and Bolanle) in the Ministry of Health in Lagos confirmed that during the Ebola outbreak community health workers played several important roles. Critically, in the process of contact tracing they engaged with community leaders and elicited their support as they went from house to house. While doing so they were able to provide useful information about the disease to communities at the same time as looking out for new cases. They also used local religious leaders to help them expand their outreach strategies (see Umukoro, 2016).

Many community-based agents, including community health workers working with NGOs, were deployed for contact tracing, community sensitisation, promotion of epidemiologically and culturally appropriate protective practices, and data collection. A group of more than 150 contact tracers was mobilised to find people who had potentially been exposed to EVD. They conducted over 18,500 face-to-face visits to check for a range of symptoms, such as fever, in each of these contacts. During the contact tracing period, anyone manifesting symptoms was immediately taken to an isolation ward for proper investigation. If an EVD case was confirmed, the patient was transferred to a designated EVD treatment centre (Shuaib et al., 2014; Umukoro, 2016).

Generally, the response to the Ebola crisis by different stakeholders was properly coordinated. Various tiers of government and agencies cooperated with one another and engaged on massive public awareness campaigns to familiarise everyone with the dangers associated with EVD. This included the effective use of social media. The cooperation of institutions at the different levels of government (federal, state, and local) was encouraged by the then-president of Nigeria, Goodluck Jonathan, as a strategy for tackling the Ebola crisis. For example, he directed the Federal Ministry of Health to work in partnership with the state ministries of health, the National Centre for Disease Control (NCDC), the National Emergency Management Agency (NEMA), and other related agencies to ensure that all relevant steps were taken to contain the spread of the disease (Bureau of Public Services Reforms, 2015).

Additional government actions that contributed to the timeous containment of EVD

Other factors that contributed to the successful containment of Ebola can be classified into two categories, namely: what the government did before EVD was detected in Nigeria, and steps the government took after the first case of EVD was confirmed. On 24 March 2014, after EVD was detected in Guinea (see Figure 1), the federal government, through the FMH and NCDC, put the necessary machinery in place to manage any case of EVD in the event of an outbreak. The following were some of the steps taken by the federal government before the outbreak of Ebola: the 36 states of the federation and Abuja were notified of the outbreak in Guinea. The need to strengthen disease surveillance for haemorrhagic fevers was recommended and they were requested to report suspected cases promptly. Training on EVD surveillance and medical procedures was also provided to some health workers. This training was carried out in different parts of Nigeria on a zonal basis, that is, north-east, north-west, north-central, south-west, south-east and south-south. Port health officers were asked to ensure strict disease surveillance.

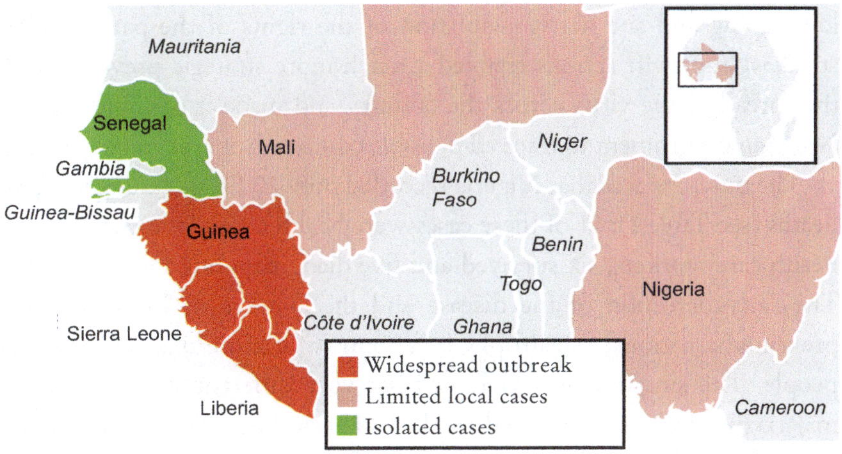

Figure 1: West Africa situation map – Ebola virus epidemic, December 2013–June 2016

Source: https://en.wikipedia.org/wiki/Nigeria

Specific factors that contributed to the successful containment of the disease

Early detection

The first two contributors to the success in handling the Ebola problem were the early detection of the disease and the prompt introduction of control measures to prevent its spread (Duric & Ilic, 2012). When the Liberian diplomat, Patrick Sawyer, who brought the EVD to Nigeria, collapsed at the airport in Lagos he was immediately taken to First Consultants Medical Centre (FCMC), where he was diagnosed with malaria. When another doctor, Dr Ameyo Stella Adadevoh, saw him during her ward round the following day, she suspected EVD. In order to confirm her diagnosis she reached out to the Lagos state and federal ministries of health and ensured that he was tested immediately for EVD. Before the test result was received by the hospital, the patient and other officials of the government of Liberia tried to insist that Dr Adadevoh discharge him so that he could attend the Economic Community of West African States (ECOWAS) conference. In spite of the pressure, Dr Adadevoh refused, even when they threatened to charge her with kidnapping and sue her for violation of the rights of the patient. Her steadfast and swift actions enabled a much more strategic prevention of the spread of the virus across the country and made it possible for the Nigerian government to trace all possible contacts from the index patient.

The outcome was that Nigeria recorded only 20 Ebola cases and eight deaths (see Table 1); 11 of these cases were health care workers. Of those health care workers, six survived and five died, including Dr Adadevoh. The early detection of the disease and the courage of Dr Adadevoh prevented a national catastrophe in a country of more than 180 million people. The situation would have been very different if Mr Sawyer's malaria diagnosis had remained and he had been allowed to travel to other parts of Nigeria.

Public enlightenment programmes

After the outbreak of the disease was announced in Nigeria, enlightenment programmes were carried out to create awareness about EVD and how it could be prevented (see Otu et al., 2018). In order to reach as many people as possible these campaigns were conducted in various Nigerian languages through radio, television, and posters. All hospitals in the country were alerted and directed to create awareness of the deadly nature of the disease and how the spread of the disease could be prevented.

Contributions of the private sector

Substantial financial resources were contributed by private sector organisations towards the containment of EVD. For example, on 14 August 2014, Alhaji Aliko Dangote contributed in the region of USD 927,007 (152,956,250) from the Dangote Foundation for the establishment of a national Ebola Emergency Operation Centre (EEOC) at Yaba, Lagos. Several private sector organisations in Nigeria supported the government's efforts through, for example, the encouragement of hand-washing and general sanitation and by providing taps in public places for people to wash their hands (Bureau of Public Services Reforms, 2015).

Cultural measures

The federal government took a series of actions pertaining to certain cultural practices in order to prevent the spread of the EVD. One such action, which was taken during the peak period of the Ebola crisis, was the banning of the transportation of corpses. The reason behind this action was because burial ceremonies bring family members and friends together and this could create the necessary conditions for transmitting the Ebola virus, particularly as some funeral traditions involve close contact with the dead (see, for example, Maxmen, 2015). This applied to the transportation of corpses not only in Nigeria, but internationally and interstate too. Bereaved families who planned to bury their loved ones during the crisis period were obliged first to get clearance from the federal Ministry of Health before they could do so. This measure assisted in curbing interstate movement of corpses, and also significantly reduced the number of burial ceremonies that took place during the crisis period.

Delay in the reopening of schools

In order to prevent the spread of EVD in primary and secondary schools the federal government directed that all schools, public and private, should remain closed until effective strategies had been put in place to prevent the spread of the disease. All tertiary institutions were also advised to suspend, until further notice at the time, the exchange of staff and student programmes, visits, and any major international seminars and workshops that had been scheduled (Bureau of Public Services Reforms, 2015).

Maintenance of public hygiene

The Federal Ministry of Health urged all Nigerians to improve their personal hygiene by washing their hands frequently with soap and running water. The use of a bucket with a tap for regular hand-washing was initiated as a strategy in places where there was no running water. The use of buckets made it possible for running water to be available in public places, even when there was no regular source of water supply such as a borehole (Ugwuanyi, 2014).

Proper health surveillance at Nigeria's entry and exit points

Another factor that contributed to the successful containment of Nigeria's 2014 EVD outbreak was health surveillance at the country's entry and exit points. This became necessary because Nigeria did not close its borders in spite of repeated calls to do so. The decision not to close the borders was because of widespread evidence that travel bans do not work; they have habitually failed to prevent the spread of disease in the past (Poletto, 2014; Khalid, 2014). To prevent importation/exportation of Ebola, therefore, it was necessary to check the health status of travellers at various points of entry. A team of health workers ensured screening of all arrivals/departures in and out of Nigeria by land, air, and sea. Screening included travellers' temperature monitoring and analysis of the entrants' contact with cases of Ebola (Otsuki & Nishiura, 2016). They also ensured that capacity was available at all border points to properly manage passengers with symptoms of Ebola, including the ability to isolate them. According to a key informant (Okeke) at the Murtala Muhammed International Airport in Lagos, 'the screening of passengers was to prevent a passenger infested with Ebola from travelling and infesting other passengers and people in the host country with the disease'. Nigeria took this measure particularly seriously because of how Ebola had first entered the country.

Suspension of the operation of certain airlines

In order to further protect Nigerians from EVD, the Nigerian Civil Aviation Authority (NCAA) suspended certain airlines from transporting passengers to Nigeria. One of these was ASKY Airlines, an Ethiopian Airlines feeder airline with a hub in Lomé, Togo. ASKY Airlines was an important player in the West, East and Central Africa region, operating 80 flights into Lagos and Abuja weekly. The airline was informed that the suspension would be lifted only when it could prove that it was capable of adequately screening passengers at all its points of operation, including the profiling of every passenger. NCCA took this action because the airline representatives could not conclusively demonstrate their capacity to prevent a recurrence of importing Ebola carriers to Nigeria. The airline's inability to give the necessary assurance was contrary to the provision of Article 14 of the Chicago Convention, 1944, which states that '(e)ach contracting State agrees to take effective measures to prevent the spread by means of air navigation of cholera, typhus (epidemic), smallpox, yellow fever, plague, and such other communicable diseases as the contracting States shall from time to time decide to designate ...' Similarly, during the Ebola crisis period Arik Air also suspended its flights to Monrovia, Liberia, and Freetown, Sierra Leone. The NCAA advised that airline to maintain the cessation of flights to the two countries until it was cleared by the authority to resume.

Government response to social media

The role that social media played after the outbreak of EVD in Nigeria could be seen as a double-edged sword. On the positive side, it made it possible for awareness about the disease to be created and ways of preventing its spread to be explained. One the negative side, social media could also be abused, with some people using its platforms to spread false information about the nature and treatment of the disease. An example was the rumour that drinking salt and warm water was a cure for Ebola. Two people died and at least 20 people were hospitalised as a result (*Vanguard Newspaper*, 2014). Since social media could easily be used to spread misleading information about the nature and treatment of Ebola, the government worked hard to respond in a timely manner to correct any false information. In order to curtail the dangerous effects of deceptive information through social media platforms, the federal and state governments engaged in different forms of public enlightenment campaigns. These initiatives helped to reduce the harmful influence of social media (see also Otu et al., 2018).

Health workers and the successful containment of EVD

Health workers in both private and public health institutions played key roles in the containment of Ebola in Nigeria. When Patrick Sawyer brought Ebola to Nigeria, health workers in public health institutions were on strike. The strike began on 1 July 2014 and dragged on even when Ebola broke out in the country later that month. It became apparent that the striking doctors were beginning to lose public sympathy when they failed to call off their strike in the face of the Ebola outbreak, but the decision was made to suspend the strike on 25 August 2014 so that all health workers could participate fully in the fight against EVD. As has been mentioned earlier in this chapter, and as confirmed by the author's aftermath research interviews, community health workers played several important roles – some health workers even risked their lives – to prevent the spread of the disease. Two key informants at the Lagos Ministry of Health (Sola and Moses) confirmed how these health workers had worked closely with community and local religious leaders. The latter were especially important in efforts to prevent or reduce transmission during funerals and burials.

Lessons from the successful containment of EVD in Nigeria

Several lessons can be learned by the Nigerian government and the governments of other African countries from the effective way in which the outbreak of EVD was contained in Nigeria. At its core, this success can be attributed not only to the early and accurate response of the different health institutions to the outbreak but also that the response was holistic and in accordance with international public health standards (Adewole, 2017). The following are specific lessons that can be learned from the successful containment of EVD in Nigeria.

The first key lesson from Nigeria's success story in combating EVD is the need to maintain strict ethical standards in medical practice. When the first EVD patient came to Nigeria and manifested symptoms of the disease, he was taken to First Consultants Medical Centre in Lagos. At the hospital, the patient claimed that he had malaria. Since malaria is not transmitted from person to person, staff at the centre did not take protective precautions at first. This contributed to health care workers becoming infected. This makes it necessary that health care workers take necessary precautions at all times whenever there is a suspected epidemic outbreak.

The second lesson is the importance of the capacity of the state in protecting its citizens through a diversity of options. In spite of the participation of the private sector in the delivery of health care services, effective participation of the government in the sector can protect citizens against public emergencies. This is because the private sector could never have done what various levels of government did during the EVD outbreak. In addition to the provision of financial resources, the government ensured that health workers were adequately trained to combat EVD and that there were enough of them, as well as sufficient and appropriate facilities to isolate those showing Ebola symptoms in treatment centres that were well equipped.

The third lesson is on the importance of financing the health sector adequately. The availability of adequate financial resources contributed to the successful containment of EVD in Nigeria. As soon as it was made aware of a potential outbreak of Ebola the federal government immediately released funds to relevant health care institutions for the establishment of EVD management facilities and other expenses. It is critically important that governments, especially of African countries, ensure adequate budgetary allocations for the health sector. Financial constraints have prevented many African countries from contributing 15 per cent of their national budgets to the health sector, as agreed in the Abuja Declaration of 2001.

The fourth lesson is that compliance with government policies and directives play a crucial role in the control of the spread of infectious diseases. The willingness of Nigerians to comply with government directives on EVD prevention contributed to the successful containment of the disease in Nigeria. The general lesson from this is that citizens should be conscious of the fact that the prevention of the outbreak or spread of infectious diseases is not the responsibility of the government alone, but rather that of the entire citizenry.

The fifth lesson concerns the need to have adequate and well-trained manpower in the health sector at all times. One of the challenges the Nigerian government had to struggle to overcome during the outbreak of EVD was the shortage of trained manpower for an appropriate response.

The sixth lesson is on the need to ensure the cooperation of religious leaders when there is an outbreak of an epidemic. Since religious beliefs and activities affect how people respond to government policies and directives, the involvement of religious leaders in giving such directives to their members can help ensure greater compliance on the part of their followers.

The seventh lesson concerns the effective use of social media in the event of an outbreak of disease, and potential epidemics. In Nigeria, the government ensured that information about EVD and how the spread could be prevented was properly disseminated through multiple platforms, including, importantly, social media. During an outbreak a country's government should be able to influence the use of the social media. This is important because both positive and negative information will be disseminated through social media. If any information that can negatively affect the control of epidemics is disseminated the government should be able to strategise ways of correcting the wrong information promptly.

CONCLUSION

Nigeria was able to manage the outbreak of Ebola in the country effectively because of adequate funding, astute medical practitioners who could diagnose accurately, collaboration between health and other authorities at the national and sub-national levels, concerted training efforts, and commitment to public education. This kind of coordinated, well-managed commitment is required to strengthen public health care in Nigeria and other African countries in order for them to be able to deal with other epidemics and work toward increasing the health status for the majority of their citizens.

In spite of Nigeria's achievement in containing EVD in 2014, much can still be done to improve the overall public health care system there. After the successful containment of the disease (using some of the infrastructure that was already in place to counter outbreaks of polio), most practical steps taken to prevent the spread of the Ebola disease disappeared. This is worrisome because there are many other diseases that afflict Nigerians, and the strategies used in containing EVD could be used in managing other diseases as well. This is important because in spite of the success the country recorded in the fight against Ebola, the health care system continues to be bedevilled by many challenges. The specific aspects of the health care sector in Nigeria that require urgent attention include medical equipment and the number of medical personnel in public hospitals. In 2009 the Nigerian national health conference identified as major challenges in the health sector a lack of synchronisation of efforts, fragmentation of services, inadequate resources (including medicine and supplies), insufficient and deteriorating infrastructure, inequity in the distribution of resources, and access to care (Menizibeya, 2011).

Health workers have regularly protested and gone on strike because of these problems. Since protests aggravate the problem of health care delivery in Nigeria, and elsewhere, lessons learned from the handling of the Ebola disease epidemic should be used to transform the health sector in Nigeria. During the outbreak of epidemics, efforts should be intensified to ensure the protection of health workers from hazards. This also applies to other African countries.

The following strategies can help improve the performance of the public health care system. First, government expenditure on health care services delivery should be increased. This will make it possible for medical facilities to be improved in public hospitals, and health workers to be adequately remunerated. The current public expenditure on health care services delivery in Nigeria is grossly below international standards. Based on the report of the World Health Organization (2014) the proportion of total GDP spent on health care in Nigeria is low in comparison with countries that have highly effective systems. Second, a social welfare system should be introduced to assist poor families who cannot pay medical bills in public hospitals. This is important because the out-of-pocket financing of health care expenses leads to problems such as reduction of expenditure on food, debt burden, preventing a sick person from seeking medical care in public hospitals, and encouraging the use of traditional medicine over, on occasion, clinically proven pharmaceutical alternatives. Third, definitive efforts need to be made to fight corruption in the health sector. Corruption contributes to problems such as a reduction in resources required for improving the performance of the health sector, lowering the overall quality of health care services (Umukoro, 2012).

REFERENCES

Abubakar, M., Anuforo, E. & Muanya, C. 20 October 2014. 'Nigeria now free of Ebola transmission, says WHO'. AllAfrica.com. http://allafrica.com/stories/201410210434.html, accessed 10 November 2017.

Adewole, I. 20 May 2017. 'Even if Ebola starts from Zamfara State, we're prepared'. *Punch,* http://punchng.com/even-if-ebola-starts-from-zamfara-state-were-prepared-prof-adewole-health-minister/, accessed 30 January 2017.

Baseler, L., Daniel S., Chertow, D. S., Johnson, K. M., Feldmann, H. & Morens, D. M. 2017. 'The pathogenesis of Ebola Virus Disease'. *Annual Review of Pathology: Mechanisms of Disease*, 12, 387–418.

Bureau of Public Services Reforms. November 2015. 'How Nigeria contained Ebola: Lessons for institutional reforms', bpsr.gov.ng/index.php/publications/bpsr-resources/evaluations, accessed 2 December 2017.

Chicago Convention/Convention on International Civil Aviation. 1944. https://www.icao.int/publications/pages/doc7300.aspx, accessed 6 December 2018.

Duric, P. & Ilic, S. 2012. 'Participation of infectious disease surveillance in primary health care'. *Sri Lanka Journal of Infectious Diseases*, 2 (2), 37–46.

Fatiregun, A. A. & Isere, E. E. 2017. 'Epidemic preparedness and management: A guide on Lassa fever outbreak preparedness plan'. *Niger Medical Journal*, 58 (1), 1–6, DOI: 10.4103/0300-1652.218414.

Federal Government of Nigeria. 2014. 'Standard operating procedures for contact tracing and follow up during Ebola Virus Disease outbreak'. http://ebolaalert.org/wp-content/themes/ebolaalert/assets/PDFS/SOPct.pdf, accessed 18 February 2015.

Khalid, K. 14 November 2014. 'Why travel bans will not stop the spread of Ebola'. World Economic Forum, https://www.weforum.org/agenda/2014/11/why-travel-bans-will-not-stop-the-spread-of-ebola/, accessed 31 January 2018.

Maxmen, A. 2015. 'How the fight against Ebola tested a culture's traditions'. *National Geographic,* https://news.nationalgeographic.com/2015/01/150130-ebola-virus-outbreak-epidemic-sierra-leone-funerals/, accessed 2 December 2017.

Menizibeya, O. W. 2011. 'The Nigerian health care system: Need for integrating adequate medical intelligence and surveillance systems'. *Journal of Pharmacy and BioAllied Sciences*, 3 (4), 470–478.

Musbau, R. 5 July 2017. 'Lagos and equitable health care services'. Lagos State Government, https://lagosstate.gov.ng/blog/2017/07/05/lagos-and-equitable-healthcare-services/, accessed 2 December 2018.

News Agency of Nigeria. 9 August 2014. 'Jonathan declares national emergency on Ebola: Approves N1.98 billion special intervention fund'. *Bella Naija,* https://www.bellanaija.com/2014/08/jonathan-declares-national-emergency-on-ebola-approves-n1-98-billion-special-intervention-fund/, accessed 31 January 2018.

Odiogor, H. 2 October 2014. 'US Sends medical experts to study how Nigeria tamed Ebola'. *Vanguard Media,* www.vanguardngr.com/2014/10/us-sends-medical-experts-study-nigeria-tamed-ebola, accessed 1 November 2014.

Ogundipe, S. & Obinna, C. 19 December 2017. 'After containing Ebola, Nigeria not prepared for disease epidemics'. *Vanguard Media.* https://www.vanguardngr.com/2017/12/containing-ebola-nigeria-not-prepared-disease-epidemics/, accessed 30 December 2017.

Osafo-Kwako, P. & Apampa, S. 2009. *Nigeria: Country Assessment Research Background Paper on the Political Economy of the Budget Process*. London: Centre for the Study of the Economies of Africa.

Otsuki S. & Nishiura H. 2016. 'Reduced risk of importing Ebola Virus Disease because of travel restrictions in 2014: A retrospective epidemiological modeling study'. *PLoS ONE*, 11 (9), DOI: e0163418. https://doi.org/10.1371/journal.pone.0163418, accessed 2 September 2017.

Otu, A., Ameh, S., Osifo-Dawodu, E., Alade, E., Ekuri, S. & Idris, J. 2018. 'An account of the Ebola virus disease outbreak in Nigeria: Implications and lessons learnt'. *BMC Public Health*, 18 (1),3. DOI: 10.1186/s12889-017-4535-x.

Poletto C., Gomes, M. F., Pastore y Piontti, A., Rossi, L., Bioglio, L., Chao, D. L., Longini Jr, M., Halloran, M. E., Colizza, V., & Vespignani, A. 2014. 'Assessing the impact of travel restrictions on international spread of the 2014 West African Ebola epidemic'. *Euro Surveillance*, 19 (42), p.e. 43.

Shuaib, F., Gunnala, R., Musa, E. O., Mahoney, F. J., Oguntimehin, O., Nguku, P. M., Nyanti, S. B., Knight, N., Gwarzo. N. S., Idigbe, O., Nasidi, A., Vertefeuille, J. F. 2014. 'Ebola virus disease outbreak – Nigeria'. *Morbidity and Mortality Weekly Report*, 63 (39), 867–872.

Ugwuanyi, S. 19 August 2014. 'Ebola: Federal Government inaugurates hand washing campaign'. *The Daily Post,* dailypost.ng/2014/08/19/ebola-fg-inaugurates-hand-washing-campaign, accessed 2 August 2018.

Umukoro, N. 2016. 'African solution to African problems and the Ebola Virus Disease in Nigeria'. *Development in Practice*, 26 (2), 149–157.

Umukoro, N. 2012. 'Governance and public health care in Nigeria'. *Journal of Health Management,* 14 (4), 381–395.

Vaz, R. G., Mkanda, P., Banda, R., Komkech, W., Olubowale, O. et al. 2016. 'The role of the polio program infrastructure in response to Ebola Virus Disease outbreak in Nigeria 2014'. *The Journal of Infectious Diseases*, 213 (Issue suppl_3), 140–146.

World Health Organization (WHO). 2014. Contact Tracing during an Outbreak of Ebola Virus Disease. Brazzaville: World Health Organization Regional Office for Africa. Geneva: World Health Organization.

World Health Organization (WHO). 12 February 2018. 'Ebola virus disease'. http://www.who.int/news-room/fact-sheets/detail/ebola-virus-disease, accessed 2 December 2018.

Section Three

Contending with Chronic Conditions in African Health Systems

The thread that runs through this section is how health systems deal with chronic conditions like non-communicable diseases (NCDs) and HIV/AIDS, and it highlights the centrality of the network of health care workers involved in delivering care. NCDs, which have previously been thought to affect high-income countries predominantly, have become more prominent in sub-Saharan Africa. Pamela Juma, Gerald Yonga, and Kenneth Juma write on the burden of NCDs in sub-Saharan Africa, citing cardiovascular diseases, diabetes, cancer, and chronic respiratory illnesses as being responsible for the greatest of burdens. The increase in unhealthy diets, higher rates of physical inactivity, increased consumption of alcohol, and addiction to tobacco all contribute to the NCD epidemic. Again, the concept of syndemics helps with understanding how socio-economic issues such as poverty and inequality, as well as environmental factors, have contributed to the increase in the prevalence of NCDs. Juma and co-authors write of the neglect of NCDs in health systems amidst the prioritisation of infectious diseases. This neglect has implications for the quality of care for chronic patients in the health system and the overall preparedness of the health system to address the NCD epidemic. The chapter also explores policy interventions that have been implemented to target major risk factors for NCDs.

Due to the widespread availability of antiretroviral treatments, HIV has shifted from being an epidemic to a chronic illness with similar care implications as other chronic conditions. Beth Vale's chapter, which draws on the care experiences of HIV-positive adolescents living in the Eastern Cape, South Africa, argues that there is an urgent need to explore practices and prospects for NCD care in African contexts. There is not enough research on how care can be best administered to chronic patients in overly burdened and under-resourced health systems in Africa. Vale thus argues that lessons can be drawn from the experiences of HIV patients who must go to great lengths to receive care.

The section ends with the chapter by Miriam Di Paola and Beth Vale. They present an analysis of the role of nurses and community health workers (CHWs) as frontline health workers in epidemics preparedness. The chapter argues for the recognition of the importance of health workers in both emergency epidemic responses and in attending to chronic patients. There are more nurses and CHWs than doctors in Africa's health workforce and thus often patients' first and primary point of health system contact is with nurses or CHWs. Di Paola and Vale argue that Africa's epidemic preparedness relies on retaining frontline health workers and empowering them to perform at their best. The authors provide systematic factors that are a barrier to health workers providing high-quality patient care, including the 'new public management', which prioritises cost-cutting and administrative tasks at the expense of the caregiver-patient relationship. This third section explores the burden that health systems in Africa carry – and the far-reaching implications this burden has – for providing care to chronic patients amidst the prevalence or threat of epidemics.

SIX

Non-Communicable Disease Epidemics

Approaches to Prevention and Control in Sub-Saharan Africa

Pamela A. Juma, Kenneth Juma, and Gerald Yonga

INTRODUCTION

Non-communicable diseases (NCDs) and their risk factors are on the increase globally. It is estimated that NCDs accounted for 72 per cent of mortality globally in 2016, with 80 per cent of these NCD deaths occurring in low- and middle-income countries (LMICs) (WHO, 2013; Forouzanfar et al., 2015). Four out of a large range of NCDs – cardiovascular diseases, diabetes, cancers, and chronic respiratory illnesses – have been identified as being responsible for the greatest share of the burden (WHO, 2013). These four diseases (or disease groups) also share a set of four risk factors, namely tobacco use, unhealthy diet, harmful alcohol consumption, and physical inactivity.

Africa has experienced the highest rate of increase of NCD-related mortality compared to the rest of the world (a 27 per cent increase between 2006 and 2015). Consistent with this trend, the WHO projects that in the decade from 2008 to 2018, the largest increase in deaths from cardiovascular disease (CVD), cancer, respiratory disease, and diabetes will occur in developing countries (WHO, 2004). In addition to the four major NCDs, Africa has a high prevalence of other conditions, such as sickle cell disease, for example, injuries and trauma, as well as mental illness.

Furthermore, the rise in NCD mortality is greatest in sub-Saharan Africa (SSA), where, by 2020, it is estimated that NCDs will account for 27 per cent of mortality, up from 23 per cent in 2000 (WHO, 2016). The impact of NCDs in African countries that are still struggling with communicable diseases is significant (infectious diseases such as malaria, HIV, and tuberculosis remain a significant burden). Addressing NCDs in these countries requires effective multisectoral policies, targeting both the main NCD risk factors and health system interventions, particularly at primary care levels, to facilitate early detection and treatment of individuals at risk and patients with chronic conditions.

A body of evidence attributes the rising burden of NCDs to factors such as globalisation, rapid and often unplanned urbanisation, which changes lifestyles (Khanal et al., 2015), and to the ageing of populations. Other factors, including international trade and urban poverty, have also contributed to shifts towards lifestyles that encompass higher consumption of unhealthy diets, higher rates of physical inactivity, the increased use of tobacco, and the consumption of alcohol – all of which contribute to the NCD epidemic.

The combined health and economic impact of NCDs in African countries is enormous. The linkages between NCDs and socio-economic development, environmental sustainability, and poverty alleviation can all be recognised (Beaglehole et al., 2011). Apart from the extreme health disabilities exerted by NCDs on patients, a range of economic losses can be seen as a result, from reduced productivity to the diversion of resources to the management of these conditions (Dalal et al., 2011; Nyirenda, 2016). Costs that families and individuals incur when it comes to seeking NCD treatment will be considerable as these conditions require long-term attention, and for the most part these costs are borne directly by patients through out-of-pocket (OOP) payments. Affected people seek health care services from health systems that are already over-strained, with the complications of unmanaged NCDs placing an even greater burden on the health system.

African health care systems, where the focus is predominantly on curative clinical services, are not well prepared when it comes to dealing with NCDs. On top of this the quality of care is also not guaranteed, given the multiple challenges these systems generally have to contend with: inadequate financing, poor infrastructure, inadequately trained and poorly motivated health care providers, and the unavailability and poor affordability of NCD medicines, including those on the WHO List of Essential Medicines (Robinson & Hort, 2012).

Health promotion has been advocated as an important vehicle to reorientate investment in health so that health systems are not only more effective but also sustainable (Demaio et al., 2014). In the context of NCDs, cases of health promotion targeted at behavioural risk factors are the most cost-effective interventions for prevention and control; they constitute a significant number of the WHO 'best buys'. Such cases of health promotion can be achieved at community level through well-coordinated multisectoral action. There is, however, a more urgent need if the rising NCD epidemic is to be curtailed and reduced. This is the need to strengthen systems at the primary health care level. Most of the reorientation efforts in primary health care have focused only on communicable diseases (such as HIV, TB, and malaria) and maternal and child health. Little attention is given to non-communicable diseases.

It is in this context that this chapter analyses the approaches to NCD prevention and control in selected sub-Saharan African countries. The authors draw insights from relevant literature, including WHO documents and additional literature from select African countries on mechanisms applied to address NCD prevention. We further synthesise qualitative data and reports from two major studies conducted by the authors to analyse NCD interventions in selected African countries. One study was implemented from 2014 to 2016 and focused on five African countries (Kenya, South Africa, Malawi, Cameroon, and Nigeria) (Juma et al., 2016). Another review focused on NCD actions in East African countries, including Kenya, Uganda, Tanzania, and Rwanda (Juma, 2018). Both studies examined the extent to which the countries were implementing the global NCD commitments. The studies highlighted the extent of implementation of NCD-prevention approaches in these low-resourced settings, and also identified important lessons learned in the process. Some of these lessons emphasised the need to enhance multisectoral coordination, the need for better strategies to reinforce the policies and enhance implementation, and the need for strategies to enhance monitoring and evaluation of NCD prevention and control actions. The chapter concludes by highlighting possible challenges to the implementation of policy interventions for NCD prevention in Africa.

TRENDS OF NCDS IN AFRICA

From 2000 to 2016, NCD-related deaths increased from 23 per cent (2.2 million) to 34 per cent (3.0 million) of total deaths in Africa (WHO, 2016). During the same period, the total NCD burden expressed in disability-adjusted life years (DALYs) increased by 35 per cent (Forouzanfar et al., 2015). While deaths were reported from across all NCD groups, CVDs (including rheumatic heart diseases (RHDs), ischemic heart diseases (IHDs), hypertensive heart disorders, and stroke) were the greatest contributors. CVD deaths in Africa experienced the greatest increase between 2000 and 2016 (8.9 to 13 per cent). Cancers (mainly breast, cervical, and prostate cancers) were the second most prevalent cause of death from NCDs (at 6 per cent) in 2016; this was up from 3.8 per cent in 2000. Tragically, survival from cancer in sub-Saharan Africa is lower than in the rest of the world. For many cancers, the risk in sub-Saharan Africa of getting cancer and dying from cancer are nearly the same (Sankaranarayanan & Swaminathan, 2011). Chronic respiratory diseases and diabetes are each responsible for about 2 per cent of total deaths in sub-Saharan Africa (see Table 1).

Table 1: Trends in NCD burden in the WHO Africa Region (2000–2016)

	% of total deaths (2000–2016)			
Year	2000	2010	2015	2016
Non-communicable diseases	22.8	28.9	33.2	34.2
Cardiovascular diseases (RHD, IHD, hypertensive heart disorders, stroke, and others)	8.9	11.1	12.6	13.0
Malignant neoplasms (breast, prostrate, cervical, liver, colon and rectum, and esophagus cancers and, others)	3.8	4.9	5.7	5.9
Diabetes mellitus	1.0	1.5	1.8	1.9
Mental and substance use disorders	0.2	0.2	0.3	0.3
Respiratory diseases (COPD, asthma, and other respiratory diseases)	1.5	1.8	2.0	2.1

Source: WHO, Disease burden and mortality estimates, 2000–2016
Abbreviations: RHD: Rheumatic heart disease, IHD: ischemic heart disease, COPD: Chronic obstructive pulmonary disease

Notably, key NCD risk factors have also been shown to be rising in Africa. Among the top ten risk factors for death, as reported in the global burden of studies (see WHO, 2018), are high blood pressure, poor diet, air pollution, high body mass index, tobacco smoking, alcohol and drug use, high fasting plasma glucose, high total cholesterol, and low physical activity. These are the same risks responsible for NCDs (Forouzanfar et al., 2015). Various African countries that have conducted NCD STEP surveys for risk factors have reported high, and rising, prevalence of these leading risk factors, especially for overweight and obesity, high blood pressure, physical inactivity, and smoking (Msyamboza et al., 2011; Kavishe et al., 2015; MoH-Kenya, 2015).

Most importantly, the significant rise in NCDs' morbidity and mortality in Africa threatens the important milestones attained in health and development over the last three decades. Projections by the WHO (in 2008 for the period 2008–2030) show that in the approximate decade to 2030, NCD-associated DALYs will surpass those contributed by infectious diseases, perinatal and maternal conditions combined (see Figure 1).

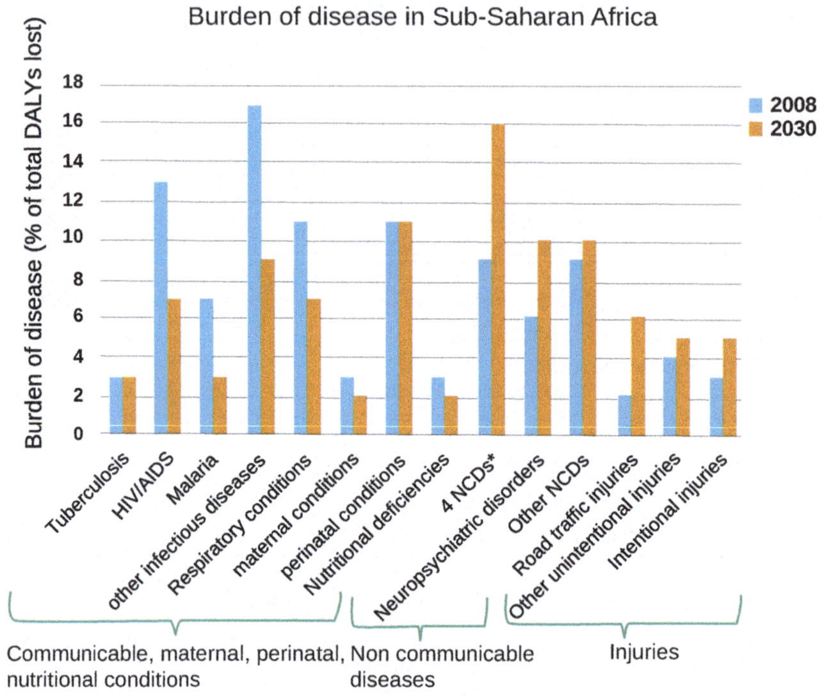

Figure 1: Projected burden of disease in SSA, 2008 and 2030

Source: World Health Organization, 2004
NCDs: Cardiovascular diseases, cancer, diabetes, chronic respiratory diseases

GLOBAL NCD POLICY CONTEXT

The United Nations' Political Declaration on the Prevention and Control of NCDs (resolution A/RES/66/2), followed by the 66th World Health Assembly endorsement of the WHO Global Action Plan for the Prevention and Control of NCDs 2013–2020, marked the beginning of active global level action to address NCDs (see WHO, 2017). The WHO Global NCD Action Plan has six priority areas: (1) raising NCD priority through international cooperation and advocacy; (2) strengthening national capacity, multisectoral action, and partnerships for NCDs; (3) reducing NCD risk factors and social determinants; (4) strengthening and reorientation of health systems; (5) promoting national capacity for research and development; (6) monitoring and evaluating progress on

NCDs (WHO, 2013). The Action Plan emphasises the need for member countries to embrace multisectoral action in policy development and implementation. Governments across the sub-Saharan African region have endorsed the WHO Global Action Plan for the Prevention and Control of NCDs. They have also committed themselves to setting national NCD targets that are in line with global targets, and to embedding multisectoral action in developing and implementing their national NCD action plans.

Policy interventions to target the major risk factors stand tall among the approaches to NCD prevention. Other interventions aim at strengthening health promotion and service delivery at the level of health systems interventions (Robinson & Hort, 2012).Deaths from cardiovascular disease, cancer, chronic respiratory disease and diabetes accounted for 63 per cent of global mortality in 2008, of which 80 per cent was in LMICs. The NCD burden is projected to increase: by 2030, NCDs will be the greatest killer in all LMICs. Thus, governments of these countries cannot afford to overlook policies in relation to NCDs. Several cost-effective measures exist to prevent and control NCDs. These include both population-wide interventions such as tobacco control and targeted treatment for individuals at high risk. Experience from high-income countries that have been able to control NCDs shows that responses must be comprehensive and multisectoral, integrating health promotion, prevention and treatment strategies, and involving the community as well as the health sector. Such a multifaceted approach requires well-functioning health systems. In the majority of LMICs, however, health systems are fragile and will need to be adapted to address NCDs appropriately, while also continuing to tackle communicable diseases. We propose that the reform of health systems can occur in a four-phased approach in four areas: building political commitment and addressing health systems constraints, developing public policies in health promotion and disease prevention, creating new service delivery models and ensuring equity in access and payments. Several policy issues will also need to be addressed, including financing of NCD programmes and the broadening of concepts of health and responsibilities for health. Adapting health systems to respond to NCDs will require a change in mindset and practices in programming for health, as well as substantial financial resources. There is scope for development partners and global health initiatives to support LMICs in addressing NCDs. (Robinson and Hort, 2012). WHO identifies a set of evidence-based interventions that are highly cost effective, feasible, and appropriate to implement within the constraints of the local LMIC health systems. The interventions are known as 'best buy' interventions (WHO, 2013). These interventions exist to reduce the burden of chronic NCDs at the population level by targeting the shared risk factors. The 'best buy' initiatives include raising tax on tobacco and alcohol products, reducing access to and enforcing bans on tobacco and alcohol advertising, reducing salt consumption, eliminating trans-fats in the food supply chain (WHO, 2013), promoting physical activity, and projects to detect and treat NCDs at an early stage. Projections have shown that in 23 LMICs, 5.5 million deaths could be averted over ten years from a 30 per cent relative reduction in tobacco use alone by 2025. This level of reduction will reduce the burden of cardiovascular disease within one year from onset, and will dramatically cut health expenditures (Beaglehole et al., 2011; Maher et al., 2012). Similarly, lowering population salt consumption by only 15 per cent would avert 8.5 million deaths in those countries by lowering the impact of hypertension on cardiovascular disease. Promoting healthy diets and encouraging physical activity would impact obesity and diabetes. Providing multi-drug combinations to those at risk for cardiovascular events or those people who have experienced a cardiovascular event would reduce deaths over ten years by 18 million and cost no more than USD 1.08 per person per year (Beaglehole et al., 2011).

Further global policy efforts are geared towards achieving the global development goals. Unlike the Millennium Development Goals (MDGs), which covered 2000–2015 and paid less attention to NCDs, the Sustainable Development Goals (SDGs), which cover 2015–2030, have several NCD-related targets. Linked to these targets, WHO has developed a global monitoring framework to enable the global tracking of progress in preventing and controlling major NCDs and their key risk factors (WHO, 2013). The framework is expected to drive progress in prevention and control of NCDs and provide the foundation for advocacy, raising awareness, reinforcing political commitment, and promoting global action to tackle these deadly diseases. The framework is intended to shape a new development agenda which advances the three dimensions of sustainable development: economic development, environmental sustainability, and social inclusion. The framework comprises nine global NCD targets and 25 indicators for countries to adopt. Other than the WHO global action plan, other policy interventions targeting the major risk factors have been available to help guide countries in developing their own prevention strategies (as elaborated in, for example, Msyamboza et al., 2011; Kavishe et al., 2015; MoH Kenya, 2015).

IMPLEMENTATION OF NCD PREVENTION AND CONTROL INTERVENTIONS IN THE SELECTED COUNTRIES

Most of the current NCD prevention and control interventions focus on addressing the major risk factors and strengthening health systems to enhance service delivery for those who live with NCDs. This section assesses the extent to which the selected sub-Saharan African countries are implementing interventions to address tobacco control, control of harmful alcohol consumption, unhealthy diets, and physical inactivity. Other interventions, like health system strengthening, as well as improvement in governance and multisectoral action for NCDs, are also highlighted.

Tobacco control interventions

Tobacco use is associated closely with several types of cancers, as well as with the risk for cardiovascular disease and diabetes (Bump & Reich, 2013) claiming over 5 million lives annually, and this toll is rising. Even though effective tobacco control policies are well researched and widely disseminated, they remain largely unimplemented in most low- and middle-income countries (LMICs). Tobacco policy development and implementation in most countries has been influenced by the WHO Framework Convention on Tobacco Control (FCTC) developed in 2003 (WHO, 2003). The objective of the framework was to protect present and future generations from the devastating health, social, environmental, and economic consequences of tobacco consumption and exposure to tobacco smoke. Recommended tobacco control interventions include tax increases, smoke-free indoor workplaces and public places, bans on tobacco advertising, promotion and sponsorship, as well as health information and warnings (WHO, 2013). These measures are aimed at reducing tobacco consumption and hence the occurrence of NCDs.

Many African countries have ratified and developed tobacco legislation that is compliant with the FCTC. Kenya, Nigeria, South Africa, and Uganda all have tobacco legislation which addresses most of the WHO's 'best buy' interventions for tobacco control (Juma et al., 2017; Juma, 2018). Rwanda and Cameroon do not have comprehensive tobacco policies but tobacco control elements have been addressed through ministerial orders and circulars published by the government. Due mainly to economic reasons, neither Tanzania nor Malawi currently have developed comprehensive tobacco control policies which address the 'best buy' interventions. Malawi generates a high percentage of its revenue from tobacco exports and so the government's concern has been that controlling tobacco production and usage will reduce the general revenue. Some countries do have tobacco laws in place, but have not adequately implemented the recommended actions. For instance, WHO recommended tobacco excise tax to be 75 per cent of the retail price of the tobacco. By 2015, South Africa had the highest percentage (52 per cent), Kenya was at 35 per cent, Cameroon at 34.6, and Nigeria at 20.63 per cent (Juma et al., 2017; Juma, 2018). Table 2 shows the implementation of other elements.

Table 2: Tobacco control across eight African countries, 2014–2017

Interventions 2014–2017	Cameroon	Kenya	Malawi	Nigeria	Rwanda	South Africa	Tanzania	Uganda
Tobacco legislation	√	√	X	X	√	√	X	√
Pack labelling and pictorial health warnings	Partial	√	Partial	X	√	√	X	√
Tobacco taxation policy	√	Partial	Partial	X	Partial	√	X	X
Smoke-free public policy	Partial	√	X	√	X	√	X	√

Interventions 2014–2017	Cameroon	Kenya	Malawi	Nigeria	Rwanda	South Africa	Tanzania	Uganda
Bans on tobacco advertising and sponsorship	Partial	√	X	X	X	√	X	√

Sources: Juma, 2018; Juma et al., 2017

Case Study: Tobacco control in Kenya (see Juma et al., 2017)

Kenya developed a comprehensive tobacco policy in 2007. The Tobacco Control Act restricts smoking in public places, prohibits tobacco advertisement, promotion and sponsorship, requires health warnings and messages on tobacco products, and recommends raising tobacco excise taxes to 70 per cent of retail prices. Some of the interventions have been implemented, although others still require re-enforcement. There have been tax regimen changes since the 2007 act came into effect. Recently, the Finance Act raised the excise duty on tobacco products at a rate of KSH 1,200 per 1,000 (or 35 per cent of the retail selling price), although it is still lower than the WHO tax recommendation of 70 per cent. Bans on tobacco advertising and sponsorship of tobacco products have largely been implemented, but there are still some gaps. Outdoor advertising on billboards and buildings, for example, still occurs in several parts of the country. Health information and warnings on tobacco packaging have been implemented. These texts now cover 30–50 per cent of the front and back display of tobacco product packages. Although there are periodic television advertisements on the harmful effects of tobacco and the need to avoid its use, these are not very frequent and are not aired across many TV and radio stations. The government has also undertaken the training of enforcement officers, and media and civil society organisations are encouraged to support the implementation efforts. Increasing awareness due to the training has led to the removal in major cities of billboards with tobacco brand advertisements. The tobacco industry has tried to interfere with the implementation of some elements of the act through court cases. The areas of concern have been mainly around taxation methods (differential taxation), the size of warning labelling on packets, and consumptions of non-cigarette products such as shisha and others. Kenya's tobacco policies have contributed to demand reduction, supply reduction, awareness creation, prohibition of illicit trade, taxation charges for tobacco products, creation of smoke-free environments, and a total ban on smoking in public areas. The main challenges to be addressed include industry interference, financing for implementation at decentralised levels, and coordination of stakeholders for implementation at decentralised levels.

Alcohol control

High alcohol consumption is linked to cancer, cardiovascular disease, and liver disease. Recommended WHO 'best buy' interventions to reduce alcohol consumption include tax increases, bans on alcohol advertising, and restricted access to retailed alcohol (WHO, 2013). The WHO global strategy to reduce harmful alcohol consumption was initiated in 2008 and endorsed in May 2010 at the World Health Assembly (WHO, 2010). All member states were urged to take appropriate action in their respective jurisdictions towards reducing the harmful use of alcohol. In September 2010 African health ministers endorsed the Regional Strategy to reduce harmful use of alcohol in the African region, which takes into account the specificities of the region, such as the need to address illegal and informal alcohol production, as well as laying emphasis on integrated approaches to prevention and treatment.

Unlike tobacco, where the majority of countries have developed legislation, many countries in sub-Saharan Africa remain slow in developing alcohol control policies and programmess. By 2017, only Kenya, South Africa, and Malawi had developed comprehensive alcohol control policies which addressed the WHO 'best buy' interventions for alcohol (Juma et al., 2017); others, like Tanzania, Nigeria, and Uganda, had only developed draft policies that were yet to be completed (Table 3). These countries had put in place certain measures, including a minimum age (18) for the purchase and consumption of alcohol, retailers requiring a licence to sell alcohol, and a drink drive law (which was not well enforced). Some countries – Cameroon, for example – had no comprehensive alcohol policy document, but instead had different regulations; included in these were restrictions on alcohol access, increased tax on alcohol, and restrictions on alcohol advertising (Table 3).

Table 3: Alcohol control across eight African countries

Elements	**Cameroon**	**Kenya**	**Malawi**	**Nigeria**	**South Africa**	**Rwanda**	**Tanzania**	**Uganda**
Comprehensive alcohol control legislation	X	√	√	X	Partial	√	X	X
Special tax on alcohol	√	√	Partial	X	√	X	-	X
Taxation for domestic brew	X	X	X	X	X		X	X
Restriction on alcohol advertising	X	Partial	X	X	√	X	-	X
Restrictions on times at which alcohol can be purchased	Partial	√	√	X	√	X	X	X
Licensing system for retailers	Partial	√	√	X	√	√	√	√
National drink driving law	X	√	X	X	√	√	√	√
Established minimum age for purchase and consumption	√	√	√	√	√	√	√	√

Sources: Juma, 2018; Juma et al., 2017

Case Study: Alcohol Control in Kenya (see Juma et al., 2017)

Kenya has the Alcoholic Drinks Control Act (ADCA) 2010, amended in 2014. The Act addresses the WHO 'best buy' interventions for the control of harmful alcohol consumption such as taxation, bans on alcohol advertising, and restricted access. Although the specific figures for taxation were not provided, the annual increase in taxes on beer and spirits in the past few years has been slow. There is a decline in the producers and importers of alcohol sponsoring events like sports tournaments and music concerts. Alcohol advertising in media is restricted; adverts can only be aired from 8.30 pm on TV and from 2 pm on radio to reduce exposure to young people. Restriction has been made on the sale of alcohol to children under the age of 18 years. Restricted access is also being achieved through the regulation of bar opening hours. The legislation restricts the sale of alcohol in bars to between 5 pm and 11 pm. Alcohol is also sold in separate sections of shops and supermarkets where children are not allowed to enter. Alcohol from supermarkets or retail outlets is only sold within certain daytime hours. Issuing of licences to alcohol sellers is ongoing. With the implementation of devolution the alcohol licensing role was transferred to the county governments, which are now responsible for issuing licences to alcohol dealers, including manufacturers, wholesalers, and retailers. Drink driving policy exists but is only being implemented in big cities like Nairobi. Further implementation involves campaigns and education aimed at the public, warning them about the effects of drugs and alcohol. Some NGOs have been organising public education activities, including campaigns targeting the youth, in partnership with the ministries of Health and Education. A significant proportion of the Kenyan population consumes local brews, which do not lend themselves to regulation or taxation. The regulation of these drinks is vested in other trade and criminal laws but they are not adequately enforced. Even though the alcohol policy is in place, the implementation of various aspects remains inadequate and requires better coordination and enforcement at all levels.

Nutrition and diet

With regard to nutrition and diet, initial global advocacies led to the development of food and nutrition security policies. The push for food and nutrition policies was also largely influenced by the need to achieve the MDGs. The WHO Global Strategy on Diet, Physical Activity and Health was developed in 2004 (WHO, 2004). In the document, recommendations for individuals included: achieve energy balance and a healthy weight; limit energy intake from total fats; shift fat consumption away from saturated fats to unsaturated fats and towards the elimination of trans-fatty acids; increase consumption of fruit, vegetables, legumes, whole grains, and nuts; limit the intake of free sugars; limit salt consumption from all sources and ensure that salt is iodised. WHO 'best buy' interventions for nutrition and diet include addressing salt reduction and replacement of trans-fat with polyunsaturated fat, and public awareness on what constitutes a healthy diet (WHO, 2013).

From 2007 to 2016 many African countries, among them Kenya, Rwanda, Cameroon, Malawi, and South Africa, developed food and nutrition security policies (Juma, et al 2017; Juma, 2018). These policies tended to be broad and their focus was on food production rather than on nutrition. Countries like Kenya, Tanzania, Uganda, and Malawi have health sector nutrition action plans but for the most part these address undernutrition, especially among children under five years of age. There have been attempts to put strategies in place to increase fruit and vegetable consumption as dietary action for NCD prevention, but primarily these strategies are intended to address prevailing micronutrient deficiencies such as vitamin A deficiency. Fruit and vegetable interventions have been taken up in LMICs, but also primarily to address prevailing micronutrient deficiencies.

Table 4: Unhealthy diet across eight African countries

Elements	Cameroon	Kenya	Malawi	Nigeria	Rwanda	Tanzania	South Africa	Uganda
National food and nutrition security policy	√	√	√	√	√	X	√	√
Nutrition strategy/action plan	X	√	√	X	√	√	√	√
Overweight/ obesity/diet-related NCDs included in nutrition plan				-	X	√		X
Taxation of unhealthy food/ beverages	X	X	X	X	X	X	Partial	X
Implementation of subsidies to incentivise healthy food consumption	X	X	X	X	X	X	Partial	X
National food-based guideline	X	X	X		X	X	Partial	√
School food policies						X		√
Reformulation targets	X	√			X	-		X
Salt reduction legislation	X	X			X	X		X
Policy to replace trans-fat with polyunsaturated fat	X	X	X	X	X	X	X	X
Public awareness about healthy diet promotion – via mass media	X	Partial	Partial	X	√	√ Once a month	Partial	X

Sources: Juma, 2018; Juma et al., 2017

Nutrition policies addressing over-nutrition, salt, sugar, and fat reduction in the context of NCDs have not been developed in these countries. Some countries have developed nutrition guidelines for prevention and management of dietary related non-communicable diseases. South Africa is the only country in sub-Saharan Africa where there is legislation for salt reduction in processed foods; this was passed in 2013. The salt reduction policy targets industries involved in the packaging of processed foods.

Case study: Salt reduction interventions in South Africa (see Juma et al., 2017)

South Africa passed salt reduction legislation in 2013 as a measure to prevent NCDs caused by unhealthy diets, particularly those attributed to high salt intake like hypertension, heart attacks, and vascular dementia. The overall objective of the policy is to reduce sodium levels in 13 processed categories of foodstuffs identified in the policy. This reduction comes in two phases, with the first phase being implemented in 2016 and the second phase in 2019. For example, it is stipulated in the act that salt levels in bread should be reduced to 400 mg Na by 30 June 2016 and to 380 mg Na by 30 June 2019; this is important because the indicators and measurables are very clear, which makes for effective monitoring and evaluation. The policy stipulates the maximum amount of sodium that each type of foodstuff may contain per 100 grams. The listed maximum grams of salt are a reduction from what has previously been used in the specified foodstuffs. Baseline data before the implementation of the policy was generated to monitor and evaluate the reductions over time and establish the impact of the salt reduction legislation. To understand the impact of salt intake and how its reduction in the diet would require behaviour change the Department of Health (DoH) convened a multisectoral stakeholder group reflective of the social, economic, health, and political contexts. The group comprised producer groups, consumer groups, retailers and trade association, and scientists. Furthermore, drawing from best practices in preventing and controlling NCDs related to unhealthy diets, the South African government drafted a policy on taxation of sweetened sugary drinks; it began taxing sweetened sugary drinks in April 2017. The main gap in this intervention is that while food manufacturing industries are targeted, interventions targeting awareness creation among the population are less robust.

Physical activity

Physical inactivity is among the major causes of mortality globally and a risk factor for NCDs such as cancer, diabetes, and cardiovascular diseases (WHO, 2013). WHO recommends at least 30 minutes of regular, moderate-intensity physical activity on most days throughout a person's life. In addition it is recommended that countries should enhance public education and awareness about physical activities and put in place measures to enable the public to engage in physical activities, such as providing conducive built environments (WHO, 2004).

Most of the African countries under review have not developed physical activity policies. Most have sports policies that promote sports for competition but do not address physical activity in relation to NCD prevention. In some countries, like Kenya, Tanzania, South Africa, and Uganda, physical activity is reinforced in schools through the inclusion of physical education in the school curriculum. South Africa also has a strategy to promote physical activity among the elderly to include awareness creation.

Table 5: Physical activity across eight African countries

Elements	**Cameroon**	**Kenya**	**Malawi**	**Nigeria**	**Rwanda**	**Tanzania**	**South Africa**	**Uganda**
National physical activity policy/ strategy	X	X	X	X	√	√	Partial	X

Elements	Cameroon	Kenya	Malawi	Nigeria	Rwanda	Tanzania	South Africa	Uganda
Provision for physical education in schools	√	√	√	√	√	√	√	√
Promotion of public awareness about physical activity (via mass media)	√	X	X	X	√	√	X	X
Workplace physical activity policy	X	X	X	X	X	X	X	X

Sources: Juma, 2018; Juma et al., 2017

A few other government policies like the NCD strategic plans in these countries mention the need for physical activity but do not provide comprehensive guidance on how to ensure that the public engages in physical activity. Cameroon has no comprehensive physical activity policy but has enhanced public awareness for physical exercises in open space in the cities. Tanzania is also conducting health promotion activities; these includes public sensitisation on physical activity through the media. Even though Rwanda has no written comprehensive physical activity policies, the country is a good example in the region: certain days are set aside for physical activity and the population is encouraged to participate.

Case study: Physical activity and health promotion in Rwanda (see Juma, 2018)

Since 2013, the government of Rwanda, with different partners, has been implementing various activities to increase awareness of physical activity and other interventions to prevent NCDs. To encourage physical activities, by order of the prime minister all public servants engage in sports every Friday afternoon and gym fees are paid for them. Rwanda has a car-free day every first Sunday of the month, when Kigali citizens are involved in walking and other sports activities; at these events people are screened for NCDs for free. With support from organisations such as the Rwanda Diabetic Association, the Rwanda Pharmaceutical Association, and the Young Professionals Chronic Disease Network, about 20 educational campaigns are carried out per year to create awareness and where free NCD screening is conducted. The campaigns include education on the prevention, treatment, and management of diabetes, awareness on cancers, including children's cancers, as well as the importance of physical activities. Campaigns have also been carried out at higher levels, where ministry staff are screened for NCDs and referred for treatment. Media houses have also been educated on the NCD situation and the risk factors in Rwanda so that they may spread the information and reach out to the masses in the community. Awareness activities are being scaled up to the rural districts. Students' associations work with the Rwanda NCD Alliance to raise awareness during organised walks, and also through social media (Twitter and Facebook). Other awareness programmes include the education on NCDs of children in school. These activities are implemented in partnership between the government institutions, the private sector, various youth groups, religious groups, businesses, the Rwanda NCD Alliance, and other civil society organisations. While the uptake of these activities has been high, there was no report at the time of this review on whether the activities have reduced NCD incidence.

Health systems strengthening

Health systems interventions include identifying and addressing modifiable risk factors, early detection through screening, treatment and follow-up of patients with NCDs, as well as referrals from primary care facilities to higher level facilities. Early detection and management is intended to prevent complications, reduce the need for hospitalisation and costly high-technology interventions, as well as prevent premature deaths. Implementing these interventions requires the presence of evidence-based national guidelines/standards for the management of major NCDs, the training of health personnel on NCD prevention and management, and also the availability of affordable essential medicines and technologies for NCD management and control. Disease prevention and health promotion at primary health care level has been emphasised as a critical approach in addressing NCDs. There are recommended NCD drugs that should be available at primary care levels. It is recommended that cardiovascular disease drugs are at least 'generally available' in primary care facilities in the public health sector, and at least 50 per cent of primary health care facilities should offer cardiovascular risk stratification for the management of patients at high risk for heart attack and stroke (Robinson & Hort, 2012; Demaio et al., 2014).

Uganda, Tanzania, and Zanzibar have all developed various care guidelines, including guidelines for the management of diabetes. Kenya has its National Clinical Guidelines for Management of Diabetes Mellitus 2010, National Guidelines for Prevention and Management of Cervical, Breast and Prostate Cancers 2012, National Guidelines for Cancer Management 2013, and guidelines for tobacco cessation. Tanzania, Uganda, Kenya, and Malawi have started training health workers on NCD management. These countries also run NCD clinics in tertiary and district hospitals. Many countries are implementing disease-specific programmes for diabetes, cancer, sickle cell, and cardiovascular diseases from primary to tertiary care levels. Some are establishing specialised care centres, such as heart centres and cancer centres.

Case study: Improving health systems for NCD care in Tanzania (see Juma, 2018)

Tanzania has implemented several initiatives to strengthen its health systems for NCD prevention and management. Guidelines for the management of cancer, cardiovascular disease, and sickle cell disease have been developed and palliative care guidelines are also in place. The development of guidelines for renal care is ongoing. The available guidelines have interventions for all levels of care from primary to tertiary levels. Training of health care workers on NCD management has been done widely with support from the Tanzania Diabetes Association. In 2003 the government, with support from partners, trained staff and strengthened the diabetes clinic at the National Referral Hospital Muhimbilo National Hospital (MNH), and three other zonal referral hospitals. In 2005 the country embarked on training health workers and establishing diabetes services at all regional hospitals – 21 in total – and at 25 district hospitals in Dar es Salaam. The government also reviewed and developed a training curriculum for diabetes and other NCDs for different levels of health care. The health sector is implementing disease-specific programmes for diabetes, cancer, sickle cell, and CVD from primary to tertiary care levels. Cervical cancer screening is ongoing, with support from partners like PATH and Jhpiego, among other NGOs. Cancer outreach services are also ongoing.

GOVERNANCE OF NCD PREVENTION AND CONTROL

The governance of NCD prevention and control requires the recognition of NCDs as a health priority in the national development and the health sector strategic plans, as well as the establishment of structures to enhance multisectoral action – WHO refers to this as a 'whole of government' approach (WHO 2013; Beaglehole et al., 2013; Horton, 2013).

All the countries reviewed addressed NCDs in their most recent health sector strategic plans as one of their national priority areas. By 2017, Kenya, Tanzania, Malawi, Nigeria, and South Africa had developed and launched their NCD action plans. Other countries have draft NCD plans which are yet to be launched. All the countries have established NCD units/departments within their ministries of health (Juma, 2018). The units coordinate NCD policy development, resource generation, and monitoring and evaluation, with support from NGOs. The presence of the coordinating units has led to improvement of NCD coordination at health sector levels. However, staffing and financial support for the units are a problem in most of the countries.

Multisectoral action in NCD prevention is still inadequate. South

Africa, Zanzibar, and Uganda have established multisectoral committees for NCD prevention and control. However, there is no tangible evidence on how other sectors contribute to NCD interventions in these countries. Civil society engagement in NCD prevention is increasing. There are funded NGOs that are implementing some NCD prevention and care interventions. National NCD alliances exist in most of the countries and they work closely with the ministries of health. However, the engagement is not well structured or coordinated.

Case study: Improvement of NCD governance and coordination in Uganda

In Uganda both the National Development Plan II (Vision 2040) and the Health Sector Development Plan 2015/16–2019/20 emphasise the need to reduce premature deaths due to NCDs as well as the need for enhanced multisectoral action in addressing NCDs. The plan has NCD objectives that include the promotion of healthy lifestyles that contribute to the prevention of NCDs, improving management of NCDs at all levels of care, and establishing a functional surveillance, monitoring, and research system to support the prevention and control of NCDs. While the plan does not mention specific NCD targets or indicators of progress, several NCD prevention and control strategies are outlined, under three key objectives. In addition, the Uganda Health Sector Investment Plan mentions efforts to address NCDs through three priority thematic areas – NCD prevention, capacity building, and management interventions – which are key to the achievement of its health outcome targets. Uganda's NCD strategy has been under development since 2013 and although by 2017 it had not yet been launched it was at an advanced stage, awaiting sharing with stakeholders for final input. The draft addresses both prevention and management of NCDs. Despite the efforts to implement the NCD interventions, financing for NCDs is still low in the country. To enhance multisectoral action Uganda had constituted a National NCD Coordination Committee with several relevant line ministries, civil society, and academia representatives. Civil society is well represented on the National NCD Coordination Committee and the MoH NCD Technical Working Group Uganda NCD Alliance representative.

MONITORING AND EVALUATION, AND RESEARCH

From the WHO review report 2016 and the available data, most of the countries have set up some mechanism to undertake periodic surveillance of NCDs and their risk factors. STEPS surveys have been conducted in many of the countries (this excludes Nigeria, which did not complete its STEPs survey). On international reporting, the countries covered in this chapter have been reporting on NCD prevalence, mortality, and morbidity to the WHO progress monitoring framework. They have also reported on risk factor exposure and country capacity. In some countries, for example Kenya, specific diseases such as diabetes and cancers are under surveillance through the integrated disease surveillance and response programme by the MoH Division of Disease Surveillance and Response.

Generally, the countries have not established strong national information systems with surveillance mechanisms monitoring all the key risk factors, morbidity and mortality, and health system capacity for NCDs. Nor have governments set up NCD research priorities or set aside funding for NCD research. Some NCD research is going on in some countries, however, through academic and research institutions.

CHALLENGES TO THE IMPLEMENTATION OF THE NCD PREVENTION-AND-CONTROL INTERVENTIONS

Various challenges affect NCD interventions, resulting in limited geographical coverage and, in some instances, failure to implement planned interventions or enforce existing laws and regulations. The first challenge is inadequate resource capacity. There is no or very low government allocation of funds for the implementation of NCD intervention. Low NCD financial allocations result in real paralysis and the inability of even committed actors to advance a cause in NCD prevention and control. Consequently, many African countries tend to rely on NGOs to support implementation.

The funding challenge is compounded by the fact that implementing institutions, NGOs, and other entities often do not seem to be pooling their resources. Thus different, sometimes duplicate, activities may take place without synergy and complementarity and this leads to disjointed or inadequate implementation of prescribed interventions. Innovative and sustainable resource generation is needed to ensure the effective implementation of NCD interventions. Although governments are seeking external resources to strengthen their health care systems, it is imperative for domestic resource allocations to health to be increased. Universal health coverage (UHC) has been recognised as a major health goal and strategy for LMIC, a programme that requires adequate and sustainable health care financing (Beaglehole & Bonita, 2016; WHO, 2016). However, allocation of resources to health care in most African countries remains very low, despite most of them being signatories to the Abuja Declaration where they pledged to allocate at least 15 per cent of government expenditure to health. Most countries allocate less than half of this. There are a few exceptions: Rwanda, for example, allocates 16 per cent.

There is also great potential for more efficient financial flows through the health care system, especially from the household direct (out-of-pocket) expenditures, which could instead be channelled into an insurance system to provide wider coverage to individuals. This could also be a vehicle for health promotion. The allocation to health promotion and health care of part of the revenues collected from taxes on tobacco, alcohol, and unhealthy foods and drinks is another possible source of funding for NCD control.

Second, implementation is hampered by weaknesses in the health care systems that are supposed to take leadership in NCD prevention and control. One of these weaknesses concerns health care providers (there are not enough of them) and human resource allocation (too few in number and not adequately trained), for both intervention coordination and care provision at health facility levels. Those who require medical care often do not get quality care because the country's public health facilities lack not only various specialist and high-level diagnostic equipment, but are consistently out of the drugs and supplies essential for NCD management. Primary health care facilities still lack the capacity to provide effective NCD preventive and care services. In some countries traditional healers who claim they treat all NCDs are mushrooming. Many patients tend to default from medication as they seek the cheaper services of traditional healers, who are not well regulated. In most of the countries, community members cannot afford most of the NCD services, which are considered expensive; hence they turn to traditional healers. It has been suggested that for LMIC health systems to address NCDs in addition to the prevalence of other health problems, integration of NCDs into health promotion and primary health care is the way to go. This requires training of health care providers, task sharing, and integration of care pathways and guidelines. There have been a variety of pilot studies with different degrees of integration, and suitable, feasible, and scalable models need to be developed for increased efficiency of the limited health resources available.

Third, while a multisectoral approach has been advocated to enhance the implementation of NCD prevention interventions (Horton, 2013), such approaches are hindered by poor governance and the absence of functional and effective coordination structures. The role of partnerships and collaborations across the sectors is crucial in realising the goals of NCD control. The private sector has to be involved in a suitable regulated and coordinated framework. African governments need to take the lead in being the primary investors in health and create a regulatory and coordination framework that enables other stakeholders to participate and contribute to the realisation of the health goals articulated in their individual national policies and action plans.

Lastly, while most of the proven interventions are in place, implementation might further be challenged by the prevailing contextual factors in the countries. Apart from epidemiological and economic contexts, which are well understood for most countries, socio-cultural factors, which are most often not well understood or well addressed, might affect both the prevalence of NCDs and the uptake of interventions. For a long time NCDs were viewed as an affliction of the affluent; in some places they are even viewed as a status symbol. Prevailing attitudes towards risk factors such as diet, alcohol consumption and levels of physical activity contribute to the higher incidences of NCDs and to the slow progress in uptake of preventive interventions. For example, uptake of physical activity interventions might be hindered by the fact that some communities view being overweight as a desirable condition, even though this is a risk factor for several NCDs. In several African contexts, people living in rural areas typically live an active lifestyle which involves walking and physical labour. When they move to urban areas and start earning higher incomes, they are less likely to engage in physical activity such as walking as it does not correspond to their new status. Limited examination of socio-cultural factors may also result in the low use of potentially powerful channels to reach community members with existing interventions. For instance, in some countries traditional healers have a lot of influence in rural communities and could become powerful allies in NCD prevention. However, to date they have not been effectively engaged; this is a wasted opportunity to achieve meaningful impact. An improved understanding of such contextual factors would lead to more effective implementation and uptake of interventions that target adoption of the behavioural changes required for NCD prevention.

CONCLUSION

This chapter has explored the situation of NCD prevention and control in the African context and reviewed interventions that are being implemented in a selection of African countries. Most of the reviewed countries in sub-Saharan Africa have taken steps to develop policies and implement practical interventions to address NCDs. Progress in the implementation of these interventions, which are expected to show success, given positive experiences in some localities, is slow, however. Much needs to be done to enhance counter-measures and effect the scale-up of these interventions – to a scale that will achieve the global targets for addressing NCDs.

Most of the interventions reviewed in this chapter have only been implemented partially, with poor geographical coverage. Implementation science frameworks which adequately contextualise the methods that have been proven to be effective and gradual scaling to achieve the NCD national goals are priorities moving forward. To enhance implementation of the interventions there is a need for more resource allocation and actor mobilisation for multisectoral action in the implementation of the interventions. There is a need as well for improved governance, coordination, and multisectoral engagement in NCD prevent-and-control interventions. In addition, there is a pressing need to address multiple other existing problems, including weaknesses in the health systems and other contextual, country-specific factors.

REFERENCES

Beaglehole, R. & Bonita, R. 2016. 'Economists, universal health coverage, and non-communicable diseases'. *The Lancet*, 387 (10021), 848.

Beaglehole, R., Bonita, R. & Horton, R. 2013. 'Independent global accountability for NCDs'. *The Lancet*, 381 (9867), 602–605.

Beaglehole, R., Bonita, R., Horton, R., Adams, C., Alleyne, G., Asaria, P., Baugh, V., Bekedam, H., Billo, N., Casswell, S. & Cecchini, M. 2011. 'Priority actions for the non-communicable disease crisis'. *The Lancet*, 377 (9775), 1438–1447.

Bump, J. B. & Reich, M. R. 2013. 'Political economy analysis for tobacco control in low- and middle-income countries'. *Health Policy and Planning*, 28 (2), 123–133, DOI: 10.1093/heapol/czs049.

Dalal, S., Beunza, J. J., Volmink, J., Adebamowo, C., Bajunirwe, F., Njelekela, M., Mozaffarian, D., Fawzi, W., Willett, W., Adami, H. O. & Holmes, M. D. 2011. 'Non-communicable diseases in sub-Saharan Africa: what we know now'. *International Journal of Epidemiology*, 40 (4), 885–901.

Demaio, A. R., Nielsen, K. K., Pinkowski Tersbøl, B., Kallestrup, P. & Meyrowitsch, D. W. 2014. 'Primary Health Care: A strategic framework for the prevention and control of chronic non-communicable disease'. *Global Health Action,* 7 (1), 24504.

Forouzanfar, M. H., Alexander, L., Anderson, R. H., Bachman, V. F. & Biryukov, S. 2015. 'Global, regional, and national comparative risk assessment of 79 behavioural, environmental and occupational, and metabolic risks or clusters of risks in 188 countries, 1990-2013: A systematic analysis for the Global Burden of Disease Study 2013'. *The Lancet*, 388 (10053), 1659-1724, DOI: 10.1016/S0140-6736(15)00128-2.

Horton, R. 2013. 'Non-communicable diseases: 2015 to 2025'. *The Lancet*, 381 (9866), 509–510.

Juma, P. A. 2018. *Non-communicable disease benchmark survey in East African*

Countries. Report. East Africa NCD Alliance 2018. Kampala, Uganda.

Juma, P. A., Shurki, M. & Kyobutungi, C. 2017. *Analysis of NCD Prevention Policies in Five sub-Saharan African Countries Synthesis Report*. Unpublished. Nairobi, Kenya.

Juma, P. A., Mohamed, S. F., Wisdom, J., Kyobutungi, C. & Oti, S. 2016. 'Analysis of Non-communicable disease prevention policies in five Sub-Saharan African countries: Study protocol'. *Archives of Public Health*, 74 (1), 25. DOI:10.1186/s13690-016-0137-9, available at https://www.ncbi.nlm.nih.gov/pubmed/27335640, accessed 2 October 2018.

Khanal, S., Veerman, L., Hollingworth, S. & Nissen, L. 2015. 'Shift in disease burden from communicable to noncommunicable diseases: Aiming to achieve Universal Health Coverage in Nepal'. *Perspectives in Public Health*, 135 (4), 177–178.

Kavishe, B., Biraro, S., Baisley, K., Vanobberghen, F., Kapiga, S., Munderi, P., Smeeth, L., Peck, R., Mghamba, J., Mutungi, G., Ikoona, E., Levin, J., Bou Monclús, M. A., Katende, D., Kisanga, E., Hayes, R. & Grosskurth, H. 2015. 'High prevalence of hypertension and of risk factors for non-communicable diseases (NCDs): A population based cross-sectional survey of NCDS and HIV infection in Northwestern Tanzania and Southern Uganda'. *BMC Medicine*, 13 (1), 126, DOI: 10.1186/s12916-015-0357-9.

Maher, D., Ford, N. & Unwin, N. 2012. 'Priorities for developing countries in the global response to non-communicable diseases'. *Global Health*, 8 (1), 14. DOI: 10.1186/1744-8603-8-14.

Maimela, E., Alberts, M., Van Geertruyden, J.P., Meulemans, H., Fraeyman, J., Wens, J. & Bastiaens, H. 2015. 'Evidence based interventions for improving management of chronic non-communicable diseases in Dikgale in Limpopo Province, South Africa'. *Tropical Medicine & International Health*, 20, 357.

Ministry of Health (MoH) Kenya. 2015. 'Kenya STEPwise Survey for Non Communicable Diseases Risk Factors, 2015 Report'. Nairobi. www.health.go.ke/wp-content/uploads/2016/04/Executive-summary-6-2.pdf, accessed 2 December 2018.

Msyamboza, K. P., Ngwira, B., Dzowela, T., Mvula, C., Kathyola, D.. Harries, A. D. & Bowie. C. 2011. 'The burden of selected chronic non-communicable diseases and their risk factors in Malawi: Nationwide STEPS survey'. *PLoS ONE*, 6 (5), 20316.

Nyirenda, M. J. 2016. 'Non-communicable diseases in sub-Saharan Africa: Understanding the drivers of the epidemic to inform intervention strategies'. *International Health*, 8 (3), 157–158.

Robinson, H. M. & Hort, K. 2012. 'Non-communicable diseases and health systems reform in low- and-middle-income countries'. *Pacific Health Dialog*, 18 (1), 179–19.

Sankaranarayanan, R. & Swaminathan, R. (eds.) 2011. *Cancer Survival in Africa, Asia, the Caribbean and Central America*. Lyon: International Agency for

Research on Cancer.
World Health Organization (WHO). 2003. *WHO Framework Convention on Tobacco Control.* Geneva: World Health Organization.
World Health Organization (WHO). 2004. *Global strategy on diet, physical activity and health*. Geneva: World Health Organization.
World Health Organization (WHO). 2008. *WHO global strategy on diet, physical activity and health: a framework to monitor and evaluate implementation.* https://www.who.int/dietphysicalactivity/DPASindicators/en/, accessed 30 November 2018.
World Health Organization (WHO). 2010. *Global strategy to reduce the harmful effect of alcohol.* Geneve: World Health Organization.
World Health Organization (WHO). 2013. *Global Action Plan for the Prevention and Control of Noncommunicable Diseases 2013-2020.* Geneve: World Health Organization.
World Health Organization (WHO). 2016. *World Health Statistics 2016: monitoring health for the Sustainable Development Goals (SDGs).* Geneve: World Health Organization.
World Health Organization (WHO). 2017. *WHO Global Coordination Mechanism on the Prevention and Control of Noncommunicable Diseases.* Progress Report, 2014-2016. Geneve: World Health Organization.
World Health Organization (WHO). 2018. *Non-communicalble diseases.* http://www.who.int/news-room/fact-sheets/detail/noncommunicable-diseases, accessed 26 November 2018.

SEVEN

Care, Context, and Chronic Illness

Lessons from HIV-positive Adolescents and their Families in South Africa's Eastern Cape

BETH VALE

INTRODUCTION

HIV/AIDS HAS BEEN THE most devastating epidemic in recent history. Since the early 1980s, over 78 million people worldwide have been infected with HIV (UNAIDS, 2014). The worst of the epidemic is in Eastern and Southern Africa, where 19.6 million people were living with HIV in 2018. Since the early 2000s, we have seen a dramatic scale-up of biomedical HIV treatment in Eastern and Southern Africa. The roll-out of antiretroviral therapy (ART) has made it possible for people living with HIV to suppress the virus and live long lives on medication. As the epidemic of HIV/AIDS is increasingly classed as a chronic condition the diagnosis of other, non-infectious chronic conditions has been on the rise. Africa is experiencing the highest increase in premature deaths from non-communicable diseases (NCDs) worldwide. Consequently, there is an urgent need to explore practices and prospects for NCD care in African contexts, where health systems are under-resourced and heavily burdened by infectious diseases. How has care been constituted in these contexts and how might this inform our response to long-term illness?

In South Africa, this growing concern with NCDs emerges amidst the world's largest HIV epidemic and its largest ART programme. Drawing on the care experiences of 23 HIV-positive adolescents and their families living in the Eastern Cape, this chapter considers broader implications for chronic patients in under-resourced settings. It makes three interrelated claims about care in these contexts: first, where health facilities are overburdened, the quest for care entails a quest to 'be seen' by health providers, both literally and metaphorically. Second, care for chronic patients spans clinic and home, involves both family and health workers, and is often enacted within pre-existing structures of authority. These caring relationships are regularly expressed through generational hierarchy and mutual obligation. Third, where livelihoods are precarious, securing medical care forms part of a wider, and often hostile, pursuit of survival and support. NGOs, government departments, homes, and communities all constitute a complex economy of care in which power and resources are unevenly distributed and social stakes are high. The ways in which homes, communities, and health facilities have enacted care in response to long-term HIV can inform responses to other chronic illnesses.

While the concept of care is now widely and varyingly used, it retains important analytic utility. By being precise about how care articulates in different contexts, we might also trace geographic and temporal change in how it is understood and practised. Part of what this chapter aims to do is situate care in – and as a response to – context. How care is enacted is informed by flows of power and resources in clinics, homes, and communities. Claiming, providing, and sustaining care is about navigating these flows: working within constraints, making oneself visible in the right ways and to the right audiences, and strengthening social ties.

METHODS

The empirical components of this chapter are situated in the context of a broader consideration of the outbreak and relative containment of HIV as epidemic, and the coexistence of HIV care with the management of multiple NCDs. The empirical components draw from an eight-month ethnographic study, exploring the practice of antiretroviral therapy among a cohort of 23 HIV-positive adolescents (age 10–19 years) in South Africa's Eastern Cape. By 'practice' I mean the precarious, situated, and relational 'work' that goes into young people's everyday achievement of ART, including taking daily medication, regularly attending health appointments, and participating in HIV treatment support groups. Data for this study was gathered through multi-method ethnographic fieldwork with HIV-positive youth, their families, and local health workers. Fieldwork was conducted alongside a research assistant, Mildred Thabeng, who played an invaluable role in data collection and concurrent analysis.

Research was conducted in two Eastern Cape sites: one rural and one peri-urban. By making this selection we hoped to cover the contexts in which most South Africans experience care, while also comparing rural and urban experiences. Between August and December 2013, we conducted fieldwork in five rural villages of an Eastern Cape municipality I call Mtembu. Mtembu has a population of approximately 72,000 residents. Among the 13 Mtembu families with whom we worked, only one household had a permanently employed member. She was employed as a domestic worker in her village but lost her job towards the end of the research period. Most of the households survived off a combination of social grants, subsistence farming, and irregular remittances from relatives working in nearby towns or farms.

Peri-urban fieldwork was conducted between January and April 2014 in the informal settlements of a small town I call Ridgetown. Including its informal settlements, Ridgetown has an estimated population of 125,000 people. At the time of the research, 66 per cent of working-age (15–64) residents in the municipal area were thought to be jobless (Stats SA, 2014). Among the nine Ridgetown families in our study, many adult members struggled to access stable jobs. Those fortunate enough to find contract work were employed on local farms and municipal projects, or as domestic workers.

Adolescent participants for this study were recruited through NGO-run ART support groups, as well as public health clinics. The length of time adolescents had spent on ART varied (from 1–11 years). Since all adolescent participants were enrolled in ART programmes, and most were receiving additional NGO support, this sample is likely to represent an especially compliant group of young treatment-takers. Recruitment did not reach those who had long fallen out of ART care, and those receiving inadequate treatment support are under-represented in this sample.

Within the research cohort, there was an almost equal distribution of male and female, as well as older (> 15 years) and younger (< 15 years) adolescents. The few adolescents in this study who had ongoing struggles with treatment adherence were often older adolescents, who were less subject to the authority of adult caregivers. One of these older adolescents, for example, had stopped taking treatment altogether, another only took treatment when food was available, and a third found he forgot his pills when he was out with his friends.

Fourteen of the adolescents in this study had lost at least one parent to AIDS illness; three had parents killed in violent crime; and eight had a parent who was either absent or estranged. As a result, most young participants were not living with biological parents, but instead with relatives. In addition to child support grants, a few adolescents in our study benefitted from care dependency or disability grants on the basis of their HIV-positive status. Grandmothers on state pensions were most frequently household heads. Eleven of our adolescent participants lived with at least one other person on HIV-treatment and many elderly caregivers took diabetes or high blood pressure medication. During one of our conversations with Nurse Kani in Ridgetown, he commiserated about the number of medications that could be found in a single household: 'Medication for high blood pressure, medication for diabetes, antiretrovirals, TB-pills …' (interview, 3 March 2014, Ridgetown). The extent of chronic illness requires families, like those in this study, to visit public health facilities regularly and follow their prescriptions diligently. This requirement shapes when households wake in the morning, what and when they eat, and how they demonstrate and enact care for one another.

Throughout fieldwork, Ms Thabeng and I visited young people and their families regularly, engaging as far as possible in their everyday lives. Hours of informal conversation were had while cooking, washing clothes, sharing food, walking, and playing with friends. This was complemented by more structured research methods, including semi-structured interviews with both adolescents and their caregivers. These interviews centred on adolescents' HIV diagnosis, treatment-taking, family life, and interactions with clinics. In addition to spending time in participants' homes and communities, we also observed their interactions with health facilities. Over the course of our fieldwork, we visited nine community clinics and four hospitals, accompanying young people and their families to appointments. While observing participants' consultations, we also had informal discussions with health workers, and in some cases conducted formal interviews.[i]

The small ethnographic study from which this chapter draws formed part of a larger, interdisciplinary research collaboration called Mzantsi Wakho (Your South Africa). Mzantsi Wakho is a research partnership between the universities of Oxford and Cape Town. In collaboration with UNICEF, the South African departments of Health, Social Development, and Education, as well as local NGOs, it aims to inform future policy and programming for HIV-positive youth.[ii]

---

i Fieldwork was carried out using a combination of both English and isiXhosa. Translation occurred in situ to allow for immediate, follow-up probing. These complex on-site translations have subjectively coloured the data and may have produced misinterpretation. Structured interviews were audio-recorded, while informal interviews, observations, and ethnographic interactions were documented in fieldnotes. Throughout fieldwork, Ms Thabeng and I were involved in ongoing, concurrent analysis, adapting the data collection to further our understanding of emerging themes. Data was then thematically coded, comparing and contrasting themes that revealed adolescents' interpretation and practice of HIV treatment.

ii Ethical approval for this study was granted by the universities of Oxford and Cape Town, and the Eastern Cape departments of Health, Social Development, and Education. Written informed consent was given by all adolescents and their primary caregivers, and consent information was read aloud in case of low literacy. Consent materials were written and discussed in English and/or isiXhosa, depending on the preference of the participant. There were no financial incentives, but we often brought refreshments to meetings and assisted adolescents with transport, grant applications, and other referrals. Confidentiality was maintained except in cases of risk of harm: if adolescents reported abuse, suicidality, rape, or severe illness. In these cases, referrals were made to relevant social or health services and followed up to ensure that services were received.

RISING CHRONICITY

Although South and Eastern Africa accounts for only 6.2 per cent of the global population, it is home to half of all people living with HIV (UNAIDS, 2017a). In 2016, the region suffered nearly half a million AIDS deaths (UNAIDS, 2017a). In the same year, South Africa accounted for one third of the world's new HIV infections, with a further 50 per cent of new infections attributable to these countries: Kenya, Mozambique, Zambia, Tanzania, Uganda, Zimbabwe, Malawi, and Ethiopia (UNAIDS, 2017b).

The human impact of HIV/AIDS in Southern and Eastern Africa has been immeasurable. The virus is borne most heavily by adult women and men in the prime of their lives, stripping economies of workers and households of important caregivers. The epidemic has deepened inequality in the region, burdened public institutions, destabilised family livelihoods, and amplified tensions in our most intimate lives. Its impact has been felt across generations, affecting children, parents, and grandparents, regardless of whether the virus itself is shared by all (Scherr et al., 2014).

The extraordinary impact of HIV/AIDS has prompted an unprecedented global effort to guarantee access to ART in order to treat HIV among those living with it. This has resulted in significant declines in AIDS-related deaths worldwide, and a related rise in global HIV prevalence (Kharsany & Karim, 2016). Despite the continued severity of the HIV/AIDS epidemic in the region, immense progress has been made, particularly over the past decade. Sixty per cent of people who live with HIV in East and Southern Africa are now receiving treatment (UNAIDS, 2017c). Between 2010 and 2016, new HIV infections among adults declined by 29 per cent, while the number of children being newly diagnosed more than halved (UNAIDS, 2017c).

A key feature of Africa's HIV/AIDS pandemic is 'that it appears as both a crisis and a systemic condition' (Poku & Whiteside, 2004). It is now widely acknowledged that, in order to curb the HIV/AIDS epidemic in Southern and East Africa, we need more than a crisis response: we need a systemic one. Encouraging people to practise safer sex, test for HIV, or adhere to their treatment is not sufficient on its own. We must also address the social and environmental conditions that support or constrain their choices and abilities. This means focusing on health systems – practices and places of care, as well as the conditions that constrain them.

With access to ART having increased dramatically in this region over the past decade, the urgent, acute aspects of the disease have slowly been de-emphasised in favour of a focus on long-term survival. The certainty of death is incrementally being replaced by 'the uncertainties of life on HIV treatment' (Whyte et al., 2014: 69). One of the most devastating infectious diseases of the last century, HIV/AIDS is increasingly framed not as an acute, terminal condition, but as one that is made both treatable and less infectious through life-long chronic medication. As with other forms of chronic illness management, 'good' HIV care is now frequently defined by adherence to treatment, regular check-ups, 'lifestyle' changes, and self-regulation (McGrath et al., 2014).

Like much of the world, South Africa is increasingly orientating its primary health system towards long-term illness, and high rates of co-morbidity. Compounding the country's burden of HIV and TB are the rising numbers of patients suffering from NCDs (Lawn & Kinney, 2009; Coovadia et al., 2009). Indeed, the arrival and mass distribution of HIV treatment is concomitant with the unprecedented roll-out of other long-term medication, particularly for high blood pressure and diabetes (Magadzire, 2016). While ART availability transforms HIV into a chronic (rather than a terminal) illness, it also increases overall chronicity and the risk of co-morbidity. This is not only because HIV-positive patients live longer, but also because they do so at increased risk of additional chronic conditions.

Experiences of NCDs in Africa are markedly different from the global north: health systems in Africa are under-resourced, heavily burdened by infectious diseases, and, consequently, poorly orientated towards non-communicable chronic conditions. And yet, 'HIV programmes are, in fact, the first large-scale chronic disease programmes in many [Southern and East African] countries' (Rabkin & El-Sadr, 2011). These programmes have had to develop effective systems of care with very few resources. The continent's HIV/AIDS response holds many lessons about the practices and stakes of long-term care in these contexts, which might inform our response to rising chronicity (Rabkin & El-Sadr, 2011).

This chapter draws on a small South African case study to explore what the HIV/AIDS response can teach us about health systems in Africa. The case study emerges from an ethnographic study with 23 HIV-positive adolescents, and their families, living in rural and peri-urban Eastern Cape. In South Africa, adolescents who contracted HIV in infancy are some of our longest-surviving HIV-treatment users. They have been taking medication and regularly attending clinics most of their lives. Yet they are the only population group for whom AIDS-related deaths have risen since 2001 (WHO, 2013; UNAIDS, 2013). This is attributed in part to a lack of retention in care and poor adherence to HIV treatment (Denison et al., 2015). Their experiences hold relevance for the challenges and possibilities of chronic care in African settings.

Drawing on practices and experiences of care among HIV-positive adolescents, their families and their health workers, the chapter makes three claims about what constitutes 'care' where illness is long-term and resources are scarce:

1. **Where health facilities are overburdened, the quest for care entails a quest to 'be seen' by health providers.** A rising burden of chronic, routine patients – together with high rates of acute illness – means that health facilities in under-resourced settings are frequently overcrowded and understaffed. Those who visit clinics and hospitals, particularly those who are not acutely ill, can expect to spend hours queueing. In an effort to secure a consultation ('be seen'), adolescents and families in this study employed a variety of tactics to make themselves visible ('be seen') to health staff. This included building personal relationships with staff, finding means to jump the queue, demonstrating good behaviour, or acquiring supporting documents. Similarly, in her examination of hospitals in Papua New Guinea, Alice Street (2012) found that there was a power in 'making oneself seen' particularly where the state was deemed weak or absent.

2. **Treatment and care for chronic patients spans clinic and home, involves both family and health workers, and operates within pre-**

existing structures of authority. Caring relationships are regularly expressed through hierarchy, mutual obligation, and entitlements. The work of 'being seen' highlights the relational nature of care in these settings. Adolescent participants and their families were interested in bolstering relationships of care, both in health facilities and their own homes. The obligations and entitlements associated with HIV treatment helped to strengthen reciprocity and caring roles. The 'proper' provision of care was often framed in terms of 'disciplining' the ART-user, thereby reinforcing the moral authority of the care provider. Conversely, the 'proper' reception of care frequently entailed forms of deference, respecting and thereby cementing bonds of mutual obligation across generations. As observed in other Southern African contexts, 'the work of nourishing and extending relations, whether as patient or caregiver, professional or volunteer, becomes an important means through which caring futures are constituted' (Mkhay, 2018).

3. **Where livelihoods are precarious, securing medical care forms part of a wider, and often hostile, pursuit of survival and support.** Rather than being about recovery, chronic care is about living well with illness. Adolescents and families in this study participating in HIV-treatment programmes formed part of a wider moral economy of survival, linking them to a range of NGO and state support services, which not only provided biomedical treatment but also sustenance and social support. Indeed, research with ART patients in Western Kenya has shown that although HIV-treatment programmes often medicalise survival they have also created linkages to other crucial forms of sustenance and support that become essential to how care is constituted (Prince, 2012). While adolescents and families in this study lived in neighbourhoods in which poverty was generalised, HIV (along with other chronic conditions) could make one visible to funders, government agencies, and non-governmental support in particular ways. Where resources for care are scarce and unequally distributed, the pursuit of care becomes both more urgent and more contested, since who is cared for, and who is not, can become a source of injury, resentment, and even persecution.

COMPARING HIV/AIDS AND NCDS

Before exploring what might be drawn from experiences of the HIV/AIDS response to tackle rising chronicity on the continent, it is worth signalling some of the similarities and differences between HIV and NCDs. The most immediate difference is that HIV is classed as a 'communicable' condition, while NCDs, by definition, are not. However, this dichotomy is murkier than it seems. While the HI virus is of course infectious, adhering to ART makes it possible to achieve viral suppression, in which a person with HIV is in fact relatively uninfectious. Second, although NCDs are technically not 'communicable', in some places the dramatic 'spread' in the number of diagnoses and rising awareness of conditions like hypertension and diabetes can feel like 'contagion' (Whyte, 2012). As a result of shared life conditions (poor diet, pollution, physical inactivity, alcohol — even genetics), which enhance vulnerability to NCDs, household members can also share non-communicable ailments, just as HIV/TB have often affected multiple family members.

Both HIV/AIDS and NCDs are 'chronic' in the sense that they can be managed through long-term treatment and monitoring. Both demand a health system in which continuity of care (between clinic and home), as well as retention in care, are paramount. In both cases, what is needed is a sustained commitment by patients, in the form of regular clinic attendance and adherence, and regular monitoring from the health system. These are lifelong commitments (Rabkin & El-Sadr, 2011). But this does not mean that HIV and NCDs are always experienced as chronic: left untested, or untreated, both HIV and NCDs can arrive in a person's life as acute (McGrath et al., 2014). Indeed, both NCDs and HIV can remain asymptomatic for long periods.

HIV has been highly stigmatised (partly due to its infectiousness), with severe implications for people's willingness to be tested and treated. This stigma has been significantly less prevalent for NCDs. Yet in most Southern and East African settings people are less likely to be tested and treated for NCDs than they are to be tested and treated for HIV. This is partly due to a lack of awareness about NCDs, and partly because access to screening is limited (Whyte, 2012). Finally, while it is primarily young people, and children, who have contracted HIV, the aged are more likely to be diagnosed with, and die from, an NCD. This is notwithstanding rising NCD rates among young adults (Kaba, et al., 2017).

Drawing from the HIV/AIDS experience in order to frame and better respond to NCDs is not simply a public health recommendation (Rabkin & El-Sadr, 2011). It has also been observed in lay practice on the continent. Research from Southern Africa suggests that local understandings of NCDs are often framed in relation to HIV. In a Ugandan study, *plesa* (high blood pressure) and *swekile* (diabetes) were described as 'new sicknesses', while HIV was understood as 'old' (Whyte, 2012). Similarly, in a South African study HIV was described as 'ordinary', while diabetes was 'new' (Mendenhall & Norris, 2015). Patients across studies compared possibilities for managing and controlling these conditions long term. What this research suggests is that in many parts of Africa HIV and NCDs are not experienced in isolation but as parallel epidemiological patterns. Households and communities experience both infectious and non-infectious conditions simultaneously, and in relation to one another. The experience is one of lifelong, compounding illness concerns with implications for how families, communities, and clinics practise care. Understanding what constitutes chronic HIV care is therefore immensely relevant for how we tackle chronicity in the region.

ART AND SOCIALITY

AIDS has taught us both the power of science and its limitations. It has given us incredible technologic successes. But fully implementing those successes still escapes us (Dr Gerald Friedland, Yale University, in Zuger, 2003).

The HIV/AIDS epidemic has taught us that, however exceptional our medical technology may be its efficacy depends on the ways in which it is interpreted, and taken up, in local contexts. At its heart, this chapter is about the forms of sociality entailed in the ways that HIV-positive adolescents, their families, and health workers practise and claim care.

It suggests that these forms of sociality, and the implications they hold for care, are born out of the experience of long-term illness in under-resourced settings and therefore have broader implications for chronic illness in Africa. Anthropology has a rich legacy of theorising health socialities, including biosociality (Rabinow, 1996), illness identities, biological disruptions, and forms of health citizenship (Nguyen, 2005; Robins et al., 2008). Much of this literature has centred on chronic and not acute conditions.

To access ART is not simply to seek treatment 'here and there'. It entails affiliation to a programme through check-ups, monitoring, and refills. In the words of Richey (2012) and Whyte et al. (2014: 58), the new generation of ART users in sub-Saharan Africa is a generation of 'clients'. A client, they argue, is not merely a customer the way a patron in a private pharmacy might be. Nor is a client simply a patient. Instead, clients *participate* in institutions of care with associated expectations and entitlements.

In a context of rising chronicity, interactions with medical facilities are less ad hoc and less determined by desperately sick bodies. Instead, an estimated 70 per cent of patients in South Africa's health facilities are regular attendees.[iii] Their experience of care is increasingly characterised by the ritualised collection and consumption of medicines, and lifelong participation in health surveillance. More and more, patients do not *visit* health facilities: they *enrol* in them.

Within the anthropological literature on (predominantly adult) ART users, some authors have sought to distinguish 'clientship' from articulations of therapeutic 'citizenship'. Therapeutic citizenship is frequently understood as a form of rights-based sociality (Nguyen, 2005). People formulate group identities based on their shared biological status, mobilise their treatment narratives to make empowered claims on state and donor resources, and are transformed into 'expert', 'self-reliant', and 'responsibilised' patients. Yet, in rapidly expanding treatment programmes across sub-Saharan Africa, the production of ART adherence has also articulated in less empowered forms of 'getting by' (Mattes, 2011; Meinart et al., 2009; Richey, 2012). Rather than

---

iii Extrapolated from District Health Barometer 2016/17, Health Systems Trust.

drawing on communities of solidarity to confront public and private donors, many people have played to their patrons, instrumentally adopting the language of funders. They have participated in tactical competitions for donor spoils, negotiating multiple relationships of hierarchy and dependency (Beckmann & Bujra, 2010: 1051). While learning to speak as 'HIV-positive', many also learn to articulate this identity in different moral registers: sometimes as responsible health citizens, sometimes as needy and suffering (Prince, 2012: 549).

Indeed, there is another meaning of clientship at play: clientship invokes hierarchical dependence between a patron and a beneficiary, where the former offers the latter scarce resources in exchange for less tangible forms of loyalty and discipline (Whyte et al., 2014). In a recent compilation of case studies from Uganda, Whyte et al., (2014) examine the experiences of the country's first generation of ART users. The authors recount a story in which one of their respondents, Robinah, tellingly described her relationship to her home-based care programme, saying: 'I am their person' (Whyte et al., 2014: 56). In ART programmes, the personal, emotional quality of these 'lop-sided friendships' (Pitt-Rivers in Wolf, 1963: 17–19) is often mediated through a nexus of paradoxically impersonal, bureaucratic procedures.

In their study of ART participation in Tanzania, Beckmann and Bujra (2010) articulate these socialities historically. They argue that, along with the increasing availability of ART, the focus of debate among those living with HIV has shifted from physical survival in the face of a deadly disease to economic survival and integration into society. ART prompts people's struggle for work, partners, and a 'normal' life, rather than necessarily encouraging them to foreground their HIV identities as 'therapeutic' or 'responsibilised' citizens. Biehl (2007: 94) has argued that the 'patient-citizenship' of ART users in the developing world frequently articulates within a global 'politics of survival', combining struggles for food, housing, and social security with a new political economy of pharmaceuticals.

In South Africa, the mass distribution of antiretroviral drugs has been carried out alongside a grand-scale project of social welfare delivery. Over 18 million people – that is one in every three South Africans – benefits from a state grant (Bundy, 2015: 1). While the growth of social welfare preceded 1995, the extraordinary expansion of the number of people on state benefits has been the most striking characteristic of policy and practice since democracy and has had a significant impact on alleviating poverty (Bhorat & Cassim, 2014).

A context of mass unemployment and social exclusion has arguably provoked new kinds of dispositions towards the authority of the state (White, 2012). Many people are seeking less mediated, paternalistic relationships with government patrons – a relationship that is sometimes imagined through welfare. This growing 'politics of distribution' (Ferguson, 2013) highlights the increasing materiality of the civil link between citizens and state. Insufficient anthropological attention has been given to large-scale redistribution 'as a distinct mode of exchange and sociality' (Bähre, 2011: 375).

One of the characteristic features of state–citizen relations in an era of mass health and welfare programmes is the centrality of bureaucratic technology in signifying membership, distributing resources, and enacting surveillance. Bureaucracy becomes a central feature of care. Birth certificates, death certificates, identity documents, and blood test results form part of the litany of documents required to demonstrate eligibility for social grants. Once registered as grant recipients, people continue to interact with state welfare through technology. A high-tech system of biometric identification and smart-card transactions facilitates a complex interchange between state and citizens, carried out millions of times every month (Donovan, 2013: 23).

ART users are similarly involved in regularised, technologically mediated interactions with the state. And as in the social welfare system, membership to an ART programme is indexed through paperwork. Records of treatment history, medical prescriptions, and appointment dates not only register patient entitlements, they also document and attempt to induce compliance. As beneficiaries of foster child, disability, and child support grants, as well as regular users of ART services, the young people in this study are uniquely located in state health and welfare programmes. The technologies and bureaucracies of these systems have therefore had important implications for how they imagine their life and livelihoods in contemporary South Africa.

Questions of sociality have been central to anthropological and social science literature on ART in Africa. The labels of 'clientship' and 'citizenship' are now widely and varyingly used. Their distinctions have at times become murky. Regardless of the labels attached, attempts to understand ART as a social relation nevertheless signal something important about the meaning of life on HIV treatment. To be an ART user involves a sense of belonging to a programme and often an intricate network of personal relationships, expectations, and entitlements (Whyte et al., 2014: 58). Increasingly, HIV-positive patients enrol in organisations which register their information, offer regular services, and have expectations of their users. Whether as 'therapeutic citizens', 'patient-citizens' or 'clients', ART users enter into 'local moral economies' – communities of care, which offer resources, services, and networks, but which also have their own rules and systems of privilege. Each of these communities calls on 'networks of obligation and reciprocity' which become part of what it means to negotiate life on ART (Nguyen, 2005: 126).

In some situations, HIV can be an asset, opening up spaces for recognition and entitlements, and making one visible to the organisations that distribute material resources. In other situations, HIV can be a source of stigma, a threat to belonging and sociality, and a status best kept hidden. As people negotiate life with HIV, they also 'move between these different registers of invisibility and visibility' (Prince, 2012: 549). Those participating in contemporary ART programmes negotiate highly ambivalent social worlds in which openness and solidarity are idealised, while secrecy, fear, and discrimination persist (Comaroff, 2010: 26).

FINDINGS

Health facilities: being seen rather than swallowed

In mid-November 2013, Ms Thabeng and I accompanied 18-year-old Thembakazi to a scheduled hospital appointment. We travelled 50km, on predominantly dirt roads, from her rural Eastern Cape village to the nearest town where the hospital was located. Like most other adolescents in our study, Thembakazi had been born with HIV. When we met her, she had been taking HIV treatment for nine years. While receiving state-sponsored HIV treatment, Thembakazi also benefited from a care dependency grant,[iv] and her grandmother from a state pension. These were the only sources of income in her home.

Thembakazi's ability to access the more lucrative care dependency grant, as opposed to a child support grant, is testament to the strong, long-term relationships she and her family had built with NGO workers throughout the course of Thembakazi's life. Thembakazi was one of the first children in her village to be initiated onto ART, which was privately sought through the NGO in 2003. In order to qualify her for a care dependency grant, Thembakazi's family, alongside the NGO doctor, would have needed to make a case for Thembakazi's long-term 'severe disability' and navigate a host of bureaucratic procedures.

For Thembakazi, enrolling in HIV treatment served as an ambivalent form of social inclusion. It was not simply a matter of initiating biomedical treatment: rather it meant being encompassed into a number of care institutions spanning NGO and state. Thembakazi is recognised as an entitled state dependent, NGO beneficiary, and recipient of life-saving resources. But she is also an object of discipline, subject to blood tests and pill counts. Wrapped up in the care she receives, then, are deeply intertwined forms of validation and support, compliance and obligation.

On this particular day, Thembakazi hoped her doctor would be referring her for a disability grant. Having just turned 18, she now met the age requirement, although age is only one of a number of eligibility criteria. After collecting Thembakazi from school, we stopped first at the village clinic to collect her folder and then at the social services office for the grant application forms. Before three o'clock, we were seated in the hospital waiting room, holding the necessary documents.

In a context where health facilities are overcrowded, and many will not be seen by a nurse or doctor, these documents play a significant role in making oneself 'visible' in the correct ways. To be documented is to demonstrate one's legitimacy and one's compliance with the procedures for welfare access, and to call upon state obligations towards you. In one Ridgetown clinic, for example, access to a doctor's appointment was dependent on getting one's name onto a waiting list,

iv Intended to provide support to caregivers of any child with severe mental and/or physical disabilities up to 18 years, requiring full-time home care.

marshalled by two female health workers. I observed one afternoon as they announced to the queue: 'You need to make an appointment with the doctor and if you are not on the list you cannot see the doctor' (fieldnotes, 7 March 2014). Two older women in the queue protested that they had made a booking, although their names did not appear on the list. 'I don't see your name here,' said one of the health workers, agitated. 'You didn't book. You'll have to book for next time.' Without bureaucratic visibility, the claims of the two older women were invalidated and they were barred from health care access.

In his effort to skip hospital queues, another adolescent from Thembakazi's village, named Siya (age 18), had taken possession of his hospital folder, which is supposed to be kept on site. 'The hospital always loses it,' he told us, and a lost folder could keep him waiting for hours. Instead, Siya sneaked his folder home with him, and then brought it along to each appointment. Already having his folder meant his visibility in the system was assured, saving him the time and the frustration of having it located and given to him.

When Thembakazi, Ms Thabeng and I were finally called to the nurses' desk, we were told the doctor had left, and then reprimanded for having arrived at the hospital 'so late'. I asked what time we should return to secure a doctor's appointment. 'It depends,' one nurse replied, her eyes still fixed on her paperwork. I persevered: 'We don't want to come here again, using time and petrol money, if we aren't going to see a doctor.' We were well aware that many people in this area spent precious resources travelling to clinics and hospitals and could not afford to be turned away. 'Come by 11 or 12 [o'clock] at least,' said the nurse.

I followed with another line of questioning about whether school learners, like Thembakazi, would be expected to miss their classes in order to attend doctor's appointments, but I was quickly silenced by Thembakazi and Ms Thabeng, who hurried me out of the hospital doors. I continued to grumble about the barriers to access, while Thembakazi and Ms Thabeng pleaded that we stop pressing the hospital staff and resign ourselves to leaving without having seen the doctor.

Back in the car, Thembakazi explained that by 'causing trouble', she risked being punished or denied treatment at her next visit. 'But patients should stand up for their rights!' I insisted. 'You are entitled to this health service. It's [intended] for you!' As we journeyed home, Thembakazi and Ms Thabeng argued that 'rights' and the ability to assert them were reserved for those with 'money and power'. By challenging state patrons on the basis of rights-based claims, the less fortunate risked losing the few services available to them.

Thembakazi's strategic submission to the hospital nurses, which she believed protected her access to care, was not uncommon. Not long before, another rural family in our study had told us that, when confronted or reprimanded by nurses, they 'just keep quiet, otherwise they won't get what they need' (fieldnotes, 16 October 2013). This tactic is far from that of the imagined 'empowered' ART-user. While the agency exercised here is not devoid of power, it is an agency that aims to protect fragile relationships with health officials. Rather than being a once-off, rights-based claim, accessing care meant protecting long-term social ties with health staff, however hierarchical these might be. Researchers in Zimbabwe also found that ART patients perform within the confines of the 'good patient' in order to access 'good care' and ensure continued access to treatment (Campbell et al., 2015). 'Good patients' were characterised as obedient, polite, patient, and grateful.

The ethnographic vignette I recount here is one in which I, as the researcher, am on the scene. On this occasion, I was attempting to straddle dual roles – as an anthropologist and as an advocate for Thembakazi's health care and rights as a citizen. While our study did not offer adolescents or families monetary compensation for research participation, we did occasionally assist with referrals or transport to health facilities. On this day, I attempted to negotiate access for one such adolescent participant, Thembakazi, but in the process, I also unintentionally provoked a significant moment of analytical development and researcher reflexivity. In our encounter at the hospital, both Thembakazi and Ms Thabeng would challenge my rights-based, individualistic assumptions about health access. In doing so, they also helped frame the nature of 'care' in the health facility. In our peri-urban fieldwork, too, we witnessed adolescents and their families attempting to nurture relationships with health providers.

Although Ridgetown clinics only opened at 8 am, patients could be seen queuing as early as 5 am. It was around 5.30 am on 13 February

2014 when Ms Thabeng and I sat with Saki (aged 13) and his mother, waiting for the clinic gates to be unlocked. While we sat in the car, Saki's mother explained the rhythms of the clinic:

> *Gates open at 7.30 for the cleaner. That's when everyone goes inside, but the nurses won't see anyone until 8 am. The clinic usually opens with a prayer. Then the nurses say who should stand in which queue. Often, they will make an announcement about staff shortages – the fact that they are supposed to have six nurses, but only have two. At 10 am the nurses usually break for tea. At 1 pm there is a full lunch break: all the nurses will stop for an hour and there is no rotation. At 2 pm, the school children arrive for the contraceptive injection as do the high blood pressure patients, and the clinic becomes full. Sometimes the nurses send you home at this point even if you have been there since the early morning.*

Contained in this description are a number of assessments about the nature and constraints of care at the clinic. Saki's mother describes the various ways in which opportunities to be 'seen' and cared for are delimited. She references persistent staff shortages and the volume of patients. By describing staff shortage announcements as routine, she suggests that shortages are the norm, rather than the exception. Reflecting on overcrowding, Saki's mother makes particular reference to other routine visitors, like those coming for contraceptives or high blood pressure treatment. Like Saki, these patients will visit the clinic regularly regardless of whether they feel sick that day. Saki's mother's description also makes implicit judgements about 'uncaring' health professionals. She references nurses' apparent refusal to rotate shifts or to begin work before 8 am. She also notes the injustice of a system in which you can be turned away despite having waited a full day.

Despite this, one can also read in this account efforts by the nurses to enact care in different forms. Starting with a prayer gives clinic operations a sense of earnestness and invokes a moral code. Nurses make an attempt to create order and fairness, and to induce acceptance, in an overcrowded system, allocating people into different queues and setting specific times for teenage or high blood pressure patients. By announcing staff shortages, nurses are also appealing to patients for patience and understanding. In response to patients' protests at being sent away at the clinic's closing time, a Ridgetown pharmacist once said:

> *You guys think we don't do anything. We are so tired. It's almost four o'clock and we still have to go home and cook. I'm also a mother and have a family that's waiting for me. You think I have nothing to do but be at the clinic (fieldnotes, 6 March 2014).*

The very description of the clinic routine suggests that caring relationships are fraught, demanding ongoing nurturing. Both patients and nurses are operating in a system that makes the provision and reception of care very difficult to achieve. Attempting to 'be seen' in the right ways is a central part of these operations.

Mastering the clinic queue becomes an important site in the struggle to 'be seen'. We saw patients pay friends R15 to stand in the queue for them, others skipped the queue by taking a seat alongside someone they knew, while others used our presence as noticeable 'visitors' to get faster access to nurses. Similarly, in rural hospitals, we saw NGO workers lobby for their adolescent patients to skip the queue. On one occasion, this required that a community health worker disguise herself as an ambulance driver. In her bid to skip the clinic queue that day, Saki's mother appealed to one of the nurses by pointing out that she and her son shared the nurse's surname. By doing this, she was attempting to call upon a family-type obligation, which demanded that she and her son be privileged (fieldnotes, 13 February 2014).

Many sought to 'work' the queue. Some succeeded. But patients also protested about those cheating the system. On one occasion, we saw a Ridgetown patient request a clinic transfer because he was not satisfied with the long queues, or nurses' relatives getting special assistance. In order to protect their moral authority, and avoid the collective anger of those queueing, it was important that nurses be seen as fair. For this reason, many nurses were wary of being seen to give special assistance. For this reason, Saki's mother's appeal to the nurse who shared her surname had no impact.

After many hours of waiting, we, along with Saki and his mother, were finally called into Nurse Mtambo's consultation room. A moment later, a young female patient arrived at the door begging for the nurse's attention. Nurse Mtambo turned to her and said: 'These people have been waiting in their car since early this morning for Sister Mtambo. Where were you?' By responding in this way to the woman at the door, Nurse Mtambo implicitly recognises our patience and understanding, and demonstrates her own sense of fairness. Both patient and provider are deemed to have 'done their part' in making care possible under difficult circumstances: the patient has waited patiently and the provider has protected their entitlement to 'be seen'. This mutual recognition, in which obligations are shared even if power is hierarchical, was fundamental to what constituted care in these settings.

On the day we travelled with Thembakazi, we (like the young woman who interrupted Saki's consultation) had been reprimanded by nurses for arriving 'so late'. Indeed, in clinics and hospitals throughout our study, we regularly witnessed nurses scolding patients for their 'lateness' and 'impatience'. These reprimands might be read as a way for nurses to show offence: it is an offence to demand care, rather than wait for it. Rather than simply being callous, nurses are often trying to engender, protect, and even enforce a semblance of order in a context in which injustices abound.

Building connections with health workers through displays of deference was central to the practice of showing and receiving care. Adolescents took on similarly deferential roles with caregivers in their homes. Indeed, adolescents' treatment-taking, and caregivers' attempts to support it, were located in practices that reinforced family roles and obligations. In doing so, these care practices entailed a bolstering of social ties. Where illness is long term, and there is a scarcity of material and human resources for care, these social ties become central to how care is constituted.

ART AS A PRACTICE OF SOCIALITY IN THE HOME

A large majority (19) of the adolescent participants in our study had contracted HIV at birth. Many had since been orphaned by AIDS, while others were estranged from their biological parents. Eighteen adolescents in our study had mothers who were either dead or absent. Of these, all but two also lived without their fathers. As a result, 11 of the 18 are now cared for by grandmothers, often in combination with other relatives.

HIV treatment enters these homes after the family has undergone significant trauma. Our findings suggest that it is often adolescents' dead or absent mothers who are blamed under these circumstances. In South Africa, caregiving has for centuries been a responsibility borne disproportionately by mothers. Initially, years of migrant labour kept many men from their homes. In the post-apartheid context, escalating unemployment has limited men's ability to afford lobola and provide for families. Female-headed homes have been further entrenched, not only by declining marriage rates, but also increased access to social grants (for which women are the primary recipients). Hence, in many households grandmothers have replaced wage-earning men as economic linchpins (Bank, 2002: 641). The immense responsibility, shouldered by women, to run households and raise future generations also exposes them to blame should they be considered to have 'failed' in their duties. In relaying family narratives both to us as researchers and to their HIV-positive adolescents, older female relatives were often engaged in attempts to position themselves as morally capable care providers, sometimes shifting blame onto other (younger) women (Vale & Thabeng 2016; Vale et al., 2017). Although men were rarely on the scene, and the majority of homes in the study were female headed, the context in which care was constituted was nevertheless deeply patriarchal.

Some grandparents, uncles, and aunts in our study told stories of adolescents' dead and absent mothers having flouted tradition, behaved recklessly, or abandoned their responsibilities – with their child's inherited illness being one of the consequences. Some mothers had been completing school during their pregnancy and were considered too young to care for their babies. Others were demonised for having had a child outside of wedlock, their purported promiscuity, or their heavy drinking (Vale & Thabeng, 2016). Absent mothers were regularly accused of neglecting their children and negating their responsibilities. Bongani's (age 17) paternal aunt, for example, said: 'I would never give him [Bongani] away to his mom because she never really looked after him' (5 March, 2014).

Among those mothers who had died were those who had started

ART but were said to have failed in taking their treatment properly. Andile's (age 13) aunt told us: 'He [Andile] knows about his mother's death. I sometimes tell Andile when he doesn't take his pills that his mom also didn't take her pills and that's why she died' (7 March 2014). In these instances, dead mothers were held up as a 'warning' and an indication of what not to do. By referring to their mothers' mistakes, adolescents were encouraged to live responsibly with HIV. Wandi (age 19) told us this: 'She [my aunt] explained that my mom did not last long because she did not accept her status. She said if I also don't accept my status I won't last' (10 December 2014).

Many of these guardians described adolescents' adherence to ART as a way for them to demonstrate obedience and good discipline to their elders, and thereby avoid their mothers' fate (Vale & Thabeng, 2016). By diligently taking their medication, adolescents were offered the chance to 'redeem' the memory of their mothers who, despite their failings, were ultimately 'good' and 'loved them'. Thus, taking treatment would serve as a means to suture familial wounds and restore intergenerational forms of care and respect.

Like many other absent mothers in our study, Naledi's (age 18) mother was accused, by her grandmother, of having been sexually reckless, abandoning her AIDS-sick child and failing repeatedly on HIV treatment. During our interview with her, however, Naledi's grandmother was eager to illustrate to us that Naledi was not like her mother. She showed us this by referencing her ART-taking: 'She [Naledi] loves her treatment. She understands. She has learnt. She loves the treatment a lot. It's her mother who is bad at taking treatment. She throws them down the toilet. And that's why she got sick' (interview, 11 September 2013). Naledi's grandmother then went on to talk about other examples of Naledi's obedience and her contributions to the home: 'She cleans, she cooks, she put in the tiles in the doorway.' In this way, Naledi's grandmother aligned ART with other practices of care, home-making, and intergenerational respect.

Indeed, taking ART diligently was often narrated as an act of care and deference towards one's elders, rather than an act of autonomous empowerment. When Anele (age 13) was resisting taking his medication, his grandmother described him as 'not listening to her' (fieldnotes, 2

April 2014). Relatedly, when we asked Xolani (age 11) about why he took his pills so well, he said 'because Makhulu (grandmother) tells me to take them' (fieldnotes, 3 October 2014). Treatment-taking was firmly located within pre-existing structures of care, which needed to be nurtured in order to sustain care and support long term.

Adolescents in this study often expressly included discipline and protection as part of their articulation of care. Some adolescents described the act of 'checking up' on pill-taking as a form of positive caregiving. Nonkosi (age 17) said he appreciated that his grandmother 'guarded' him when he took his medication, describing how she would watch as he swallowed his daily dose (fieldnotes, 10 March 2014). Bongani (age 16) described, with affection, how his aunt did weekly pill counts to ensure that he was taking his pills properly (fieldnotes, 3 April 2014). When Lisa (age 19) told us about her deceased mother, she remembered fondly that her mother was 'always someone who knew where I was. Even when I went to play, she looked where I was playing [...]' (interview, 10 December 2014). As we saw in the clinic, to 'be seen' becomes essential to the experience of care. Not only are routine monitoring and constant oversight essential to the very nature of chronic illness management, but more so, in social contexts where the risk of feeling abandoned is great – perhaps due to overcrowded clinics, parental loss, or poverty – being 'seen' is a rare commodity, and an important source of dignity.

Hence, in both clinics and homes, relationships of care were often defined by consensual, hierarchical dependencies and forms of deference and discipline. The relationships were defined by mutual obligations and entitlements. Care had moral and material valence for both the caregivers and the cared for. Tied up with 'making a life' on ART was making a life with others — one that embedded itself in existing structures of care, respect, and authority.

COMMUNITIES: CARE AND SURVIVAL

Living with HIV, as with other long-term conditions, means locating biomedical treatment within the wider project of 'making a life' – sustaining health, livelihood, and sociality. Where resources are scarce, and survival precarious, building and sustaining networks of care becomes even more critical. This chapter has already discussed the ways in which adolescent participants and their families secured and experienced care in clinics and homes. In both spaces, being 'seen' and protected by caregivers in ways that might nurture caring relationships was important. But ART also linked adolescents and their families to other sources of care. Not only were adolescents in this study visiting clinics on a regular basis for pill collection, monitoring, and blood tests, many had also been enrolled in NGO-run support groups. In Mtembu's rural areas, this meant quarterly weekend-long gatherings filled with treatment literacy and psychosocial support. In Ridgetown, some of our participants attended weekly support group meetings. Both rural and peri-urban support groups dealt not only with the challenges of ART, but also assisted adolescents with schooling and family troubles. To add to this, all of the adolescent participants in our study had a community health worker or 'treatment buddy' occasionally visiting their home.

Beyond this system of ART support was a larger social services system. Participation in the former often helped one gain entry to the latter. Community health workers mediated access to a range of social grants on families' behalf: foster child grants, child support grants, and care dependency grants. Some families were referred for food parcels. For adolescents in this study, to initiate HIV treatment was to slowly enter into a web of caring connections that provided for their life and their livelihoods.

South Africa's expansive social welfare system is the largest in the region. The organisation of state assistance in South Africa aims to alleviate the plight of the country's poorest citizens by targeting those among them who are either unfit to work or are caring for children. The result is an arbitrary divide between the poorest households that have no state support at all and the otherwise very similar households that receive comparatively generous support simply because they include grant-eligible children, elderly persons, or disabled persons (Ferguson, 2013: 78). In many other homes, it is perversely the sick, the orphaned, the disabled, or the elderly who generate income, rather than young adults in the prime of their lives (Bähre, 2011: 383). Some families may rely on their youngest children for material support – those in whose names grants are available (Henderson, 2012).

In addition to childcare assistance, a few adolescents in our study also benefited from care dependency or disability grants on the basis of their HIV status, with many more hoping to apply. Thus, in this study, it is the youth, chronic illness, and sometimes orphan status of young participants that brings them under multiple forms of state paternalism. While these categories signal marginalisation and exclusion, at the same time they also bring youth on ART under unique state protection.

HIV-positive adolescents in this study have negotiated both the burdens and potential resources of HIV, as they work to make a life on ART. Some adolescents and their families have been able to mobilise their HIV and orphan status to tap into the resources and networks of a burgeoning AIDS industry, often with significant social stakes. Their ability to do this is historically located during a time in which the category of HIV orphanhood carries significant clout, both in the social grants economy and in the NGO industry.

This is not to say that illness and orphanhood do not place immense strain on the lives of adolescents and their families, but rather that the dynamics of making a life on ART are often complex and contradictory. I have written elsewhere (Vale & Thabeng, 2015) about how it is not simply in presenting themselves as HIV-positive that young people are stigmatised. Instead, the receipt of seemingly privileged care can itself provoke resentment in a context in which resources for care are scarce. The ability of HIV-positive adolescents to access HIV-targeted resources provoked conflict within, and between, families. Some also felt vulnerable to resentment from neighbours. This was attributable both to a context of generalised poverty and the uncomfortable confluence between desirable care and a stigmatised illness.

In our study, the worry that accessing care might attract community resentment was a source of significant stress among caregivers and adolescents alike. Aware of the perception that she was using Thembakazi (age 18) to add to her income, Thembakazi's grandmother made sure to tell us that she 'loved Thembakazi deeply', not because 'she's sick and getting a grant' (interview, 10 September 2013). She feared that her care for Thembakazi would be perceived as self-interested and exploitative because of the state support she received.

Similarly, Siya's (age 18) grandmother told us that when she returned home with a sick grandchild after her daughter's death, neighbours accused her of 'liking money' (fieldnotes, 7 October 2013). Amanda (age 13) said that since joining her HIV-support group, other children in her village had bullied her, saying she thought she was 'too big for her shoes'.

Fear of neighbours' 'jealousy' made some of our participants feel vulnerable to witchcraft. Indeed, two adolescent participants were, at the time of our study, consulting healers about the threat of neighbours' resentment. Both adolescents felt that their neighbours were jealous of their 'success' and survival, *despite* and perhaps *because* of HIV (Vale & Thabeng, 2015). Hence, for some adolescents and families in our study, the pursuit of care could be volatile and double edged. Accessing HIV-related care could threaten community relationships. For these adolescents and families, sustaining care meant managing a delicate balance: pursuing HIV care and wider networks of support, while also maintaining relationships with neighbours.

CONCLUSION

NCDs pose a growing threat to African health systems, which are already heavily burdened by infectious diseases, among others, and are often severely under-resourced. Rising chronicity has important implications for how we think about the provision of care on the continent: care will increasingly be long term and routine; it will necessarily span clinics, communities, and homes; it will need to encompass biomedical treatment, nutrition, and social support; and it will include both those who are acutely sick and those who are ostensibly well.

Despite growing rates of NCDs in Africa, little research has been conducted on what this might mean for the nature of care in these settings. This chapter suggests that there are lessons to be learned from experiences of HIV care, which is increasingly framed in terms of chronic illness management. It draws on ethnographic research with HIV-positive adolescents and their families, living in rural and peri-urban areas of South Africa's Eastern Cape. These adolescents and families have long-term experience managing HIV, and have found ways to claim and sustain care under volatile health system conditions.

Indeed, this chapter shows that where resources for care are scarce, unequal, and precarious, this has significant implications for how care itself is constituted. In overburdened health facilities, 'being seen' became a significant component of what it meant to access and experience care. Adolescents and families employed different tactics to gain the attention of health professionals, document their entitlements, and ultimately secure a consultation with a nurse or doctor. It was also important that one 'be seen' in the right ways: as patient, respectful, and compliant. Acts of deference bolstered the moral authority of health staff, boosting their sense of competence in a context where their own capacity to care was regularly called into question. In order for patients and health staff alike to 'be seen', we will need to increase the numbers of health workers in clinics and reduce waiting time to every extent possible. This will mean improving the efficiency and accessibility of pill collection and monitoring for chronic patients.

As in the clinic, sustaining care in the home entailed significant relational work and mutual obligation. Adolescents' disciplined pill-taking formed part of the myriad ways to obey and respect one's elders, contribute to the household, and strengthen familial ties. Reinforcing familial roles became particularly important in households where a generation had been lost and relations of care had been unsettled. Thus, larger contexts translated into how care was enacted. To provide a strong continuum of care for chronic conditions, we must view health systems as extending into homes, and find ways to support families in grappling with both the emotional and physical labour of chronic conditions in their homes.

The larger context also reflected in the moral economy of HIV care in adolescents' communities. While the stigma (and indeed the deaths) associated with the HIV/AIDS epidemic have placed strain on everyday social relationships, HIV/AIDS has also been attendant with a multitude of care responses at the household, local, national, and international level. ART, like any other chronic illness treatment, forms part of this everyday politics of survival and repair. Achieving care entailed that adolescents and their families mastered the bureaucracies of health systems and social services and built relationships with important gatekeepers, while also maintaining intergenerational and neighbourly ties. Making a life with chronic illness often required that adolescents repaired, appealed to, and guarded their attachments. This was made all the more complicated in that their ability to access HIV-specific resources, in a context of generalised poverty, could fuel resentment and threaten neighbourliness. We would do well to locate chronic care in Africa within a wider economy of material and social survival, in which there are significant stakes and inequalities.

REFERENCES

Bähre, E. 2011. 'Liberation and redistribution: Social grants, commercial insurance, and religious riches in South Africa'. *Comparative Studies in Society and History*, 53 (2), 371–392.

Bank, L. 2002. 'Beyond red and school: Gender, tradition and identity in the rural Eastern Cape'. *Journal of Southern African Studies*, 28 (3), 631–649.

Beckmann, N. & Bujra, J. 2010. 'The politics of the queue: The politicisation of people living with HIV/AIDS in Tanzania'. *Development and Change*, 41 (6), 1041–1064.

Bhorat, H. & Cassim, A. 27 January 2014. 'South Africa's welfare success story II: Poverty-reducing social grants'. *Brookings: Africa in Focus*, https://www.brookings.edu/blog/africa-in-focus/2014/01/27/south-africas-welfare-success-story-ii-poverty-reducing-social-grants/, accessed 8 November 2018.

Biehl, J. G. 2007. *Will to Live: AIDS Therapies and the Politics of Survival.* Princeton: Princeton University Press.

Bundy, C., 2015. 'The ANC and social security: The good, the bad and the unacknowledged', in Oxford: Department of Social Policy and Intervention, *Annual Zola Skweyiya Lecture*, 13 May 2015.

Campbell, C., Scott, K., Skovdal, M., Madanhire, C., Nyamukapa, C. & Gregson, S. 2015. 'A good patient? How notions of "a good patient" affect patient-nurse relationships and ART adherence in Zimbabwe'. *BMC Infectious Diseases*, 15 (1), 404.

Cohen, K. & Meintjes, G. 2010. 'Management of individuals requiring ART and TB-treatment'. *Current Opinion in HIV and AIDS*, 5 (1), 61–69.

Comaroff, J. 2010. 'Beyond bare life: AIDS, (bio)politics, and the neoliberal order', in Dilger, H. & Luig, U. (eds.) *Morality, Hope and Grief: Anthropologies of AIDS in Africa*, New York: Berghahn Books.

Coovadia, H., Jewkes, R., Barron, P., Sanders, D., & McIntyre, D. 2009. 'The health and health system of South Africa: Historical roots of current public health challenges'. *The Lancet*, 374 (9692), 317–834.

Denison, J., Banda, H., Dennis, A., Packer, C., Nyambe, N., Stalter, R., Mwansa, J., Katayamoyo, P. & McCarraher, D. 2015. '"The sky is the limit": Adhering to antiretroviral therapy and HIV self-management from the perspectives of adolescents living with HIV and their adult caregivers'. *Journal of the International AIDS Society*, 18 (1), 19358.

Donovan, K. 2013. 'The biometric imaginary: Standardization and objectivity in post-apartheid welfare'. CSSR Working Paper. Centre for Social Science Research, University of Cape Town.

Ferguson, J. 2013. 'Declarations of dependence: Labour, personhood and welfare in Southern Africa'. *Journal of the Royal Anthropological Institute*, 19 (2), 223–242.

Glasgow, S. 2012. 'The politics of self-craft: Expert patients and the public health management of chronic disease'. *Sage Open*, 2 (3), 1–11.

Henderson, P. 2012. 'AIDS, metaphor and ritual: The crafting of care in rural South African childhoods'. *Childhood*, 20 (1), 9–21.

Kaba, Z., Khamisa, N. & Tshuma, N. 2017. 'Age-group differences in risk perceptions of non-communicable diseases among adults in Diepsloot township, Johannesburg, South Africa: A cross sectional study based on the Health Brief Model'. *South African Medical Journal*, 107 (9), 797–804.

Kharsany, A. & Karim, Q. 2016. 'HIV infection and AIDS in Sub-Saharan Africa: Current status, challenges and opportunities'. *Open AIDS Journal*, 10, 34–48.

Lawn, J. & Kinney, M. 2009. 'Health in South Africa: An executive summary for the Lancet series'. *The Lancet*: http://allafrica.com/download/resource/main/main/idatcs/00011852:fa2b1f5c0a6f138890b44318c9328677.pdf, accessed 2 October 2018.

Magadzire, P. 2016. *Understanding the Dynamics of Accessing Chronic Medicines in the Public Sector: Implications for policy in South Africa*. PhD thesis. Cape Town: University of the Western Cape.

Mattes, D. 2011. '"We are just supposed to be quiet": The production of adherence to antiretroviral treatment in urban Tanzania'. *Medical Anthropology*, 30 (2), 158–182.

McGrath, J., Winchester, M., Kaawa-Mafigiri, D., Walakira, E., Namutiibwa, F., Birungi, J., Ssendegye, G., Nalwoga, A., Kyarikunda, E., Kisakye, S., Ayebazibwe, N. & Rwabukwali, C. 2014. 'Challenging the paradigm: Anthropological perspectives on HIV as a chronic illness'. *Medical Anthropology*, 33 (4), 303–317.

Meinart, L., Mogensen, H. & Twebaze, J. 2009. 'Tests for life chances: CD4 miracles and obstacles in Uganda'. *Anthropology and Medicine*, 16 (2), 195–209.

Mendenhall, E. & Norris, S. 2015. 'When HIV is ordinary and diabetes new: Remaking suffering in a South African township'. *Global Public Health*,

10 (4), 449–462.
Mkhay, R. 2018. *Medicine in the Meantime: The Work of Care in Mozambique*. Durham: Duke.
Naik, R. & Kaneda, T. 2015. 'Non-communicable disease in Africa: Youth are key to curbing the epidemic & achieving sustainable development'. *Population Reference Bureau*, https://assets.prb.org/pdf15/ncds-africa-policybrief.pdf, accessed 2 October 2018.
Nguyen, V. 2005. 'Antiretroviral globalism, biopolitics and therapeutic citizenship', in Ong, A. & Collier, S. (eds.) *Global Assemblages*. London: Blackwell, pp. 124–144.
Prince, R. J. 2012. 'HIV and the moral economy of survival in an East African city'. *Medical Anthropology Quarterly*, 26 (4), 534–556.
Poku, U. & Whiteside, A. (eds.) 2004. *The Political Economy of AIDS in Africa*. Farnham: Ashgate.
Rabinow, P. 1996. 'Artificiality and enlightenment: from sociobiology to biosociality', in *Essays on the Anthropology of Reason*. Princeton: Princeton University Press.
Rabkin, M. & El-Sadr, W. 2011. 'Why reinvent the wheel? HIV scale-up to confront non-communicable diseases'. *Global Public Health*, 6 (3), 247–256.
Richey, L. A. 2012. 'Counselling citizens and producing patronage: AIDS treatment in South African and Ugandan clinics'. *Development and Change*, 43 (4), 823–845.
Robins, S., Cornwall, A. & Von Lieres, B. 2008. 'Rethinking "citizenship" in the postcolony'. *Third World Quarterly*, 29 (6), 1069–1086.
Sherr, L., Cluver, L., Betancourt, T., Kellerman, S., Richter, L. & Desmond, C. 2014. 'Evidence of impact: Health, psychological and social effects of adult HIV on children'. *AIDS*, 28, 251–259.
Statistics South Africa (Stats SA). 2014. *Poverty Trends in South Africa: An Examination of Absolute Poverty Between 2006 and 2011*, Pretoria. http://beta2.statssa.gov.za/publications/Report-03-10-06/Report-03-10-06March2014.pdf, accessed 2 September 2018.
Street, A. 2012. 'Seen by the State: bureaucracy, visibility and governmentality in a Papua New Guinean hospital'. *The Australian Journal of Anthropology*, 23 (1), 1–21.
UNAIDS. 2013. *Report on the Global AIDS Epidemic: Joint United Nations Programme on HIV/AIDS*, http://www.refworld.org/docid/50eebaf52.html, accessed 2 October 2018.
UNAIDS, 2014. *The GAP Report 2014*, Geneva. Available at: http://www.unaids.org/sites/default/files/media_asset/UNAIDS_Gap_report_en.pdf.
UNAIDS. 2017a. 'AIDS info', http://aidsinfo.unaids.org/, accessed 2 October 2018.
UNAIDS. 2017b. 'Data Book', http://www.unaids.org/sites/default/files/media_asset/20170720_Data_book_2017_en.pdf, accessed 2 October 2018.

UNAIDS. 2017c. 'Ending AIDS: Progress towards the 90-90-90 targets'. http://www.unaids.org/sites/default/files/media_asset/Global_AIDS_update_2017_en.pdf.

Vale, B. & Thabeng, M. 2015. 'Mobilising AID(S)? Contesting HIV as a social and economy resource among youth in South Africa's Eastern Cape'. *Journal of Southern African Studies*, 41 (4), 797–813.

Vale, B. & Thabeng, M. 2016. 'Redeeming lost mothers: Adolescent antiretroviral treatment and the making of home in South Africa'. *Medical Anthropology*, 35 (6), 489–502.

Vale, B., Hodes, R. & Cluver, L. 2017. 'Negotiations of blame and care among HIV-positive mothers and daughters in South Africa's Eastern Cape'. *Medical Anthropology Quarterly*, 31 (4), 519–536.

White, H. 2012. 'A post-fordist ethnicity: Insecurity, authority and identity in South Africa'. *Anthropological Quarterly*, 85 (2), 397–427.

Whyte, S. R. 2012. 'Chronicity and control: Framing "noncommunicable diseases" in Africa'. *Anthropology and Medicine*, 19 (1), 63–74.

Whyte, S. R., Etyang, G., Kajubi, P., Kyaddondo, D., Meinart, L., Mogensen, H., Twebaze, J. & Whyte, M. 2014. *Second Chances: Surviving AIDS in Uganda*. Durham: Duke University Press.

Wolf, E. 1963. 'Kinship, friendship and patron-client relations', in Banton, M. (ed.). *Pathways of Power Building: An Anthropology of the Modern World*. London: Tavistock.

World Health Organization (WHO). 2013. *HIV and Adolescents: Guidance for HIV Testing and Counselling and Care for Adolescents Living with HIV*, http://www.who.int/hiv/pub/guidelines/adolescents/en/, accessed 2 October 2018.

World Health Organization (WHO). 2017. 'Non-communicable diseases: Key facts'. http://www.who.int/mediacentre/factsheets/fs355/en/, accessed 2 October 2018.

Zuger, A. 11 November 2003. 'What did we learn from AIDS?' *New York Times*, https://www.nytimes.com/2003/11/11/science/what-did-we-learn-from-aids.html, accessed 2 October 2018.

EIGHT

Knowledge, Power and the Role of Frontline Health Workers for South Africa's Epidemic Preparedness

Miriam Di Paola and Beth Vale

INTRODUCTION

Nurses and community health workers (CHWs) far outnumber doctors in Africa's health workforce. They are on the frontlines when epidemics strike. Investing in these frontline health workers has been identified as a key strategy for strengthening health systems and preventing future outbreaks (for example, of Ebola) (Perry et al., 2016; Sagar, 2015). During the 2014–2015 outbreaks of Ebola in Liberia and Sierra Leone, frontline health workers played important roles in screening and educating communities about the disease, at the same time as tracing active cases and contacts (Perry et al., 2016; Sagar, 2015), often at immense risk to their own lives. A substantial body of evidence further demonstrates the effectiveness of nurses and CHWs in managing malaria cases at community level (Corley et al., 2016; Paintain et al., 2014). Finally, despite early scepticism that an understaffed health system could effectively administer antiretroviral treatment (ART) in response to the HIV/AIDS epidemic, treatment programmes led by nurses and CHWs have halved AIDS death rates in South Africa since 2005 (Setswe, 2016). While initiating patients on ART, these frontline health workers have also led support groups to bolster treatment adherence and ensure long-term health (Mottiar & Lodge, 2018).

In multiple African contexts then, nurses and CHWs have played essential roles in bolstering epidemic responses at a community level. Nurses, in particular, also play an invaluable role attending to critical cases in hospitals, since doctors are often in short supply. Africa's epidemic preparedness rests heavily on its ability to retain frontline health workers, and create enabling environments so that they are able to perform at their best. Drawing on South African case studies of nurses in tertiary hospitals and CHWs in primary health care clinics, this chapter describes key systemic factors that constrain frontline health workers' ability to provide high-quality patient care.

Whether as nurses in hospitals or CHWs in clinics, the health workers we discuss in this chapter are patients' first and primary point of contact, and it is on this basis that we refer to them as 'frontline'. Yet, relative to other health workers in their facilities, they are also on the lowest rung of the professional hierarchy. Indeed, the under-recognition, and subordination, CHWs experience in relation to nurses in primary health care clinics mirrors what nurses in tertiary hospitals report experiencing from doctors. Both nurses and CHWs are overburdened and poorly paid, and their unique knowledge and experience of patients are often undervalued. Despite these similarities, there are also key differences between these two sets of frontline health workers: nurses have professional status (and their own professional hierarchies), accredited training, an established labour union, and full employment. In contrast, CHWs, who are recruited from the communities they serve, operate as lay workers, with highly tenuous job security and varying levels of training. Growing state reliance on CHWs to shoulder the burden of primary health care has been attended by a growing call for proper remuneration, accreditation, and employment benefits (Trafford et al., 2017). In Gauteng, and elsewhere, CHWs have publicly protested for labour rights (Molelekwa, 2016; Swartz & Colvin, 2014). As the scope of work for CHWs at a primary care level continues to expand, research needs to consider how CHWs accrue and deploy workplace knowledge, and under what constraints.

While much of the literature, and indeed the public media focus, has been on the need to improve skills among frontline health workers (Dawson & Joof, 2005; O'Donovan et al., 2018; Wu et al., 2017), this chapter argues that these workers are often constrained in their ability to deploy their knowledge. Beyond their training (which is comprehensive for nurses, and variable for CHWs), frontline health workers have unique expertise in enhancing the patient–provider relationship. Nevertheless, they are often diverted from this core area of their expertise. This is not only due to unmanageable workloads and struggles for workplace recognition, but is exacerbated by the interests of the 'new public management' that has attended the emergence of neoliberalism in public health systems; elevating cost cutting and administrative tasks at the expense of the caregiver–patient relationship has had a deleterious effect on health care.

The chapter draws on studies conducted by two researchers: Di Paola conducted ethnographic research with public hospital nurses in Johannesburg, from April to September 2017 and then in September and October 2018. She spent five months observing in two different wards – pulmonology and postnatal – in an academic hospital and, in addition, conducted 16 in-depth interviews with nurses[i] and key informants, including academics, nurse educators, one policy maker, and representatives from the health labour movement. Di Paola investigates what Sawchuk (2017, drawing on the work of Smith, 1987) calls the everyday knowing, working and judgement-making of nurses. Methodologically, she combines observation with the analysis of nursing labour process and with the political economy of health care provision (as in Valiani, 2012; White, 1993; and Norrish & Rundall, 2001).

Vale draws on a long-term (the past seven years) research engagement with CHWs: beginning with fieldwork conducted between 2011 and

i Health workers' and key informants' identities have been protected through the use of pseudonyms; only in the case of Dr Armstrong was a real name used.

2012 with CHWs in two Western Cape public health clinics (see Vale, 2012a; 2012b; 2012c), and later in 2013 with rural village health workers in the Eastern Cape (see Vale et al., 2017). This was complemented by a scoping review of the community health worker landscape, produced in 2018, for the DG Murray Trust's Zero-Stunting Initiative. While Vale's fieldwork is some years old now, South Africa is still in the process of formulating a national CHW programme. Vale's 2018 review reveals that challenges facing CHWs when the research was conducted have not changed very much. This has significant implications for the 'Re-engineering of Primary Health Care' and the formulation of the country's National Health Insurance (NHI).

The chapter begins with a description of the structure of the South African health system, which is characterised by stark inequalities, a heavy burden of disease, as well as class, race, and gender dynamics that mirror wider South African society. We then locate the challenges of frontline health workers who are positioned as 'mediators' between 'the community' and the 'health system', struggle to assert workplace authority, and must regularly negotiate professional, gendered, and race-based power relations.

Following this, we define the 'new public management' and describe how it has affected the everyday practice of frontline health workers. In public hospitals, cost-cutting imperatives associated with new public management worsen staff shortages and can result in patients' early discharge. Meanwhile, in primary health care clinics, the scope of work expected of underpaid CHWs is ever expanding. Frontline health workers find themselves overwhelmed by duties, struggling to juggle time spent on patients and paperwork.

As evidenced in both popular and academic literature, South Africa's frontline health workers are often described as incompetent, uncaring, or abusive (Honikman et al., 2015; Kruger & Schoombee, 2010; Khumalo, 2011; Seid, 2017; Zwane, 2017; Makhubu, 2016; Berquist et al., 2018). Without excusing patient mistreatment, this chapter illustrates how systemic pressures on health workers constrain and erode care. Frontline health workers in both Di Paola and Vale's studies felt that the core of their work, the caregiver–patient relationship, was displaced by heavy workloads, pressure to meet cost-cutting goals and therefore rush care, managerialism, and under-recognition of their specialised contribution.

SOUTH AFRICAN HEALTH CARE SYSTEM

Despite significant progress made in granting access to health care to the majority of the population, 25 years after the fall of apartheid South Africa is still battling with health outcomes that are similar to those found in lower-income countries.

Progress can be seen in that child mortality in South Africa reduced significantly from 74 deaths by the age of 5 per 1,000 live births in 2000, to 44 in 2013 (UNICEF, 2014). This may have been the result of the introduction of large-scale antiretroviral treatment post-2005 (Stats SA, 2018), but it has to be noted, nevertheless, that these results are similar to the low-income Democratic Republic of Congo (49 in 2013) and much higher than those reported by other upper-middle-income countries, e.g. Brazil (14 in 2013) or Algeria (25 in 2013).

South Africa is a country where access to health care is significantly unequal and overall inadequate when compared to the country's economic development (DoH, 2014). High levels of inequality, unemployment, persistent poverty, and a migrant labour system still in place characterise the socio-economic context.

The public hospital setting, which serves the majority of the population, is historically underfunded and beset by health worker shortages and patient overcrowding (Coovadia et al., 2009). Racial policies adopted during colonialism and apartheid led to a race-based division of health services into segregated establishments, subsequently exacerbated by the institution of separated Bantustans, each with its own health department and professional bodies. These had a great impact on the historical maldistribution of health professionals and on the unequal access to health services (Van Rensburg, 2014).

In 1994, the democratic government inherited a country marked by racial segregation, acute socio-economic inequalities, and highly unequal access to health. Major achievements have been made in the past two decades in the provision of health care: first, in transforming a segregated system into an integrated, comprehensive national health service (McIntyre & Thiede, 2007); second, in terms of a more equitable provincial funding distribution; third, in financing and provision of primary care (through the use of funds previously used in tertiary care rather than availing additional funds); and finally, yet highly significantly, affirmative action policies which made the public sector workforce more race representative (Baker, 2010). Policies aiming to redistribute health professionals towards primary health care have been implemented, for instance through compulsory service of post-secondary graduates. The result has been an overall increased use of health facilities by the most disadvantaged groups in society, most of whom rely on primary health care. In the past few years, the Department of Health (DoH) has been formulating plans to 'Re-engineer Primary Health Care' in South Africa (Barron et al., 2010; Morrell et al., 2011). These plans situate CHWs as drivers of primary health care services, offering peer education, treatment support, screening, and home visits, as well as referrals to social services. Often, the work of CHWs is supervised by a nurse.

These improvements have nevertheless been overshadowed by other shortcomings. Primarily this can be seen as the failure to address the fallacies of the private/public mix and the restriction in public spending (McIntyre & Thiede, 2007; Baker, 2010). Of the 8.7 per cent of South Africa's GDP that goes towards health, 4.5 per cent is spent subsidising the narrow segment on medical aid (16 per cent of the population) (Motsoaledi, 2018). This means that although South Africa spends as much as many European countries on health care, its health outcomes are not comparable, since much of its resources are diverted to a privileged minority of the population. As argued by McIntyre and Ataguba (2018), a macroeconomic policy that puts redistribution rather than discipline at the centre, and allows for the development and implementation of comprehensive social policies that modify living and working environments, is pivotal to address the failures of the health system and the maldistribution of health workers between private and public institutions, and between rural and urban settings.

Compounding, and in many ways emanating from these challenges is South Africa's quadruple burden of disease: HIV/AIDS and tuberculosis (TB); high maternal and child mortality; non-communicable diseases

(NCDs); and injuries linked to significant levels of violence and crime (DoH, 2014). These factors, exemplified in the poor health of the majority of the population, have a direct impact on the heavy workloads experienced by health workers and consequently on access to health care for the black majority (Breier et al., 2008; DoH, 2014).

During Di Paola's observation, several nurses pointed to the hardship of the public hospital setting as related to the quadruple burden of disease (Breier et al., 2008). Hence, Sister Smith, a professional nurse in pulmonology, explains that many patients are recurring patients dealing with multiple morbidities:

> *Many patients here have multiple diagnoses, for instance: one or several COPDs [chronic obstructive pulmonary diseases] together with embolism, and HIV. This happens because of permanently damaged lungs resulting from recurrent or poorly treated tuberculosis. The lungs are like cardboard! They can't clear the airflows from mucus because they lost elasticity; the phlegm sits there [in the lungs] and gets infected causing all sorts of diseases. Then there's nothing you can do to fully cure the lungs (Sister Smith, interview, 2017).*

Due to the severity of this quadruple burden of disease, nurses witness high levels of fatalities and morbidities. At the same time, because of cost-cutting policies, the institution is constantly overcrowded and health professionals, including nurses, are forced to make decisions with significant ethical aspect, regularly having to weigh up the quality and quantity of care provided.

At both primary and tertiary levels of health facilities, there is awareness that patients' poor socio-economic conditions dramatically impact on the functioning of wards and clinics. In an attempt to respond to the severity of patients' socio-economic circumstances, regular meetings are held in hospitals and clinics to assess their needs and, where appropriate, to arrange for social worker intervention. Austerity measures and a culture of cutting costs run counter to health personnel being able properly to address the socio-economic needs affecting their patients' health. In particular, patients are discharged early (nurses refer constantly to the mantra of 'emptying beds') which negatively affects their care. This practice is not aligned with patients' socio-economic needs, as this example confirms:

> *During the morning round, Sister Nancy tells me about the patients in most critical conditions ... During the round the consultant keeps discharging patients without consulting with Sister Nancy. She is staring at him without saying a word. He only says, without looking at her: 'We need the beds.' Sister Nancy tells me she doesn't think the patients discharged before doing the necessary exams will come back [for the exams booked after two or more days] because most of them don't have transport and discharging them on the same day means the nurses won't have the opportunity to arrange transport with the family or the hospital (field notes, 19 July 2017).*

Frontline health workers often feel overwhelmed by the needs of their patients, and often ill-equipped to address their scope. They constantly have to find ways to come to terms with unsuccessful care – whether in the form of non-adherent patients, helpless cases, or the deceased. Of course, the experience of being overwhelmed and overburdened is not particular to CHWs and nurses – doctors experience this too – but it affects health workers in different ways. Partly this is influenced by class dynamics and workplace power.

FRONTLINE HEALTH WORKERS AND THE SOUTH AFRICAN HEALTH SYSTEM

South Africa's public health care system is severely impaired by a crisis of production, recruitment, and retention of health workers, particularly nurses (Rispel & Bruce, 2015). Addressing the health workforce 'crisis' is central to responding to the gross inadequacy of access to health care in the country.

The nursing profession has high levels of attrition both during and after training, and particularly in the public health care system. Some nurses leave the profession to seek employment in other sectors of the economy or emigrate abroad (Rispel, 2015). Moreover, since the end of apartheid there has been a significant decline in the social and professional status of nursing (Blaauw et al., 2014: 18).

While shifting tasks to lay (community) health workers has served as one strategy to address staff shortages in nursing, turnover rates among CHWs often exceed 40 per cent (Nkonki et al., 2011). Much of this is due to the precariousness of their employment. During Vale's fieldwork, for example, a passionate CHW and HIV activist left her post to work at McDonald's, where she would have a lesser workload and greater job security (Vale, 2012b).

As the current standard in health care delivery in under-resourced African settings, community health worker programmes have been widely celebrated for their ability to improve the health of large numbers of people at low cost (Igumbor et al., 2011; Kabore et al., 2010; Nglazi et al., 2011; Williams et al., 2006). But this success depends on the ability of CHWs effectively to negotiate a highly onerous scope of work, and be retained in care work.

The understaffing of health workers, rather than being the result of a 'skills shortage', is a consequence of historical under-resourcing of public health facilities. This is exacerbated by organisational and power dynamics which ultimately disempower frontline health workers, and render them unable to use their specialised knowledge of patients.

Patient care represents the core of frontline health workers' specialised knowledge. Rather than being concerned about a 'skills shortage', attention should be paid to these health workers, who express confidence about their specialised knowledge and commitment to deliver patient care, to the point of servicing patients even beyond their scope (Le Marcis & Grard, 2015). Frontline health workers' roles also routinely include cultural mediation between patients and the health care setting. In both Di Paola and Vale's research, these workers expressed concern that this unique knowledge of the caregiver–patient relationship was not valued and that their work was evaluated based on administrative outcomes (this is referred to as managerialism) rather than patient care.

While most studies of professions focus on the specialised body of knowledge that underpins each profession (Freidson, 1989), they often overlook power relations in the workplace, including class and gender dynamics. These dynamics influence the capacity of workers in professions to assert their claim over specialised knowledge (Livingstone, 2014; Sawchuk 2017). Structural dynamics informing work in public health care, including the everyday practices of frontline health workers in deploying their specialised knowledge, deserve further attention in both academic debates and policy interventions.

PROFESSIONAL HIERARCHIES

Feminist scholars have highlighted the consistent devaluing of care across countries, including in relation to salaries and social status (Valiani, 2011). It has been argued that studies of the professions, in particular those concerning health workers, have sometimes reproduced the devaluation of women's work (Davies, 1996; Halford et al., 1997).

Historically, in South Africa as well as in the United Kingdom,[ii] nurses' legitimacy to make claims over knowledge and work has been linked to doctors' control and 'permission' for them to exercise these claims (Marks, 1994). Power relations in 1880s South African hospital settings were informed by strong gender/class dynamics and were also enmeshed in racial structures. If women were to perform biological and reproductive roles in the family structure, similar tasks were given to them in hospitals. The profession was highly gendered, as exemplified by Florence Nightingale's famous quote that 'To be a good nurse one must be a good women' (Nightingale, 1881). Moreover, it has been noted that the hospital setting mirrored the archetypical Victorian family, composed of the knowledgeable father-doctor, the caring mother-nurse, and the needy child-patient (Schneider et al., 2010; Marks, 1994).

The vast majority of nurses and CHWs in South Africa are black women. More likely to be unemployed (Stats SA, 2018) and often subject to gender-based violence (Dunkle et al., 2004; Kim & Motsei, 2002), the social, cultural, and economic power of black women in South Africa is regularly and powerfully undermined. Even when

ii The first nurses working in South Africa in the mid-19th century were British citizens linked to Christian orders. The first training institutions established in the country were also started by British sisters coming to South Africa to serve the motherland. In this sense nursing in South Africa shared a similar trajectory to that of nursing in the UK.

they are educated and employed (as nurses are), black women struggle to assert social and professional clout. In the case of CHWs, a lack of professional status and precarious employment are exacerbated increasingly by generational hierarchies, as rising numbers of young women enter community health work.

Vale observed that care delivered to older male patients by younger female CHWs, which often involved instruction, reprimanding, and probing into intimate bodily and behavioural functions, was not readily accepted. While CHWs experienced fewer difficulties asserting their authority over men in the clinic, the home space presented a significant challenge. Some CHWs reported being fearful of sexual violence when visiting a male patient. While none of the CHWs in Vale's study could recall there having been an instance of sexual assault in a patient's home, some had been sexually harassed. Male patients have overtly flirted with CHWs, phoning them at inappropriate times and professing their love to them. In one instance, a patient pulled down his pants in front of a CHW, and in another, a CHW was invited into a patient's home despite him being naked (Vale, 2012a).

Workplace power is defined by Livingstone (2014) as the capacity to direct oneself and command others to achieve the goals of an organisation. This influences the ability of professionals to enclose and make legitimate claims over a specialised body of knowledge. The class position of the professional, e.g. professional owner, professional self-employed, professional manager, and professional employee, and non-professional (in the case of CHWs), impacts greatly on the level of workplace power. As professional employees (in the case of most nurses) and lay workers (in the case of CHWs), frontline health workers tend to have very little or no control over the goals or the final service of their organisations.

In the context of her fieldwork, Di Paola noticed that despite being responsible for the functioning of the ward, nurses were not consulted when strategic decisions were being made about their patients. Their autonomy was limited to the pacing of their work, but even that was further limited by heavy workloads. Sister Hlubi points to this:

The thing is, I know, by the end of the day, I should have done

> *everything; done the reports, done the books, delegations, patients' rounds, medication rounds, vital signs, done the matron's report because I also have to do a matron's report. Yah. All the admissions, all the discharges, all the beds. By the end of the day, I should have accomplished everything so that when the night staff comes I am able to hand over to them (Sister Hlubi, 2017).*

In both the pulmonary and postnatal wards in which Di Paola observed, the subordination to doctors is evident and not always justifiable by knowledge differentials. For instance, medical interns may have the same years of training as registered nurses, but their knowledge of patients – their experiential knowledge – is not as thorough as that of nurses. Nevertheless, medical interns make decisions over treatments, medications, and procedures, often without consulting nurses.

Di Paola witnessed several occasions when nurses reported that what was written in patients' folders was not correct and had to be changed. For instance, during a medication round in the pulmonology ward, Sister Moyo put a large 'X' on what was written in the folder of a patient and wrote something else. During an interview, Di Paola asked Sister Moyo whether there was a mistake on the prescription that she was supposed to administer and, if so, who had made the mistake. She responded:

> *It was the doctor. The doctor prescribes but we are also trained about the medication. We know the rules and the regulations: you can give this to this patient, you can't give this other medication. If ever the patient, let's say is hypertensive, Brufen is a no-no because it's gonna make the patient worse ... Even the fluids, if ever the patient is hypertensive you can't give Ringer's lactate because it's gonna make him sky high. So you have to give normal saline which will stabilise the blood pressure of the patient ... Sometimes they [doctors] just do things without any insight. They just ask the patient: how you feel? They don't read, they don't check the folder and then they don't consult us (Sister Moyo, 2017).*

Also expressing frustration at nurses' subordination to doctors, one midwife in the postnatal ward said:

> *I do have a problem because the doctors don't want the advice from the nursing staff. They think they're better, they know everything. They forget that they come here for a short period. We are the ones who stayed with this patient for 12 hours ... Even if you are having an emergency, you're the one, we're the ones who start by attending the patient ... before the doctor comes. They don't trust anything that we tell them. They'll be busy telling you, 'You didn't do medicine, I didn't see you in Medunsa or Wits.' They really think they [are] better than us but they aren't (Sister Sindi, 2017).*

In both wards, Di Paola encountered nurses who described their nursing cohort as being scared of doctors. An advanced midwife she shadowed in the postnatal ward talked extensively about fear among her colleagues; she said that 'the hospital should offer training on building nurses' confidence' (fieldwork notes, 6 June 2017).

Similarly, as lay workers at the bottom of the professional hierarchy, CHWs in clinics struggle with confidence and with asserting their workplace knowledge. More so, the everyday proximity of carers and cared-for makes it difficult for CHWs to assert their authority or protect workplace boundaries. One of the Western Cape CHWs, Bulelwa, said:

> *Sometimes when you pass there [by the patients], or you do education, or you [are] just standing there outside, we'll hear what they are saying about us: 'These people they think they are clever. Why should they come to our houses?' Stuff like that. (3 June 2011).*

In saying that respondents 'think they are clever', patients may be pointing to CHWs' performed and ascribed superiority, which is used as a means of manufacturing social distance despite living in the same community. Without accreditation or professional status, the expertise that might underwrite CHWs' authority is called into question, both by patients and nurses. CHWs also lack those symbolic markers of authority bestowed on their professional counterparts through uniforms and technical instruments.

In the primary health care clinics where Vale observed, health professionals continued to refer to CHWs as 'volunteers', calling their training and job security into question. Many CHWs believed a lack of professional qualifications discredited their knowledge, and some cited instances in which their expertise was undercut by clinical professionals. Some resented having to translate for other clinic staff, arguing that this was not part of their job description (Vale, 2012a: 5). Others said nurses behaved like 'bosses', rarely giving CHWs credit for their contribution to patients' well-being (Vale, 2012a: 5).

THE KNOWLEDGE OF FRONTLINE HEALTH WORKERS

In recent years, South African public opinion has pointed to nurses' poor performance and to a diminishing ethic among nurses (Hall, 1994; Armstrong & Rispel, 2015). Dissatisfaction with nurses has become a mantra in the media and in the literature (Breier et al., 2008; Armstrong & Rispel, 2015), which points to a lack of commitment and preparedness. During Di Paola's observation, she found, in contrast to popular perspective, that nurses were highly confident about the professional knowledge acquired during their studies. Moreover, and as confirmed in several interviews, nurses consider their theoretical knowledge as empowering them in relation to other health workers, particularly doctors. For instance, in relation to pharmacology and nursing knowledge, Sister Hlubi explained that knowing your subjects and the medications well may save lives and it empowers you in the workplace:

> *If you get a patient coughing up blood and severe headache, I'm not going to wait for the doctor to come and prescribe morphine. Morphine is a schedule seven, a doctor needs to prescribe that but I'm going to give morphine, and call the doctor. When he comes I'd say, 'I've started morphine, just write it down' (Sister Hlubi, 2017).*

Nurses take pride in their qualifications, particularly in terms of theoretical and practical subjects. In the following quote, Sister Raja points to two important aspects of nurses' knowledge and qualifications: first, the complexity and intensity of the degree and, second, the importance of knowledge in claiming autonomy.

> *The first two years are like the stepping stones in nursing. When you get to third and fourth year it's when you are seniors, by then you have done a lot of theory: anatomy, physiology, psychology, sociology, community nursing, and fundamentals of nursing. From third year the course is way more pressurised and compact, then you must be independent, you have to do everything yourself, you have to make decisions. If I'm being immature, unknowing [it means I] can't be independent, responsible. If you don't know things you can't be independent. Knowing your subjects gets you into looking after a patient holistically. So, theory helps with that (Sister Raja, 2017).*

The nurses Di Paola interacted with valued their knowledge as a weapon to claim autonomy and assert power within a specialised body of knowledge – that is, the knowledge required to nurse patients. These data on nurses' perceptions of their education and knowledge, supported by the researcher's observation of their challenges at work, suggest findings contrary to the skills shortage discourse: professional nurses do not see their knowledge as weak and do not point to a need to strengthen their theoretical knowledge.

In the context of the 'nursing crisis' and the government's focus on the supply of nursing skills, findings pointing to the fact that nurses are confident of their knowledge of theoretical disciplines compels us to explore power dynamics in the workplace and in society with the aim of recognising nurses' knowledge-based contribution to the hospital setting. Livingstone (2014) points to the *continuum* of disempowerment certain professions may experience in society and in the workplace: if specialised knowledge in nursing is not socially recognised, it cannot be translated into workplace power.

Staff shortages and heavy workloads, as well as the wider imperatives of new public management (described in the next section), have direct consequences for nurses' ability to deploy their specialised knowledge through activities like patient education.

As part of their scope of practice, nurses educate patients on health, hygiene, nutrients and, in the case of postnatal care, how to breastfeed, monitor a caesarean section wound, and other important aspects of the mother's and child's health (see Esterhuizen, 2016). During Di Paola's observation, she appreciated how educating patients was something nurses always tried to make time for, as reflected in her fieldnotes:

> *While administering the immunisation, Sister Busisiwe explains every step to the patients. She takes the immunisation round as an opportunity to educate patients about the importance of early pregnancy detection and testing; she explains that they advise mothers to register at hospitals or clinics after the first period missed and to get tested straight away; in this case whether they are RVD or RPR positive, which may suggest HIV and syphilis respectively, they can start treatment and the child will be healthy. If they don't get tested they won't know if they are positive; in the case of syphilis, if they don't take medications the child may be born blind or have severe skin disorders (field notes, 16 August 2017).*

Today, due to shortages of doctors in South Africa's public health institutions, nurses' scope of work has extended to meet the needs of the population. In general terms, although South African nurses undergo longer training, due also to structural shortages of other health professionals, a tension remains as to what they are formally requested to perform in terms of nursing practice, and what they find themselves doing, the latter being more complex than what is institutionally acknowledged.

Educating patients takes a specific form in South African public health facilities. Nurses play the role of educators as well as translators. Their role blurs into one of cultural mediators reflecting the socio-economic inequalities, as well as the differences in terms of languages, and cultural beliefs between nurses and doctors in hospitals.

Nurses describe their role as facilitators in the communication between doctors and patients, first in terms of language, but also in terms of values and beliefs. This role is rooted in the history of nursing in South Africa, in which nurses were identified as conduits between Western and traditional medicine (Horwitz, 2013). In the ward, they play a highly specialised, albeit unrecognised, role as cultural mediators, as their predecessors did during colonial and apartheid times.

In order to understand this aspect of the work and knowledge of nurses, it is important to appreciate certain specific characteristics of the South African public hospital setting. It reflects society's divisions and inequities which are enmeshed with racial and class relations. The majority of patients in the hospital Di Paola conducted research in are black African and coloured people from disadvantaged socio-economic backgrounds, whereas doctors are mostly white, Indian or black foreign nationals. Communication between doctors and patients is impaired not only by language, but also by socio-economic and cultural divides. The nurses' mediator role between doctors and patients entails the mastering of scientific knowledge, English and African languages, as well as cultural differences. This is reflected in the following example:

> *During the patients' round in pulmonology the doctor was explaining to a 54-year-old woman, suffering cardiovascular diseases and lungs malfunctions, that she had to stick to a low-fat and low-carb diet. The patient would understand and speak English but she was visibly perplexed by the core message the doctor was trying to convey. Sister Hlubi, who was accompanying the doctors on their round, decided to explain to her what the doctor meant and gave her several examples of 'good food' and 'bad food'. By the time she was finished the doctors had already visited two more patients without Sister Hlubi (field notes, 26 June 2017).*

Combined with their language versatility, the knowledge nurses acquire during their studies gives them a unique ability to convey the required information in ways that patients can grasp more easily. At the same time, nurses share, or at least are profoundly aware of, patients' values and beliefs. They are positioned in a liminal space between scientific and cultural knowledge and because they master both they can mediate between the hospital setting's protocols and patients' needs.

Similarly, CHWs in Vale's study (see Vale, 2012c) felt confident in their ability to know and understand the needs of patients better than their nurse counterparts in the clinic. This is partly because they are recruited from the same communities as patients, and because they spend significant time in patients' homes. One CHW, Caroline, remarks: 'It is good [to work in the community where you come from] because you know your community. You know [...] their belief[s], their religions. [...] You must understand most of your people' (8 June 2011). CHWs believed their knowledge of their target population aided in the delivery of quality care.

As will be explored in the sections that follow, such unique caregiving skills are not part of the evaluation and auditing system. Instead, they are largely taken for granted or brushed off by other health professionals. Nurses find themselves in a position where they are asked to perform tasks that are not technically part of their scope of practice, even though they have become essential to delivering on this scope, e.g. translating and mediating. Yet these tasks are sidelined by the system, significantly undervalued, and go largely unrecognised. This lack of recognition of their expanded role aggravates nurses' low morale and stress levels.

NEW PUBLIC MANAGEMENT

Management reforms in health care, which have been taking place internationally since the 1980s, and in South Africa since the 1990s, have allocated greater power to managers. This has elicited concerns among health professionals, as efficiency and financial soundness goals have seemingly surpassed the need for patient care. Under the new public management, public services have been increasingly encouraged to behave like businesses, aimed at efficiency and performance management measured in terms of administrative rather than clinical goals.

New public management and managerialism have been a global feature of the restructuring of the state under neoliberalism (Saad-Filho & Johnston, 2005; Eagleton-Pierce, 2016), including the restructuring of health care provision (Norrish & Rundall, 2001; Valiani, 2012; Sawchuk, 2017). Public sector reforms started in South Africa with the first democratic Public Service Act, promulgated in 1994, and are still ongoing (Pearson et al., 2016; Naidoo, 2016).

Over the course of the 1990s and 2000s, several legislative and policy measures have been adopted to achieve new public management principles of efficiency, effectiveness, and accountability. Performance-based and results-orientated principles have been adopted, while market-based mechanisms to implement accountability have replaced democratic devices based on professionals' authority (Chipkin & Lipietz, 2012). These reforms have implied that managerial structures as well as the following of rigid procedures have gained importance in the running of the hospital, while professional employees are subjected to stricter accountability measures to achieve cost-containment and efficiency goals. As a result the role of managers, at different levels, acquired unprecedented importance (Klikauer, 2013) at the expense of the role of professional employees. In terms of labour relations and organisational structures, hospital employees, including health professionals, have been organised into a silo system of accountability and subjected to a management and evaluation system based on outcomes (Von Holdt, 2010; Carvalho, 2014; Chipkin & Lipietz, 2012). As a result, power relations in the workplace are altered by the adoption of new public management devices: while managers and managerial procedures acquire greater importance, clinical care drifts away.

As Di Paola's research indicates, the reforms that the public hospital sector has undergone internationally and in South Africa have had a profound influence on the labour process in terms of the nursing model adopted (Sawchuk, 2017). Nursing models included the total patient care model used in many institutions until the mid-1990s when it was largely replaced by task-based nursing when shortages of registered nurses began to be felt (Dr Armstrong, interview, March 2018).

Historically, there has been an assumption that professional health workers only look after patients, somewhat overlooking the cost impacts of clinical activities, while administrators focus on the financial and organisational soundness of hospitals and overlook clinical results. Recently, clinicians have critiqued the growing power of managers and 'managerialism' for focusing on financial orthodoxy thereby compromising the quality of their clinical practice (Doherty et al., 2014). The displacement of the nurse–patient relationship that nurses point to may result from an over-emphasis on efficiency at the expense of quality care.

The nurse–patient relationship has always been a fundamental aspect of nursing (Henderson & Jones, 2017). Nurses establish and maintain this relationship, drawing on their professional knowledge and skills and, at the same time, applying the fundamental ethical principles of nursing care. The main ethical principles, as defined by the nurses' scope of practice, relate to the protection of the patients' rights (as human rights) and the empowerment of patients, even beyond their stay in the hospital setting, specifically through patient education (DoH, 2013). Always having been centred on the nurse–patient relationship, the nursing profession in South Africa underwent a significant broadening of its scope in the last three decades of the 20th century, as reflected in the regulations to the Nursing Act of 1978, issued in 1984 and amended in 1987, 1990 and 1991 (SANC, 1978) in relation to the nursing curriculum and the nursing practice.

Structural dynamics, such as organisational and managerial reforms ascribing to new public management, have greatly impacted on the running of the public hospital setting and on nurses' work (Von Holdt, 2010; Carvalho, 2014). These dynamics may not be mirrored in the formal scope of practice, yet they have prompted significant change in nurses' actual work and knowledge. The material and organisational conditions under which nurses work are reshaping their practice away from the nurse–patient relationship and towards a greater emphasis on administrative and managerial tasks, based on efficiency and cost containment.

Vale's (2012c) research suggests that the mandate of efficiency, cost containment, and administration has placed similar pressures on CHWs in primary health care clinics. This is exacerbated by the fact that many CHW programmes, including the one studied by Vale, are co-funded by major international donors who set their own targets and reporting standards.

In the sections that follow, we outline how cost cutting, along with the prioritisation of particular performance measures, have delimited frontline health workers' ability to provide quality care and fully utilise their expertise.

Cost cutting

Although much of the debate on the nursing crisis is tilted towards skills shortages, austerity measures and cost-containment goals at the provincial level, and consequently at the hospital level, are major contributors to the crisis. In fact, despite the greater role acquired by hospital managers and managerial structures, hospital CEOs have little autonomy when it comes to budgets. In his research on the role of hospital CEOs under new public management, Naidoo (2016: 115) argues that:

> *As far as staffing is concerned, CEOs in the majority of provinces can replace staff that leave during a financial year, but any new staff appointments have to be motivated for at head office*[iii] *... All new posts and unfunded vacant posts need to be approved by head office before filling them.*

Budget cuts for tertiary hospitals, like the one in which Di Paola conducted fieldwork, are aggravated by the shifting of resources from tertiary to primary health care, in order to redress the legacy of apartheid without increasing expenditures. As a result, Von Holdt and Maserumule (2005) argue that in tertiary care institutions shortages of nurses are rampant, and today public health workers are subjected to workloads that are, overall, far greater than those experienced by those who work under market pressures in manufacturing and other private industries.

Nurse shortages in an institutional environment marked by new public management translate into heavy workloads and stressful conditions, which add to nurses' emotional labour (Schneider et al., 2010). Shortages in the health profession, particularly the shortage of nurses, have significant consequences on workloads, nurses' work satisfaction, and, ultimately, service delivery (Khunou & Davhana-Maselesele, 2016). In Di Paola's interaction with nurses, she observed that they perceive the workloads they are subjected to as unbearable:

> *This week I did night shifts. I worked 84 hours ... in a week ... and it's too much for a normal human being, it's too much. And they expect you to excel in everything (Sister Busisiwe, 2017).*

---

iii Head office refers to the provincial Department of Health, which liaises directly with the National Treasury.

Health worker shortages at the hospital level are exacerbated by poor information systems on recruitment and retention of health professionals, particularly nurses (Rispel & Bruce, 2015). This was confirmed by one of my key informants, a health researcher, who said:

> *Major shortages of health workers that affect public health are only partly documented because of a lack of updated standards and norms on the minimum number of health workers required for each clinical setting (Dr Armstrong, interview, April 2017).*

This key informant had been involved in a study on nursing norms commissioned by the Department of Health; the study was indeed aiming at identifying the right number of nurses needed in a hospital setting, considering the population to cater for. The informant explained that:

> *When the study released the first figures to head office, those figures were dramatically higher than the number of nurses actually employed. As a result of the discrepancy between the number of nurses needed and the capacity of the national or provincial departments to release additional funds to create more posts, the recommendations were not implemented. The study was interrupted (Dr Armstrong, March 2018).*

Cost-cutting measures remain pervasive not only at the provincial DoH head office but also at the level of the hospital. A culture of austerity may trigger the early discharge of patients. During Di Paola's observation, early discharge was suggested several times in order to make space for new patients and to meet cost-saving goals. Often patients were discharged even when not fully recovered and asked to come back to do the exams necessary to establish a medical therapy. This is reflected in the fieldwork notes:

> *During the morning round, a patient suspected to have a lung tumour is waiting for a CT scan. The consultant asks the registrar (and not Sister Nancy) if they have enough beds to keep the patient*

> *until he gets the scan. The registrar responds: 'We're just surviving.' Hence, the consultant tells the patient she can go home and come back in two days for the CT scan (field notes, 19 July 2017).*

This excerpt reveals a practice in which nurses are asked to arrange early discharges in order to meet cost-cutting goals. Such a practice creates ethical dilemmas for nurses as they are, according to the Nursing Scope of Practice (South African Nursing Council, 2005), fully responsible and accountable for 'the provision of comprehensive nursing treatment and care', 'protection of the human rights of individuals and groups within the health care environment', as well as for 'the creation and maintenance of an enabling environment for ethical practice'.

Cost-cutting and staff shortages have also been central to the debates surrounding a national level community health worker Policy Framework (DoH, 2017), which will be a crucial component of delivering on primary health care. On the one hand, government, which has often outsourced the employment of CHWs to NGOs, has been encouraged to employ CHWs more directly to standardise the programme across the country and grant decent wages. This would also be a cost-efficient way to deliver on many of the ambitious primary health care goals. But cost-cutting incentives will also limit the number of CHWs that can be employed. Already, draft policy prescriptions about household coverage and CHW workload are of major concern. Most recent suggestions are that each CHW will be responsible for 250 households, with little indication as to how often these homes should be visited. To add to this, CHWs' scope of work is intended to include HIV/TB care, maternal and child health, chronic illness support, lay counselling, household screening, health promotion, palliative care, social service referrals, and administrative tasks. Many worry that the management of these tasks will result in reduced contact with patients overall (Vale et al., 2017).

The hardships incurred from cost cutting are exacerbated by the socio-economic conditions of South Africa's public health patients. The vast majority of public health care users are socio-economically vulnerable (Nambiar & Mander, 2017). From this point of view, heavy workloads in the context of cost-cutting measures, such as early discharge, expose nurses and community health workers in public health settings to renewed strains linked to emotional labour (Valiani, 2012; Smith, 1992) and related stress.

As Di Paola notes, nurses are aware of their contribution to the functioning of the ward and the fact that taking leave, including sick leave, may have a negative impact on the work of the other nurses. Moreover, shortages impact on the way in which shifts are organised and have important consequences for nurses' lives beyond the workplace, as well as affecting their morale. Sister Sindi in Di Paola's study points to: 'The worst part of our job is little family time. The shifts can be awkward and difficult to organise your time when you're not at work' (Sister Sindi, 2017).

Community health workers in Vale's study also felt a heavy emotional burden about being unable to relieve their patients from the stresses of poverty. One CHW, Miriam, said:

> *Yoh! You feel bad, man. You feel bad. It seems you can take the client with you to stay with you. But even you [...] like I'm earning this stipend. How can you take another person to stay with you? You get so little money (Miriam, 24 May 2011).*

Jacob, another community worker, described his emotional distress in this way:

> *You refer the patient [...] The social worker played his/her own role into this situation. [But] still the problem is still there [...] and there's nothing I can do about it. That is what is killing me the most (Jacob, 29 April 2011).*

In a 2017 scoping review, Vale found that this experience continues to be reported by numerous CHWs across the country, and that many spend up to 5 per cent of their small stipend assisting patients with basic household needs.

Paperwork

In the context of new public management, performance measures in the form of extensive reporting and auditing are believed to ensure the viability of health care practice. Meanwhile, the caring work of frontline health workers including their role as translators, cultural mediators, and educators often remains invisible to the health care system, hospitals, and clinics in which they work (Toffoli et al., 2011), precisely because it goes unmeasured. The reality of staff shortages and heavy workloads, described earlier, is also characterised by an emphasis on administrative tasks.

Di Paola observed the increased pressure this put on nurses, who would occasionally respond to these pressures by rushing nursing tasks in order to resume and complete administrative tasks by the end of their shifts. As a result, a causal relationship can be drawn between heavy workloads, the emphasis given to administrative tasks, and the compromise to nurses' core activities. This is exemplified in the following excerpt of Di Paola's fieldwork notes:

> *At the end of the meeting that we attend together, Sister Hlubi gets back to her morning reports: she is late in submitting them. Soon a patient arrives in a mobile bed; he's been sent from ICU without notice. Sister Hlubi has to organise for him to be admitted and to record admission before getting back to her reports. The patient suffers from asthma. He must have had a severe asthma attack. He needs to be on oxygen and has a catheter. The patient arrived naked from ICU, he needs to be dressed. Sister Hlubi helps the auxiliary nurse to find him a bed (they get one from a female cubicle). Then she approaches the patient, addresses him in isiZulu, she prompts him to stand up and seems impatient because he struggles to follow her instructions. She swiftly takes the oxygen out, helps the patient getting dressed and puts the oxygen back on. Her manners are harsh (fieldnotes, 6 July 2017).*

As Sister Hlubi would later explain, she had been under pressure to submit her reports. Yet, as the shift leader, she was also the one best positioned to admit the patient and stabilise him. Drawing on her nursing ethics and knowledge, she put aside her administrative responsibilities and attended to the patient's needs first. She wanted to make sure the patient was stable and secured on his bed. In a context of heavy workloads, the nurse decided to prioritise her core nursing tasks over her administrative tasks, and as a consequence was brisk and disrespectful to the patient.

Despite the assumption that nurses need to be upskilled to keep up with the changing needs of the hospital settings, in the course of Di Paola's fieldwork, she noticed that new public management has entailed routinisation and new forms of control over nurses' work due to the emphasis given to strict procedures, data capturing, and reporting. According to Gorman and Sandefur (2011: 282), 'rationalisation and codification also have implications for expert occupations' ability to maintain control over 'their bodies of knowledge'. In the case of nurses, strict procedure and the focus on 'paperwork' come at the expense of the nurse–patient relationship which lies at the core of nurses' specialised body of knowledge, thus challenging the scope of nurses' professionalism. An excerpt from a discussion with Sister Smith is illuminating:

> *Sister Smith tells me how much she hates her job and she states that she does it only to service the patients although nobody seems to care. 'The pay is terrible and your work is never acknowledged. The biggest problem is management, even your own area manager attacks us all the time. It doesn't matter how many people in terrible conditions we treat ... they come with health, family, and all sort of problems that make our work even more difficult but that doesn't matter, it's only about papers. "The papers aren't right, you can't write a proper report," that's what they [management] say. 'And we never stop writing, we compile reports all the time and then we have to submit a paper on each report we have written' (field notes, 21 June 2017).*

Nurses talk about ever more pressing obligations to follow strict procedures and document every single decision they make and task they perform. During their day shift, nurses take vital signs every four hours, and again three times a day when they give medications to the patients. Each and every task performed and all information collected is captured in the patients' files. In addition to writing their activities in the patients' files, nurses write three reports per day where they fill in all the tasks performed. For each report compiled they have to write a letter stating that the report was submitted. The same protocol applies to the night shift.

As a result of changes in the health system and in the institutional environment, including a new emphasis on administrative and managerial tasks, nursing professional skills as well as the founding ethical principle of the profession, of treating the sick, may be eroded. Professional nurses are constantly under pressure to make decisions as to whether they should prioritise their core nursing activities or their administrative tasks (Sawchuk, 2017).

The monitoring and evaluation system in place perpetuates fragmentation, and emphasises administrative tasks over nursing work. As results-orientated practices are adopted, results-measuring processes, such as performance management, acquire importance in the running of the hospital and in the organisation of nurses' work. At the same time, clinical activity receives progressively less attention than the following of rigid protocols. Moreover, nurses are subjected to two types of evaluation: the auditing of nursing units based on the National Core Standards for Health Facilities in South Africa (2011) and the evaluation of the individual nurse through the Nursing Records and Performance Management and Development System. According to one of Di Paola's key informants, an academic researcher in nursing, both require following long processes of recording and reporting, but fail to mirror the amount and the quality of nursing activities performed in the workplace: 'professional nurses end up nursing papers not patients' (Dr Armstrong, interview, 2018).

The ward-auditing system reinforces the emphasis on administrative tasks at the expense of nurses' relationship with patients. Wards are audited often and without warning. Audits, or inspections, may be performed by an external or internal inspection team or as part of an internal self-assessment process. The so-called five keystones of the auditing process are: the client, teamwork, focus on data, focus on system, and processes. The auditing consists of an examination of the compliance to data capturing protocols and reporting systems.

Overall, the auditing and evaluation systems contribute to the displacement of the nurse's relationship with patients. As we have shown in the previous sections of this chapter, structural changes in public health provision have had a pervasive impact on the organisational environment of the hospital as well as on the culture of clinical care provision. These changes pose new challenges to the professional power of nurses in the workplace, and in society, as they negotiate social recognition of their specialised body of knowledge. The new hospital organisational structure and its culture, and what these entail in terms of work intensification, fragmentation, and the principles underpinning work evaluation, do not stem from professional principles and values but from a managerialist approach to service provision, as it is seen in studies on professionalism in the neoliberal era (Carvalho & Santiago, 2015; Baines et al., 2010). As happened in other contexts, for instance among Ontario nurses working in public health in Canada as studied by Sawchuk (2017), new public management reforms deeply affect professional power by affecting workplace practice, even if they do not entail substantial formal adjustments to the professional scope of practice. Rather, adjustments occur in the form of 'a dynamic that changes ongoing professional judgement-making, changes the professional practice of attention and dis-attention to specific tasks, skills and knowledge in such a way that professional knowledge (and identities) as a whole become significantly reformulated' (Sawchuk, 2017: 13).

A very similar set of managerial practices have entered South Africa's primary health care clinics. As a result of funders' reporting requirements, the success of CHW care programmes, like the one Vale observed, is often measured in terms of outcomes, particularly the number of patients enrolled, visited, and retained in the system. Quantifiable proof is required in order to demonstrate work completed. 'We are told that it is important to fill in the forms because [...] it's proof [...] there are funders to the organisation, so you need the forms [...] as back up that you are doing the job,' said Jacob, a 23-year-old community health worker (28 June 2011).

While the utility and efficacy of the care provided is assessed on the basis of quantitatively reported outcomes, the content of care appears to be given less attention. Illustrating the potential consequences of this, Andile (another male CHW) spoke about the number of home visits he completes per day:

> *The most I've done on one day was 11. Because why? Sometimes you don't find the people, so there's no wastage of time. Then you*

> *go to the following [visit]. Sometimes you do find six out of those 11 [patients at home]. So four they are also visits even though [no one was home] (interview, 7 June 2011).*

Here Andile suggests that when he does find his patients at home, it is possible that time might be 'wasted' talking. But if no one is home, 'there's no wastage of time' and the visit is still recorded in daily statistics. Hence cost efficiency is measured in terms of the number of visits a CHW is able to complete (or, more accurately, report) in one afternoon. Ironically, this goal is impeded when CHWs spend quality time with patients.

Hence, in an effort to provide good care (defined by meeting measurable targets), CHWs run the risk of providing an uncaring service. While Andile's excerpts seem to imply a commitment to outcomes-based, quantity-driven care, it may be that Andile is simply expressing the pressures of working within a target-driven paradigm. His supervisors expect reports that reflect a high number of visits completed.

Similarly, while nurse supervisors and managers of the CHW programme promote a target-driven, measurable, and numbers-orientated approach to care in order to meet the reporting needs of funders, they also make claims that CHWs should be compassionate and take their time. This further highlights the tensions and complexities of the prescribed practice of care. Joan, a supervisor of the CHW programme, said this:

> *If you've been to a clinic, everything happens fast and there's very little time that this Sister and this counsellor can spend with a patient. So if we can get that relationship building [...] with the CHWs – because you do find patients saying, 'You know what, I didn't have a chance to ask the Sister this' (17 March 2011).*

The trouble is that this relationship building, which clinic-based nurses no longer have time to do (and was in this instance deferred to CHWs), is eroded regularly by the demands of managerialism. As with the hospital nurses in Di Paola's study, Vale observed that CHWs were similarly burdened by administrative work. The quantity of paperwork that CHWs were expected to process meant that 50–60 per cent of carers' daily activities were consumed by administration. The paperwork load had become overwhelming for many CHWs, who complained of having no time for their families or part-time study. 'We are not laptops,' Miriam, a CHW, remarked.

RESISTANCE

Despite relatively little power in the professional hierarchy, frontline health workers in both Vale and Di Paola's research felt a great responsibility towards patients and tried to put their patients' interests first. As Sister Nancy explained:

> *The patient doesn't know things, he cannot talk. I need to talk on behalf of the patient. When we were in college they used to tell us, 'You are the advocate of that patient' (Sister Nancy, 2017).*

In so doing, nurses draw on their professional knowledge and scope of practice to assert their specific role and related power (Carvalho, 2014). During Di Paola's fieldwork, she noted that older and highly experienced professional nurses or specialised nurses, such as advanced midwives and neonatal nurses, took very seriously the need to resist subordination to doctors. It may take a deferential form, consistent with the historical role played by nurses in hospitals, or it could also take a more confrontational form, as Di Paola observed in the postnatal ward. Here, interactions between nurses and doctors are less structured and they appear more confrontational. There are advanced midwives who feel entitled to carry out certain procedures, e.g. inserting a drip, and who express disapproval about what they perceive as under-recognition of their work and practical knowledge.

In the context of managerialist-driven adjustment to the nursing practice in the workplace, drawing on scientific knowledge to challenge subordination, and putting patients first, as in the traditional professional scope of nursing, could be seen as avenues of resistance. When nurses put the interests of patients first and use this to challenge authority they are also stating the centrality of nursing care to protect their professional boundaries and to reassert power in the workplace as based on their professionalism.

In certain instances, as seen among some nurses in Portugal in response to new public management reforms, nurses use professionalism as a tool of resistance:

> *The way care, and the scientific knowledge associated with it, is identified as the specific domain of nursing, is a strategy to retain control and autonomy over their work in the face of the presence of potential threats from management (Carvalho, 2014: 532).*

Although they are under pressure to submit reports several times a day, Di Paola observed instances in which nurses resisted the pressure and prioritised patient care. The alternative to this scenario is to accept the fragmentation and delegate a large part of their core nursing activities to nurses' auxiliaries, who have a lower level of training. Nurses were often torn between different activities and tasks and had to make constant decisions on what to prioritise. This entailed new forms of judgement-making in which they had to negotiate an ethical dilemma: continue nursing patients as they have learned to do, or give up that role and focus on the administrative tasks by which they will be evaluated. Despite the pressure to write and submit reports, nurses may try to organise their work in a way that their nursing tasks are dealt with first. This is one of the ways in which nurses assert their professional power and specialised knowledge, amid managerial pressures. The conflict between managerialism and professionalism may well affect the pace and quality of a nurse's performance.

Similarly, Vale (2012c) observed that CHWs in primary health care clinics sought strategies to resist administrative demands. Like many CHWs, Caroline felt immense anxiety at the prospect of returning to the clinic with nothing to report. Despite her supervisors having condoned it, she did not subscribe to the practice of recording as visits cases in which patients were not found. This was her subtle tactic for protecting the definition of care having been provided. Articulating his frustrations with the target-driven reporting demands, Andile, another CHW, said:

> *The most important part [of my job], they [our supervisors] say it's the visitation. But the most important part to me is not about the visits. It's about are they doing well? Are they taking their medication correctly? (7 June 2011).*

Amid a highly bureaucratised system of care, CHWs found ways to strategise and improvise, appeasing authorities while attending to other pressures (see also Livingstone, 2012). Sinazo, a Western Cape CHW, admitted that she sometimes cheated the system, choosing not to fulfil all the paperwork requirements: 'I'm not doing all the paperwork [...] I don't follow all those procedures' (17 May 2011).

CONCLUSION

Drawing on case studies of community health workers and hospital nursing professionals in South Africa, this chapter has argued that, despite the vital contribution, and unique knowledge, held by these frontline health workers, structural dynamics related to professional hierarchies, historical underfunding of public health services, and new public management have served to undermine the care that health workers provide. As a result, retention of these essential care providers is threatened along with patient care. This has indelible consequences for epidemic preparedness, both in South Africa and further afield. More so, given that nurses and community health workers are the core of health staff across Africa, the implications of these South African case studies are far-reaching.

Experience from epidemic outbreaks in resource-limited settings illustrates how essential it is that frontline health workers are able to prioritise the patient–provider relationship. When a cholera epidemic strikes in Haiti, for example, nurses are reported to be in far greater demand than any other health professional (Fisher et al., 2014). The key functions for nurses during a cholera outbreak include direct patient care, offering counselling and emotional support to patients, as well as family education. As this chapter has illustrated, these functions are also at the core of South African nursing practice, but are thwarted by underfunding, managerialism, and under-recognition (Fisher et al., 2014).

Similarly, the success of CHWs in combating the Ebola epidemic, particularly in Liberia, has been attributed precisely to the fact that they were embedded in communities. Following the height of the Ebola outbreak, public health experts recommended greater investment in CHWs (Perry et al., 2016). In order to be effective, however, these investments would need to ensure that the relationships between CHWs and communities are maintained. The same will be true to ensure the ongoing efficacy of community health worker programmes in South Africa.

Di Paola's fieldwork has provided significant insights into contemporary constraints on South African nursing practice, and specifically into factors which could affect the readiness of these frontline health workers to assume roles of countering epidemics if or when they occur. Most scholarly work on professions focuses on the specialised body of knowledge that underpins a profession, but overlooks the power relations in the workplace that influence the capacity of professionals to assert their claim over specialised knowledge (Livingstone, 2014). In the case of power dynamics between nurses and doctors, Di Paola observed a tension between the institutionalised subordination of nurses to doctors, and the practised power of nurses who often have to make decisions in the interest of patients in the absence of doctors. Nurses use their knowledge to make these types of judgements, but they may be doing so in contravention of formal regulations, stretching their scope of practice. Considering the level of biomedical scientific preparation nurses undergo in their four-year studies and the knowledge they further acquire in the workplace, extending the scope of practice for experienced nurses could be envisaged; this could aim at including powers and decision-making processes that already take place in practice.

Despite some differences between the pulmonary and postnatal wards, the labour process and the related power dynamics in both shared several similarities. Di Paola observed that nurses' daily working, making judgements, and knowledge (Smith, 1987; Sawchuk, 2017) were largely influenced by structural economic conditions due to cost-containment goals, such as early discharge of patients and 'managerialism'. The material conditions and institutional setting under which nurse employees work affected their ability to make legitimate use of their multidimensional knowledge, to establish a sense of reward and belonging to their professional work, and ultimately to do their work well. The nurse–patient relationship was affected and as a result patient treatment was impaired. The chapter has argued that, due to pressures emanating from managerialism, including diminished power in the workplace, under-recognition, and cost-cutting goals, the core of nursing knowledge is displaced and the nurse–patient relationship is affected.

Vale's (2011/2012) fieldwork, as well as her recent review (Vale, 2018), suggests that many of the dynamics that Di Paola observed among nurses in tertiary hospitals are mirrored for CHWs in primary health care clinics. These dynamics are critical considerations in ensuring high levels of preparedness of health care systems in the event of epidemics outbreaks. At the centre of CHWs' role in clinics is their unique relationship with patients. Relative to other staff in the clinic, they spend the most time with patients, and have unique knowledge of their needs, context, language, and culture. CHWs are the only members of the clinic staff who visit patients' homes. CHWs must find tactical and sensitive ways to assert their workplace knowledge and authority in contexts where they are not only intruding on patients' private lives but are also often recognised members of the patient's community. Despite what CHWs gain from the time spent in patients' homes, they often feel their expertise, and experience, are dismissed by the clinic when important decisions are being made about patients. Without accreditation, uniforms, or even secure employment, CHWs struggle to make a case that their knowledge is valuable. To add to this, the work of patient care, where their experiential knowledge lies, is often eroded by unrealistic targets for the number of patient visits to be completed per day, and the paperwork burden they have to carry.

This chapter has shown that the essential, and unique, contribution of frontline health workers to the functioning of South Africa's public health system is being undermined by a number of significant structural burdens: first, that their work is undervalued and often unrecognised. This is frequently tied up in professional hierarchies, as well as their class, race and/or gender position relative to other health staff. Second, cost-cutting imperatives, heavy workloads, and numerous administrative tasks burden frontline health workers with significant dilemmas: having to choose between direct patient care and meeting the requirements of their supervisors. These pressures have significant implications not only for the retention of frontline health workers, but ultimately for patient health outcomes in situations of outbreaks of epidemics.

Any successful strategy for the future of South African health care, and indeed epidemic preparedness across the continent, will need to nurture and strengthen frontline health worker programmes. It must prioritise patients over paperwork, pursuing clinical and care goals, rather than efficiency and cost-saving targets. In addition, it must work to address class and gender injustice, both beyond and within health facilities. Empowerment of frontline health workers should be institutionalised and governing bodies, from the national treasury to national and provincial departments of health, should come to terms with the fact that in many cases poor health outcomes and health provision failures are systemic, as outlined in this analysis. Finally, frontline health workers should be recognised, valued, and supported, since prevention, control, and treatment of epidemics rests very much on their shoulders.

REFERENCES

Armstrong, S. & Rispel, L. 2015. 'Social accountability and nursing education in South Africa'. Global Health Action, 8 (1), 27879.

Baines, D., Cunningham, I., & Fraser, H. 2010. 'Constrained by managerialism. Caring as participation in the voluntary social service'. *Economic and Industrial Democracy,* 32 (2), 329–352.

Baker, P. 2010. 'From apartheid to neoliberalism: Health equity in post-apartheid South Africa'. *International Journal of Health Services*, 40 (1), 79–95.

Barron, P., Shasha, W., Schneider, H., Naledi, T., Subedar, H., Masilela, T., Morewane, R., Asia, B., & Taole, K. 2010. 'Re-engineering primary health care in South Africa: Discussion document'. Presented at Umhlanga Rocks, Durban.

Bateman, E. & Jithoo, A. 2006. 'Lung diseases in South Africa: An overview'. *Novartis Foundation Symposium*, 279 (4-11), 216–219.

Berquist, R., St Pierre, I. & Holmes, D. 2018. 'Uncaring nurses: Mobilising power, knowledge, difference and resistance to explain workplace power in academia'. *Research and Theory for Nursing Practice*, 32 (2), 199–215.

Blaauw, D., Ditlopo, P. & Rispel, L. 2015. 'Nursing education reform in South Africa – lessons from policy analysis study', in Rispel, L. (ed.). *Global Health Action*, 7(1), 26401 2014.

Breier, M., Wildschut, A. & Mgqolozana, T. 2008. 'Nursing in a new era'. Research brief, No. 1. Institutional Repository, Human Sciences Research Council.

Carvalho, T. & Santiago, R. 'Professional autonomy in a comparative perspective', in Cavalho, T. & Santiago, R. (eds.), *Professionalism, Managerialism and Reform in Higher Education and the Health Services*. London: Palgrave Macmillan, pp. 30–63.

Carvalho, T. 2014. 'Changing connections between professionalism and managerialism: a case study of nursing in Portugal'. *Journal of Professions and Organisation*, 1 (2), 176–190.

Chipkin, I. & Lipietz, B. 2012. *Transforming South Africa's racial bureaucracy: New public management and public sector reform in contemporary South Africa*, Long Essays No. 1., Johannesburg: Public Affairs Research Institute.

Coovadia, H., Jewkes, R., Barron, P., Sanders, D., & McIntyre, D. 2009. 'The Health and Health System of South Africa: Historical roots of current public health challenges'. *The Lancet*, 347 (9292), 817–834.

Corley, A., Thornton, C. & Glass, N. 2016. 'The role of nurses and community health workers in confronting neglected tropical diseases in Sub-Saharan Africa: A systemic review'. *PLoS Neglected Tropical Diseases*, 10 (9), 4914. https://doi.org/10.1371/journal.pntd.0004914.

Davies, C. 1996. 'The sociology of professions and the profession of gender'. *Sociology*, 30 (4), 661–678.

Dawson, A. & Joof, B. 2005. 'Seeing, thinking and acting against malaria: A new approach to health worker training for community empowerment in rural Gambia'. *Rural and Remote Health*, 5 (353), https://opus.lib.uts.edu.au/bitstream/10453/35813/1/Dawson%20Joof.pdf.

Department of Health. 2013. *Regulations Regarding the Scope of Practice of Nurses and Midwives* (No. 36935).

Department of Health. 2014. *Strategic Plan 2014/15 – 2018/19* (No. 37/2014) https://www.health-e.org.za/wp-content/uploads/2014/08/SA-DoH-Strategic-Plan-2014-to-2019.pdf, accessed 7 December 2018.

Department of Health. 2017. *Policy Framework and Strategy for Ward Based Primary Health Care Outreach Teams*. Pretoria: Department of Health.

Doherty, T., Horne, T. & Wootton, S. 2014. *Managing Public Services — Implementing Changes*. London: Routledge.

Dunkle, K., Jewkes, R., Brown, H., Yoshihama, M., Gray, G., McIntyre, J. & Harlow, S. 2004. 'Prevalence and patterns of gender-based violence and revictimisation among women attending antenatal clinics in Soweto, South Africa'. *American Journal of Epidemiology*, 160 (3), 230–239.

Eagleton-Pierce, M. 2016. *Neoliberalism: The Key Concepts.* London: Routledge.

Esterhuizen, J. 2016. 'The professional nurse's scope of practice: A historical South African perspective'. *Professional Nursing Today*, 20 (1), 12–14.

Fisher, M., Wood, T. & Plyler, L. 2014. 'CE: Responding to the cholera epidemic in Haiti'. *The American Journal of Nursing*, 114 (5), 38–46.

Freidson, E. 1989. 'Theory and the professions'. *Indiana Law Journal*, 64 (3), 423–432.

Geyer, N. 2016. 'Scope of nurses' practice: Legal and ethical column'. *Professional Nursing Today*, 20 (1), 51–52.

Gorman, E. & Sandefur, R. 2011. '"Golden age", quiescence, and revival: How the sociology of professions became the study of knowledge-based work'. *Work and Occupations*, 38, 275–302.

Halford, S., Savage, M. & Witz, A. 1997. *Gender, Careers and Organisations.* London: Palgrave.

Hall, J. 1994. 'Caring for corpses or killing patients?' *Nursing Management*, 25 (10), 81.

Henderson, A. & Jones, J. 2017. 'Developing and maintaining compassionate care in nursing'. *Nursing Standard*, 32 (4), 60–69.

Honikman, S., Fawcus, S. & Meintjies, I. 2015. 'Abuse in South African maternity settings is a disgrace: Potential solutions to the problem'. *South African Medical Journal*, 105 (4), 284–286.

Horwitz, S. 2013. *Baragwanath Hospital Soweto. A History of Medical Care 1941–1990.* Johannesburg: Wits University Press.

Igumbor, J., Scheepers, E., Ebrahim, R., Jason, A. & Grimwood, A. 2011. 'An evaluation of the impact of a community-based adherence support programme on ART outcomes in selected government HIV treatment sites in South Africa'. *AIDS Care*, 23 (2), 231–236.

Kabore, I., Bloem, J., Etheredge, G., Obiero, W., Wanless, A., Doykos, P., Ntsekhe, P., Mtshali, N., Afrikaner, E., Sayed, R., Bostwelelo, J., Hani, A., Moshabesha, T., Kalaka, A., Mameja, J., Zwane, N., Shongwe, N., Mtshali, P., Mohr, B. & Smuts, A. 2010. 'The effect of community-based support services on clinical efficacy and health-related quality of life in HIV/AIDS patients in resource-limited settings in Sub-Sahara Africa'. *AIDS Patient Care and STDs*, 24 (9), 581–594.

Khumalo, G. 2011. 'The era of uncaring, impatient nurses is over'. *SA News.*, website: https://www.sanews.gov.za/south-africa/era-uncaring-impatient-nurses-over-zuma, accessed 25 November 2018.

Khunou, S. & Dharhana-Maselesele, M. 2016. 'Level of job satisfaction amongst nurses in the North-West Province, South Africa: Post occupational specific dispensation'. *Curationis*, 39 (1), 1438.

Kim, J. & Motsei, M. 2002. '"Women enjoy punishment": attitudes and experiences of gender-based violence among PHC Nurses in rural South Africa'. *Social Science & Medicine*, 54 (8), 1243–1254.

Klikauer, T. 2013. 'What is managerialism?' *Critical Sociology*, 41 (7–8), 1103–1119.

Kruger, L., & Schoombee, C. 2010. 'The other side of caring: abuse in a South African maternity ward'. *Journal of Reproductive and Infant Psychology*, 28 (1), 84–10.

Le Marcis, F. and Grard, J. 2015. 'Ethnography of everyday ethics in a South African medical ward', in Herdt, T. & Olivier de Sardan, J.P. (eds.) *Real Governance and Practical Norms in Sub-Saharan Africa: The Game of the Rules*. London and New York: Routledge, pp. 160–185.

Livingston, J. 2012. *Improvising Medicine: An African Oncology Ward in an Emerging Cancer Epidemic*. Durham: Duke University Press.

Livingstone, D. W. 2014. 'Interrogating professional power and recognition of specialised knowledge: A class analysis'. *European Journal for Research on the Education and Learning of Adults*, 5 (1), 13–29. https://doi.org/10.3384/rela.2000-7426.rela9023.

Makhubu, N. 16 May 2016. 'Nurses enraged by "nurses in white" statement'. *IOL News*, https://www.iol.co.za/news/south-africa/nurses-enraged-by-devils-in-white-statement-2022101, accessed 23 November 2018.

Marks, S. 1994. *Divided Sisterhood: Race, Class and Gender in the South African Nursing Profession*. Johannesburg: Wits University Press.

McIntyre, D. & Ataguba, J. 2018. 'How to do (or not to do) … a benefit incidence analysis'. *Health Policy and Planning*, 26 (2), 174–182.

McIntyre, D. & Thiede, M. 2007. 'Health care financing and expenditure: pooling resources and purchasing of health care'. *South African Heath Review*, (1) 35–46.

Molelekwa, T. 2016. 'Community health workers protest for better working conditions'. *Health-e News*, https://www.health-e.org.za/2016/11/12/community-health-workers-protest-better-working-conditions/, accessed 21 November 2018.

Morrell, P., Schneider, H., Lewis, J. & Mbalati, L. 16 May 2011. 'Strategic summary of issues regarding community health workers compiled from the work of three SANAC technical task team'. South African National AIDS Council. Unpublished.

Motsoaledi, A. 24 June 2018. 'NHI is the health equivalent of the land question'. *IOL News*, website: https://www.iol.co.za/news/opinion/nhi-is-the-health-equivalent-of-the-land-question-15657848, accessed 6 November 2018.

Mottiar, S. & Lodge, T. 2018. 'The role of community health workers in supporting South Africa's HIV/AIDS treatment programme'. *South African Journal of AIDS Research*, 17 (1), 51–61.

Naidoo, S. 2016. *Chief executive officers and public hospital management in South Africa*. Johannesburg: Wits School of Government, http://wiredspace.wits.ac.za/jspui/bitstream/10539/23820/1/PhDShanNaidoo30September2016.

pdf, accessed 6 December 2018.

Nambiar, D. & Mander, H. 2017. 'Inverse care and the role of the state: The health of the urban poor'. *Bulletin of the World Health Organization*, 95, 152–153.

Nglazi, M., Lawn, S., Kaplan, R., Kranzer, K., Orrell, C., Wood, R. & Becker, L. 2011. 'Changes in programmatic outcomes during 7-year scale-up at a community based antiretroviral treatment service in South Africa'. *Journal of Acquired Immune Deficiency Syndrome*, 56 (1), 1–8.

Nightingale, F. 6 May 1881. Letter to trainee nurses at St Thomas' Hospital, London.

Nkonki, L., Cliff, J. & Sanders, D. 2011. 'Lay health worker attrition: Important but often ignored'. *Bulletin of the World Health Organization*, 89, 919–923.

Norrish, B. R. & Rundall, T. G. 2001. 'Hospital restructuring and the work of registered nurses'. *The Milbank Quarterly*, 79 (1), 55–79.

O'Donovan, J., O'Donovan, C., Kuhn, I., Sachs, S. & Winters, N. 2018. 'Ongoing training of community health workers in low-income and middle-income countries: A systematic scoping review of the literature'. *BMJ Open*, 8 (4), 021467. http://dx.doi.org/10.1136/bmjopen-2017-021467.

Paintain, L., Willey, B., Kedenge, S., Sharkey, A., Kim, J., Buj, V., Webster, J., Schellenberg, D. & Ngogo, N. 2014. 'Integrated case management of malaria: A systematic literature review'. *The American Journal of Tropical Medicine & Hygiene*, 91 (3), 461–470.

Pearson, J., Pillay, S., Chipkin, I. 2016. 'State building in South Africa after apartheid. The history of the National Treasury'. Working Paper, Public Affairs Research Institute.

Perry, H., Dhillon, R., Liu, A., Chitnis, K., Panjabi, R., Palazuelos, D., Koffi, A., Kandeh, J., Camara, M., Camara, R. & Nyenswah, T. 2016. 'Community health worker programmes after the 2013–2016 Ebola outbreak'. *Bulletin World Health Organization*, 94 (7), 551–553.

Rispel, L. & Bruce J. 2015. 'A profession in peril? Revitalising nursing in South Africa', in Padarath, A., King, J. & English, R. (eds.), *South African Health Review 2014/15*, 4 (9), pp 117–125. Durban: Health Systems Trust.

Rispel, L. 2015. 'Transforming nursing policy, management and practice in South Africa'. Global Health Action, 8: 28005.

Saad-Filho, A. & Johnston, D. 2005. *Neoliberalism: A Critical Reader*. Chicago: University of Chicago Press.

Sagar, P. 2015. 'Nurses leading in the fight against Ebola virus disease'. *Journal of Transcultural Nursing*, 26 (3), 322–326. https://doi.org/10.1177/1043659615574326.

Sawchuk, P. H. 2017. 'Professions, working and knowing: Class conflict and contested hybridisation among Ontario nurses', in the Proceedings of the Canadian Sociological Association. Toronto: Congress of Social Sciences and Humanities, http://www.academia.edu/33402388/Professions_Working_and_Knowing_Class_Conflict_and_Contested_Hybridization_among_Ontario_Nurses.

Schneider, H., le Marcis, F., Grard, J., Penn-Kekana, L., Blaawu, D. & Fassin, D. 2010. 'Negotiating care: Patients tactics at an urban South African hospital'. *Journal of Health Services Research and Policies*, 15 (3), 137–142.

Seid, S. 13 June 2017. 'Rude nurses putting young women off HIV treatment'. *Sunday Times*, https://www.timeslive.co.za/sunday-times/lifestyle/health-and-sex/2017-06-13-rude-nurses-putting-young-women-off-hiv-treatment/, accessed 25 November 2018.

Setswe, G. 2016. 'Three decades of the HIV epidemic'. Johannesburg: Human Sciences Research Council. http://www.hsrc.ac.za/uploads/pageContent/7164/3%20decades%20of%20HIV%20epidemic%20in%20SA.pdf, accessed 25 November 2018.

Smith, D. 1987. *The Everyday World as Problematic: A Feminist Sociology*. Toronto: University of Toronto Press.

Smith, P. 1992. *The Emotional Labour of Nursing*. Basingstoke: Macmillan.

Statistics South Africa (Stats SA). 2018. *Quarterly Labour Survey*. Pretoria, p 37. http://www.statssa.gov.za/publications/P0211/P02112ndQuarter2018.pdf, p. xv, accessed 6 December 2018.

Swartz, A. and Colvin, C. 2014. '"It's in our veins": Caring natures and material motivations of community health workers in contexts of economic marginalisation'. *International Journal of Integrated Care*, 14 (8), 139–152.

Toffoli, L., Rudge, T. & Barnes, L. 2011. 'The work of nurses in private health: accounting for the intangibles in care delivery'. *Health Sociology Review*, 20 (3), 338–351.

Trafford, Z., Swartz, A., and Colvin, C. 2017. '"Contract to volunteer": South African community health worker mobilisation for better labour protection', *New Solutions*, 27 (4), 648–666.

UNICEF. 2014. *Levels and Trends in Child Mortality Report 2014*, from https://www.unicef.org/media/files/Levels_and_Trends_in_Child_Mortality_2014.pdf, accessed 7 December 2018.

Vale, B. 2018. 'Community health workers in South Africa: a scoping review'. Cape Town: DG Murray Trust. Unpublished.

Vale, B., Hodes, R., Cluver, L. & Thabeng, M. 2017. 'Bureaucracies of blood and belonging: documents, HIV-positive youth and the state in South Africa'. *Development & Change*, 48 (6), 1287–1309.

Vale, E. 2012a. '"I know this person, why must I go to him?" Techniques of authority among community health workers in Cape Town'. *Centre for Social Science Research Working Paper* 314. Cape Town: University of Cape Town.

Vale, E. 2012b. '"Looking for greener pastures": Locating care in the life histories of community health workers'. *Centre for Social Science Research Working Paper* 313. Cape Town: University of Cape Town.

Vale, E. 2012c. '"You must make a plan or some story": Community health workers' reappropriation of the care manual'. *Centre for Social Science Research Working Paper* 313. Cape Town: University of Cape Town.

Valiani, S. 2011. *Valuing the invaluable: Rethinking and Respecting Caring Work in Canada*. Toronto: Ontario Nurses' Association.

Valiani, S. 2012. *Rethinking Unequal Exchange. The Global Integration of Nursing Labour Markets*. Toronto: University of Toronto Press.

Van Rensburg, H. 2014. 'South Africa's protracted struggle for equal distribution and equitable access — still not there'. *Human Resources for Health*, 12 (26), https://doi.org/10.1186/1478-4491-12-26.

Von Holdt, K. & Maserumule, B. 2005. 'After apartheid: Decay or reconstruction in a public hospital?' in Webster, E. & Von Holdt, K. (eds.) *Beyond the Apartheid Workplace: Studies in Transition*. Scottsville: University of KwaZulu-Natal Press.

Von Holdt, K. 2010. 'Nationalism, bureaucracy and the developmental state: The South African case'. *South African Review of Sociology*, 41 (1), 4–27.

White, J. 1993. 'Changing labour process and the nursing crisis in Canadian hospitals'. *Studies in Political Economy*, 40, 103–134.

Williams, A., Fennie, K., Bova, C., Burgess, J., Danvers, K. & Dieckhaus, K. 2006. 'Home visits to improve adherence to highly active antiretroviral therapy: A randomised control trial'. *Journal of Acquired Immune Deficiency Syndrome*, 42 (3), 314–321.

Wu, R., Roychowdhury, I. & Khan, M. 2017. 'Evaluations of training programs to improve human resource capacity for HIV, malaria and TB control: A systematic scoping review of methods applied and outcomes assessed'. *Tropical Medicine and Health*, 45 (16), DOI: 10. 11182-017-0056-7.

Zwane, J. 21–23 June 2017. 'Wicked and greedy: Gossip and rumour around nurses in Modimolle [pseudonym] community hospital'. *South African Historical Society Biennial Conference*, Johannesburg.

Section Four

The Future of Health Systems in Africa

THE LAST SECTION OF THE book explores several interrelated issues that concern the future of health systems in Africa. A core emphasis is the potential of groundbreaking technological innovation in building strong health systems and addressing the efficient treatment of epidemics. It further addresses the issues around financing of health care, all with a view to building stable systems that will also embrace the poor and destitute. The common thread in this section is access to quality health care, first through faster and cheaper medical technologies and, second, through a form of national health insurance. To explore the potential of technological innovation in health systems, the first chapter maps briefly the state of health research in Africa and reveals the insufficient number of researchers on the continent. This is despite Africa bearing a large burden of disease.

Zamanzima Mazibuko and Steven Mufamadi explore the two

possible sides of research partnerships between Africa and international organisations – one being an extractive partnership that leaves the disadvantaged with no recognition, and the other being beneficial to Africa and promoting research relevant to the continent. Mazibuko and Mufamadi argue for the elevation of research and development and the use of technological innovation to address the burden of disease in Africa. The concept of 'disruptive' technologies is introduced as having the potential to provide affordable and efficient medical solutions. Nanotechnology is presented as the disruptive technology that has been shown to improve the efficacy of antiretroviral therapy and TB drugs. Nanotechnology has also been used for water treatment, which is essential for clean safe water and the prevention of waterborne diseases such as cholera. The chapter reveals the constraints in advancing nanoproducts from the laboratory into the market and the lack of participation from the pharmaceutical industry.

Financing of health care is crucial to achieving widespread access to quality health care. The two previous sections alluded to the gaps in financing of health care and the next chapter of this section explores health financing in the African context. Samuel Adu-Gyamfi reflects on the health financing in Ghana and Rwanda, two countries that have implemented some form of national health insurance. Adu-Gyamfi writes on the need for sub-Saharan governments to finance health care and to bridge the gap to health care access between the rich and the poor, through different forms of public health insurance. Ghana and Rwanda are used as case studies to determine the post-independence origins of public health insurance and the impact of socio-economic and political factors in the development of health insurance schemes.

Lastly, Alex van den Heever examines how prepared the South African health system is to counter epidemics. He analyses the current capacity of the health system and then assesses whether the proposed NHI framework will improve the capabilities of the existing health system. Indicators of capability are used to assess South Africa's level of preparedness for any health-related incident.

NINE

The Potential of Technological Innovation in Health Care in Africa

Lessons from Nanotechnology

ZAMANZIMA MAZIBUKO AND
STEVEN MUFAMADI

INTRODUCTION

VARIOUS HEALTH-RELATED INTERVENTIONS HAVE been implemented in Africa with the aim to decrease mortality and improve health conditions caused by epidemics (and endemics) such as HIV/AIDS, tuberculosis, and cholera. And yet epidemics are still prevalent on the African continent. Part of the reason is because access to these health-related interventions has not been widespread. Also, the interventions have not been sustainable. This leaves the most vulnerable populations with the continued burden of disease (WHO, 2010). Resourceful and equitable health systems[i] are at the core

i According to WHO, health systems are 'all organisations, people and actions whose primary intent is to promote, restore or maintain health. This includes efforts to influence determinants of health as well as more direct health-improving activities'.

of addressing both infectious and non-communicable diseases (NCDs) on the continent (Temu et al., 2014). This is a conundrum, however, as the health systems in most African countries are weak (Olu, 2017). From the six building blocks[ii] required to strengthen health systems to a standard where they can handle disease outbreaks as well as chronic illnesses, this chapter explores 'medical products, vaccines and technologies' from the research and development (R&D) perspective.

With the highest burden of disease, worldwide, low- and medium-income countries' (LMICs) contribution towards global medical research is the lowest (Franzen et al., 2017). According to a study by Rahman and Fukui (2003), sub-Saharan Africa produced only 0.8 per cent of global biomedical research publications. The Commission on Health Research for Development (COHRED) reported that less than 10 per cent of global health research funding has prioritised health conditions that account for 90 per cent of the global disease burden, an imbalance referred to as the '10/90 gap' (COHRED, 1990). This means that not only have LMICs conducted insufficient research to deal with their burden of disease, but also that high-income countries (HICs) have channelled medical research funding towards diseases affecting the least disease-burdened global population. Almost two decades later, several LMICs still have insufficient health research capacity to improve population health (Franzen et al., 2017).

Health research is exceedingly valuable to society and has an important role to play in the reduction of global health imbalances. Through medical research, crucial information on disease trends and risk factors, effects of treatment and results of public health interventions, as well as costs of health care, can be determined (Nass et al., 2009). More so, research on technological innovations which can deliver faster and economic treatment and diagnosis should be at the forefront. Indeed, the control of infectious diseases can be achieved by effectively applying knowledge that already exists and by conducting clinical investigations on existing drugs and technologies. However, the search for more efficient medications and technologies must also remain a high priority. Emerging technologies present the possibility for African countries 'leapfrogging' into improved

ii The six building blocks of health systems strengthening are: (1) Service delivery; (2) Health workforce; (3) Information; (4) Medical products, vaccines, and technologies; (5) Financing; (6) Leadership and governance health care (McConnell et al., 2008). Technological innovation that is disruptive[iii] and which overtly uses low-cost materials, methods, and applications for low-cost health care delivery is a way in which researchers can respond to the urgent need to make health care efficient and accessible in Africa. It is important, however, that the development of these new technologies considers the socio-economic challenges of African countries; in other words, it is important that the process is simultaneously gone about with sensitivity to local circumstances, goals, and capacities.

In this chapter nanotechnology is presented as an example of such a disruptive technology. Nanotechnology is an emerging and rapidly developing field. It has become one of the most important scientific fields of the 21st century (Dube & Ebrahim, 2017). In the health care sector, nanotechnology has the potential to transform medicine by creating new drug delivery systems and diagnostics (Maksimovi, 2017). Nanomedicine, as it is termed, can potentially offer real breakthroughs by providing cost-effective health care, which is a crucial factor in making medicines and treatments accessible for all (Gudimalla et al., 2017).

This chapter therefore presents African innovation, particularly in medical technologies, as a key driver for health and economic development on the continent. To build this argument, the chapter is essentially in two parts – first it reviews, broadly, the state of research capacity and research and development (R&D) on the continent, as this is at the core of innovation. The tools required to get the African region to an acceptable research status are discussed, including financial intervention through partnerships with international organisations. In these partnerships lies great potential for accelerating health research in Africa in the provision not only of funding and resources, but skills too – although some have been known to be extractive and exploitive (Boum II et al., 2018). As part of the objectives of this chapter, several partnerships that are collaborative and benefit African researchers and institutions optimally are referenced.

The second part is an assertion that research and development of emerging and disruptive technology, specifically nanotechnology, can play a major

iii Disruptive technologies have been described as scientific discoveries that transform the original product's characteristics and provide the foundation for a novel and more competitive one. According to Clayton M. Christensen (1997) in his book *The Innovator's Dilemma* disruptive technologies create new markets and value networks that ultimately disrupt traditional markets and leading firms and products.

role in providing affordable, effective medicine and disease prevention methods. It argues that it is essential to include disruptive technological innovation in research agendas. Examples of studies are presented that demonstrate nanotechnology's potential to improve current treatments of some of the epidemic diseases prevalent on the continent. Further, examples of nano-enabled water treatments are discussed, given that access to clean and safe water is crucial in preventing or containing diarrhoeal diseases such as cholera. The last part of the chapter discusses the interventions required for nanotechnology development, commercialisation, and, ultimately, its successful and widespread use in communities.

The analysis in this chapter draws on high-level scholarly insights to draw new perspectives on nanotechnology in relation to epidemics in Africa. To obtain data for this chapter, keywords and phrases such 'nanomedicine', 'nanotechnology', 'research capacity', 'research in Africa', 'science in Africa', 'research partnerships', 'nanotechnology commercialisation', 'nanotechnology research and development' etc. were subjected to systematic searches for pertinent research conducted in this specialised field. Establishing research activity in several African countries proved challenging as data was not always available. Only in countries where a defined research strategy has been implemented was the data more accessible.

HEALTH RESEARCH IN AFRICA

The need for locally driven and produced health research that is relevant for the African continent and that has cost-effective implementation remains urgent. African researchers, as scarce as they are, are better placed to outline which research issues need to be prioritised for the African population. In addition, African researchers need to be provided with an environment which allows them to conduct research efficiently. This section thus explores research capacity in Africa and the elements required to be put in place to enhance this capacity, including the partnerships that promote equitable research on the continent. It also offers nanotechnology as a possible solution for a cost-effective technological innovation that potentially has groundbreaking implications for health care in Africa.

African research institutes and research capacity

Impactful and valuable research requires good individual research skills and ability, suitable infrastructure, institutional and regulatory frameworks, investment, and the ability to contribute to global research and policy needs (Chu et al., 2014; Morel et al., 2018). To contextualise research in Africa, it is thus important to explore research capacity and availability as well as quality of infrastructure, what research is already being done, and where research is lacking. Research capacity in Africa, particularly in sub-Saharan Africa, is lagging behind other parts of the world (Morel et al., 2018). Among other reasons, this can be attributed to the loss of university staff to foreign institutions, lack of appropriate infrastructure, a policy environment that is not conducive for research, and insufficient funding. It must be noted, however, that research capacity varies widely across African countries (Morel et al., 2018).

Only 1 per cent of global investment in R&D is allocated to Africa, and only 0.1 per cent of the world's patents are in Africa's possession (Kariuki & Kay, 2017). A pilot study on the expenditure on health research in 42 sub-Saharan African countries over two years estimated that approximately USD 1.5 billion (USD 750 million per annum) was spent in this region (Kebede et al., 2014). This is approximately one-sixth of the total annual expenditure reported by the Global Forum for low- and middle-income countries in 2003 of USD 4.1 billion (Kebede et al., 2014). This dearth of investment is due on the one hand to the low numbers of researchers in Africa and, on the other, an infrastructure that is not conducive for research. In 2017, the continent had 198 researchers per million people, measured against 428 in Chile and more than 4,000 in the United Kingdom and United States (Kariuki & Kay, 2017). The percentage of Africans pursuing graduate study is three times lower than the global average. The number of researchers per capita in Africa is also unreasonably low. The continent would require an additional million new PhD graduates for it to reach the world average (Kariuki & Kay, 2017). Research capacity needs to be prioritised to improve Africa's R&D and innovation landscape.

In brief, following reports that global health research is biased towards diseases affecting HICs (COHRED, 1990), various international organisations have been undertaking research in Africa, mostly in the form of clinical trials but also, gradually, in genomics and biobanking projects (WHO, 2002; Adoga et al., 2014; Munung et al., 2017). Unfortunately, when institutions and organisations in HICs have funded research conducted in Africa, they have also largely been the lead researchers and sole publishers of this research, which is not always to the continent's advantage (Crane, 2010).

Partnerships with international organisations have great potential in accelerating health research in Africa by providing funding, resources, and skills. However, these partnerships need to be wholly beneficial to African countries. They need to put African researchers at the forefront and not just be an extractive initiative for international organisations.

Funding that does not require African researchers to take the back seat in research conducted in Africa is what we should be aiming for. The Developing Excellence in Leadership, Training and Science (DELTAS) Africa scheme, which was initiated by the Wellcome Trust[iv] in partnership with the Alliance for Accelerating Excellence in Science in Africa (AESA),[v] and other partners, is exemplary in illustrating how international organisations can invest in health research in Africa. DELTAS supports the African-led development of researchers and research leaders in Africa, thus ensuring that science for Africa is led by Africa's researchers, and that the science remains relevant to the needs of the continent (Table 1).

iv The Wellcome Trust is a global charitable foundation that supports scientists and researchers all over the world to explore ideas in science, population health, medical innovation, the humanities and social sciences, and public engagement (https://wellcome.ac.uk/about-us).

v AESA is a funding platform that aims to develop science strategies and funding research in Africa. AESA seeks to develop research leadership and promote scientific excellence and innovation to overcome some of Africa's developmental challenges that include the shortage of researchers to deal with its disease burden (https://aasciences.ac.ke/programmes/easa/alliance-for-accelerating-excellence-in-science-in-africa-aesa/).

Table 1: Health research programmes led by African researchers in African institutions (Supported by DELTAS)

Name of Programme	Aim	Lead Researcher	Institution
Training Health Researchers into Vocational Excellence in East Africa -2 (THRiVE-2)	To transform East African universities into world class research hubs for key emerging health issues in the region.	Prof. Nelson Sewankambo	Makerere University College of Health Sciences in Uganda
Developing Excellence in Leadership and Genetic Training for Malaria Elimination in Sub-Saharan Africa (DELGEME)	Training graduates, doctoral fellows, and postdoctoral fellows in the genomics and bioinformatics of malaria.	Prof. Abdoulaye Djimdé	University of Science, Techniques and Technologies in Mali
African Science Partnership for Intervention Research Excellence (Afrique One-ASPIRE)	To expand research capacity in sub-Saharan Africa by focusing on 'One Health' – the concept that the health of animals, humans, and the environment is interconnected – as an approach to tackle major challenges in ecosystem health.	Prof. Bassirou Bonfoh	Centre Suisse de Recherches Scientifiques (CSRS) in Côte d'Ivoire

Name of Programme	Aim	Lead Researcher	Institution
Consortium for Advanced Research Training in Africa+ (CARTA+)	Continue to develop a critical mass of multidisciplinary researchers who work in research-supportive environments in Africa, with the aim of improving public and population health.	Prof. Alex Ezeh & Prof. Sharon Fonn	African Population and Health Research Center (APHRC) in Kenya; University of the Witwatersrand in South Africa
Initiative to Develop African Research Leaders (IDeAL)	Keeping scientists at African institutions through a defined programme of recruitment, supervision, mentorship, multidisciplinary approaches, and clear career paths.	Dr Samson Kinyanjui	Kemri-Wellcome Trust Research Programme in Kenya
African Mental Health Research Initiative (AMARI)	Develop a cohort of outstanding mental health researchers in sub-Saharan Africa.	Dr Dixon Chibanda	University of Zimbabwe
Sub-Saharan Africa Consortium for Advanced Biostatistics Training (S2ACABT)	Address a fundamental gap in expertise in the area of biostatistics, a discipline that is essential for a broad range of research areas and crucial for developing robust research questions.	Prof. Tobias Chirwa	University of the Witwatersrand

Name of Programme	Aim	Lead Researcher	Institution
Sub-Saharan African Network for TB/HIV Research Excellence (SANTHE)	Strengthening the scientific research base for two diseases (HIV and TB) that account for a major burden of morbidity and mortality in Africa.	Prof. Thumbi Ndung'u	KwaZulu-Natal Research Institute for Tuberculosis and HIV (K-RITH) in South Africa
West African Centre for Cell Biology of Infectious Pathogens (WACCBIP)	Address the underlying causes of both communicable and non-communicable diseases in African populations.	Dr Gordon Akanzuwine Awandare	West African Centre for Cell Biology of Infectious Pathogens (WACCBIP) in Ghana
Malaria Research Capacity Development in West and Central Africa (MACARD)	Build on the achievements of the Malaria Capacity Development Consortium (MCDC) to provide PhD, early, and senior post-doctoral fellowships in areas of research relevant to malaria elimination.	Prof. Oumar Gaye	Université Cheikh Anta Diop (UCAD) in Senegal

Source: https://aasciences.ac.ke/aas/en/academy/academy-pages/developing-excellence-in-leadership-training-and-science-deltas-africa-initiative/

By 2018, DELTAS had been supporting leading African researchers based in research institutions across 21 countries on the continent. Thus far, approximately USD 100 million has been granted to these researchers to enable them to implement groundbreaking research and training programmes. The research agenda is set by African researchers and direction is given to international researchers. Regional collaboration is encouraged and reinforced through these programmes. The Training Health Researchers into Vocational Excellence in East

Africa (THRiVE) programme, for instance, aims to strengthen regional research capacity through collaborations by academic institutions from Uganda, Rwanda, Tanzania, and Kenya. This type of collaboration has not been common between African institutions, as seen in a comparative study by Pouris and Ho (2014), and individual projects that become successful do not reach their full potential because they are not linked with all the relevant expertise from Africa.

One initiative that aims to establish a well-funded, systematic, and innovative collaboration of the R&D community on the continent is the Coalition for African Research and Innovation (CARI) (Photopoulos, 2018). Led by Africans, CARI is supported by AESA, which encourages collaboration among researchers, organisations, and governments across the continent to bring resources and allow synergy among existing investments to support research and development in Africa (AESA, 2017). The investments from the various stakeholders from the African continent and international community provide a platform that enables a common discussion regarding the R&D priorities for Africa, including the areas where limited resources should be invested (Photopoulos, 2018).

Role of technology and innovation in African health care and development

Globally, access to efficient and affordable health care is one of the most pressing issues. Increased life expectancy, a growing burden of chronic disease, and significant health inequalities (Doyal & Hoffman, 2009) make this even more urgent. Health care quality is measured by efficacy, evidence basis, patient centredness, and cost-effectiveness (Russo & Adler, 2015). The epidemics affecting the African population the most, such as HIV/AIDS and tuberculosis (TB), traditionally are managed with high doses of therapeutics over a long period of time (or lifetime). These therapeutics must be taken frequently, they often cause severe adverse effects, and they are expensive. Therefore, these treatments do not always meet the health care quality criteria as patient compliance is compromised, the treatments are not affordable, and the efficacy is not optimal.

That there are major gaps that need to be filled and that there is widespread uncertainty about the most cost-effective and efficient ways of administering health care is acknowledged. Emerging technologies such as biotechnology and nanotechnology have been recognised as disruptive technologies that can change conventional health care. Disruptive technologies are innovative developments that establish new markets and standards within an existing market, therefore displacing prominent market leaders and products (Perrot, 2018). The development of these technologies should be sensitive to the syndemic nature of diseases and consider the socio-economic context of the population for whom they are being developed. HIV/AIDS patients, for instance, are likely to also suffer from other health conditions such as TB, and in several cases their ill-health will be worsened by poverty, undernutrition, or various other socio-economic factors. Technologies that diagnose multiple conditions and provide treatments concurrently would be highly valuable. Liberian biomedical scientist Dr Dougbeh Christopher Nyan developed a rapid test which can detect and simultaneously differentiate at least three to seven infections at the same time within 10 to 40 minutes (Jackson, 2018). This type of innovation would help address the management of co-infections that commonly occur in African settings.

Nanotechnology, an example of an innovative technology, promises to improve existing products and make them cheaper and more effective (Maine, 2014; Chang et al., 2015). Moreover, it has the potential to address many societal challenges experienced by developing countries.[vi] Scientists and technologists define nanotechnology as an applied science in which a material of nanoscale size (below 100 nm) presents characteristics that are unlike the bulk material (Lane & Kalil, 2005). These characteristics enable a product to be transformed into a more novel and competitive one, e.g. one that is faster, smaller, uses less material, is cheaper, etc. Several developing countries are pursuing nanotechnology strategies, proposing that nanotechnology has a role in alleviating poverty, reducing unemployment, and improving health (Perrot, 2018).

Nanotechnology research and development

A study by Woodson (2012) showed that 78 per cent of the publications on nanomedicine in Web of Science (WoS) from low-income countries

vi The term nanotechnology is derived from the prefix 'nano' in nanometre (nm), which is one billionth of a metre and is approximately the width of 10 hydrogen atoms (Bhushan, 2007).

focused on diseases affecting their populations. In comparison, only 16 per cent of nanomedicine articles from very high-income countries deal with these diseases. Therefore, even though low-income countries' nanomedicine publications are far fewer than those of high-income countries, the low-income countries' research prioritises diseases which affect their populations. Indeed, since the mid-2000s African countries have included nanomedicine in their science and technology research agendas. The South African government, for example, established a nanotechnology initiative in 2005 to promote and enhance nanotechnology research and development, with health care as one of its six focus areas, spending about R170 million (USD 26 million) on this (Claassens & Motuku, 2006). Researchers in South Africa, therefore, have been conducting nanomedicine research for some time, with a focus on its use in enhancing treatment of diseases affecting LMICs (Dube & Ebrahim, 2017). Moreover, South Africa is one of 27 African countries that constitute the Nanosciences African Network (NANOAFNET),[vii] which was created in 2005. NANOAFNET aims to improve Africa's global prominence and contribution in nanomedicine, as well as formulate cost-effective nanotechnologies to address urgent continental societal needs, including health sector needs. Among the NANOAFNET countries, South Africa, Ethiopia, Nigeria, Kenya, Morocco, Egypt, and Libya have nanomedicine publications. Tanzania and Cameroon are two other African countries that are conducting nanomedicine research.

Nanomedicine can provide solutions to conventional drug administration methods which are used broadly but provide unsatisfactory results. Research suggests that investment in the development of new and more efficient treatment is crucial in realising health care, but this is not occurring at a notable scale (Tiwari et al., 2012). The increase in R&D costs of such conventional drugs has resulted in a decline in the approval of new chemicals since the late 1950s (Tiwari et al., 2012). Investing in nanomedicine is thus an important and cost-effective alternative. Nanomedicine also has great potential for reducing the toxicity and improving the solubility and efficacy of therapeutics for infectious diseases such as TB, malaria, and HIV (Hayeshi et al., 2012),

vii http://www.nanoafnet.tlabs.ac.za/

and NCDs like cancer (Din et al., 2017). Thus, for drug discovery and development to advance to where minimal returns, if any, can be expected, new approaches such as nanotechnology must be explored.

NANOTECHNOLOGY RESEARCH IN DISEASE MANAGEMENT

Across the globe, research is underway to determine the efficacy of nanotechnology in treating infectious diseases. This research, although not always fully fleshed out, has shown improvement when compared to conventional methods of treatment. A few studies are presented to demonstrate several ways in which nanotechnology can improve health care when it comes to some of the diseases prevalent in Africa.

Nanotechnology in HIV therapy

Combination antiretroviral therapy, or highly active anti-retroviral therapy (HAART), has effectually been successful in managing HIV/AIDS. Many challenges remain, however, which can and do result in unsuccessful therapy. Some of these challenges are: lifetime administration; high costs; poor patient compliance; major adverse effects caused by high and frequent dosages; the development of multiple resistant HIV strains caused by a high mutation rate; the presence of viral reservoir sites inaccessible to current drug delivery methods; low oral bioavailability; and poor drug pharmacokinetics (Adesina & Akala, 2015; Curley et al., 2017).

Nanotechnology has the potential to address challenges presented by current treatments and possibly failed and future therapeutics as well (Curley et al., 2017). It presents the possibility of the improved safety of drugs by reducing doses or providing targeted drug delivery systems (Tiwari et al., 2012; Din et al., 2017). Nanomedicine strategies that are being explored for delivery of antiretroviral drugs range from oral nanomedicines, long-acting injectable nanomedicines, and targeted nanomedicines (Curley et al., 2017). Solid drug nanoparticle (SDN) formulations are being investigated for enhancement of the bioavailability of poorly water-soluble drugs. In vivo pharmacokinetics studies of SDN formulations containing efavirenz showed that they could achieve similar pharmacokinetics to the standard SustivaC© formulation with a 50 per cent lower dose (McDonald et al., 2014). Long-acting injectable nanomedicines aim to address poor drug-regimen compliance that results in failure of treatment (Havlir & Gandhi, 2015). A study involving 56 healthy volunteers administered a cabotegravir-containing long-acting injectable nanomedicine. The treatment sustained exposure for up to 24 weeks and cabotegravir was well tolerated with no grade 2–4 injection site reactions reported (Spreen et al., 2012).

Targeted nanomedicines are developed in HIV therapy for drugs to reach inaccessible viral reservoir sites (Mallipeddi & Rohan, 2010). The blood–brain barrier presents a challenge for therapeutics to reach the brain. For delivery to the brain, magnetic azidothymidine 5'-triphosphate liposomal nanoformulations have been developed. When a magnetic field was applied in an in vitro model of the blood–brain barrier, the transcellular apparent permeability was increased compared to a free drug (Saiyed et al., 2010).

Nanotechnology in TB therapy

As with antiretroviral treatment, TB treatment faces challenges when it comes to patient compliance, drugs that are not targeted, and side-effects. Frequent dosing and prolonged treatment duration are major considerations when nanoformulations are developed for TB treatment.

As such, in a study, rifampin (RMP), isoniazid (IHN), and pyrazinamide (PZA) were encapsulated by poly(lactide-co-glycolide) (PLG) nanoparticles (NPs) for oral delivery (Pandey et al., 2005). After a single dose of drug-loaded PLG NPs in mice for 6 to 9 days, drug levels were maintained above the least inhibitory concentration (MIC90) in the plasma. Free drugs were not found in the plasma within 12 to 24 hours after oral administration. Only subsequent to administration of 46 doses were free drugs able to generate the same effects as nano-enabled drugs (Pandey et al., 2005). In another study, ethambutol-encapsulated nanoparticles were administered simultaneously with encapsulated RMP, IHN, and PZA (Ahmad et al., 2006). Following a single dose of drug-loaded NPs to mice, therapeutic drug concentrations were retained in the plasma for 9 days, 7 days, and 11 days in the case of rifampicin, ethambutol and isoniazid/ pyrazinamide respectively. Contrastingly, the plasma did not contain any free drugs within 12 hours of intravenous or oral administration (Ahmad et al., 2006).

Injectable nanomedicines are also being developed for TB treatment. Nanoformulations of PLG drug-nanoparticles containing RMP, INH, and PZA were injected subcutaneously into mice. Sustained therapeutic drug levels were observed in plasma for 32 days and in lungs or spleen for 36 days. To achieve the same results oral free drugs had 35 doses (Pandey & Khuller, 2004). In another study, nanotechnology was incorporated with clofazimine, an anti-TB drug for mycobacterial infection, in order to address its insolubility problem. Clofazimine was formulated as a nanosuspension with a particle size of 385 nm. Subsequent to intravenous administration, colony-forming unit count in the liver, spleen, and lungs of mice infected with *M. avium* had decreased (Peters et al., 2000).

These studies established that it is possible for nanomedicine to decrease the doses required to achieve the desired effect of the drug. They have also demonstrated the importance of nanotechnology to overcome the solubility problems and toxicity of drugs.

NANOTECHNOLOGY IN THE PREVENTION OF INFECTIONS

As much as treating and containing diseases is a priority, prevention would be more efficient and in the long run more cost effective. The properties nanotechnology offer allow for the effective and economical treatment of water. This section explores the implications of water treatment using nanotechnology in preventing the spread of diseases.

Nanotechnology in water treatment

The importance of clean water in curbing epidemics, the prevention of certain diseases, or re-infections cannot be understated. Diarrhoeal diseases caused by the use of contaminated water are among the biggest causes of illnesses and death in sub-Saharan Africa (Montgomery & Elimelech, 2007; Nwabor et al., 2016; see also Chapter 3). Access to clean water remains a huge issue in sub-Saharan Africa. According to the World Health Organization (WHO), approximately half of the 663 million people in the world who lacked access to reliable and clean water in 2015 lived in sub-Saharan Africa (WHO, 2015). Thus, sub-Saharan Africa suffers from water-borne diseases, like cholera, habitually. Between 2000 and 2015, 83 per cent of cholera deaths reported by WHO occurred in sub-Saharan Africa (Lessler et al., 2018). The lack of safe and affordable water severely affects vulnerable groups, including persons with compromised immune systems such as HIV/AIDS patients (Kamminga & Wegelin-Schuringa, 2005).

The supply of clean water is thus even more imperative for HIV/AIDS patients to prevent opportunistic infections from polluted water. Preventing water-borne infections that may further weaken the immune system is crucial in reducing HIV- and AIDS-related morbidity and mortality (Makaudze et al., 2012). Adequate water supply and sanitary facilities are of the utmost importance for HIV-infected people to maintain a healthy status as long as possible. Clean water for people living with AIDS will reduce their chances of getting diarrhoea and skin diseases (which are opportunistic infections); and being able to take their medication with clean water is especially important for this vulnerable population group (Kamminga & Wegelin-Schuringa, 2005; Makaudze et al., 2012).

Centralised purification and expansion of existing piped water distribution systems are resource intensive and time consuming (World Bank Group, 2017). Realistically, therefore, providing safe water widely in sub-Saharan Africa is not going to occur speedily, so a large number of people will continue to be without safe water. Solutions that are decentralised, self-sustaining, and targeted to the most vulnerable groups in order to improve health as well as enhance development should therefore be implemented expeditiously.

One of the approaches to the provision of clean water being investigated in a number of countries is nanotechnology as it holds great potential in providing innovative water treatment. The characteristics of nanomaterials make them apposite for treating water, either as an improvement of current techniques (which are costly and time consuming) and/or as part of completely novel methods for treating domestic, industrial, and mining wastewater (Hashem, 2014; Kunduru et al., 2017). Fundamentally, nanotechnology provides advanced performance and economic water and wastewater treatment solutions (Hashem, 2014; Kunduru et al., 2017). Nano-enabled devices are durable, multifunctional, and have a large surface to volume ratio which allows for manipulation of the interaction with pollutants and/or bacteria (Chong et al., 2010; Kunduru et al., 2017). Nanotechnology can offer a customised solution for the removal of a targeted contaminant or for removing several contaminants (Kanchi, 2014; Anjum et al., 2016). The latter is optimal for water purification as water contains a variety of widely dispersed contaminants.

Examples of nanotechnology use in water treatment

Tea bag water filter: The 'tea bag' filter is a small water filter developed to fit into the neck of a bottle. It promises to provide an affordable water purification method in remote areas or where the water supply is contaminated (Smit, 2010). The tea bag filter sachets are developed from the same material as rooibos tea bags, only they contain activated carbon instead of tea (Makoni, 2010a). A thin film of biocides encapsulated within tiny nanofibres coats the inside surface of the tea bag material. This feature ensures that the filter traps the bacteria, which are then killed by the biocide coating, something that is not found in traditional water filters (Makoni, 2010a; Smit, 2010). The tea bag filter was developed by a team at the University of Stellenbosch, South Africa, to provide an innovative and effective decentralised point-of-use technology (Smit, 2010). Moreover, it is biodegradable due to the structure of the nanofibres and thus poses no risk to human health or the environment.

Capillary ultrafiltration: The capillary ultrafiltration (CUF) technology is a membrane and filter system used for potable and industrial water purification. It has a pore size of 35 nm in diameter, allowing it to remove bacteria and viruses, colour, and metal oxides (SAASTA, 2011). It can also be used for pre-treatment of seawater and the treatment of industrial water and wastewater (Zamxaka & Riley, 2010). The CUF was developed by a team at Stellenbosch University in partnership with the Water Research Council to provide cost-effective systems to replace expensive imported equivalents (SAASTA, 2011). Currently, the CUF technology provides water treatment solutions for rural areas, especially for those municipalities seeking to provide new water services (SAASTA, 2011).

Nanofilters: The nanofilter is a sand-based water filter that utilises nanomaterials to remove contaminants such as heavy metals, fluoride, and biological toxins, while the sand traps the remaining fragments (Obiukwu, 2015; BITRI, 2018). This novel technology was developed by a Tanzanian innovator, Askwar Hilonga, and offers affordable water purification (BITRI, 2018). In 2015, the nano-enabled device, which can be shared by a community and can produce up to 60 litres of safe drinking water per day, sold for USD 130 per device (Obiukwu, 2015). This is without electrical or solar power, nor any UV or chemical treatment (Obiukwu, 2015). The nanofilter can be customised according to the water condition in a particular area as water conditions differ depending on pollutants found in the water, human activities, and the geological formation of soil and rocks.

CONSTRAINTS OF NANOTECHNOLOGY

Notwithstanding the advantages of nanotechnology, there are some constraints to its research and development and also to getting the technologies onto the market. Nanotechnology is an emerging field and thus requires more research (and investment) before it can be embraced fully by governments, the private sector, and society. For instance, although formulating nanotechnology products can be economical, acquiring the initial equipment for developing these products can be costly. In this regard, this section explores some of the barriers to realising the full potential of nanotechnology.

Investment in nanotechnology

Investing in any new technology is important for its development and ultimately its commercialisation. A report compiled by the Nanotechnology Research Group indicated that African countries are slow or are not prioritising the adoption of nanotechnology despite the potential it holds. South Africa, Egypt, and Nigeria are all making strides towards nanotechnology development (Rateng, 2017), while some other African countries – Botswana being one – are at the developmental phase of nanotechnology-based solutions (*Sunday Standard*, 2017). Lack of investment by the majority of countries in Africa has been identified as the major obstacle to embracing this technology (Rateng, 2017). According to Ezema et al. (2014), if Africa is to succeed in the development of nanotechnology, there needs to be a multidisciplinary collaboration or partnership between government ministries, agencies, institutions, the private sector, and donor agencies. This will help African countries to gather the resources that are required towards nanotechnology development.

South Africa is striving to be at the forefront of nanotechnology development and commercialisation in Africa. The government has developed a strategy and allocated funding to enhance technological innovation in the country. The success of South Africa in nanotechnology development is powered by government funding, specifically the Department of Science and Technology (DST) and support programmes such as the Technology Innovation Agency (TIA) and the Industrial Development Corporation (IDC). Spanning 10 years from 2005 until 2015, the government invested over ZAR 400 million (about USD 28.6 million) towards nanotechnology R&D, human capacity building, and infrastructure (National Nanotechnology Equipment Programme). For infrastructure investment, the focus was on nanotechnology research equipment, cleanrooms, and piloting facilities (Dube & Ebrahim, 2017). South Africa's success in nanotechnology development is further supported by alliances or partners, particularly from the BRICS countries (Brazil, Russia, India, China, South Africa). These are among the major players and constitute the hub of nanotechnology (Molapisi, 2012).

Although many countries in Africa are demonstrating an interest in nanotechnology research, their national projects and financial support emanate mostly from governments (UNITAR, 2012). When it comes to financial support for nanotechnology innovation and/or commercialisation, South Africa and Morocco have a financial support structure and strategy for industrialisation. Morocco's government strategy focuses on university-industry collaboration through the InnovAct programme (UNESCO, 2016). The South African government is focusing on the establishment of nanotechnology industrialisation through the New Industries

Strategic Business Unit (SBU) from the IDC Industrial Development Corporation (IDC, 2015).

Big pharmaceutical companies are in a favourable position to finance or invest in nanotechnology-based products and to fuel the nanomedicine market, given that they have good infrastructure, big budgets, and the expertise in areas such as clinical trials, intellectual property, regulation, and marketing. However, according to the Joint Research Centre of the European Commission (JRC-EURO), big pharmaceutical companies have a low interest in investing in emerging nanotherapeutics. This is due to the high acquisition costs, which can result in low financial rewards and/or negative returns. Attracting investment in nanomedicine from big pharmaceutical firms will therefore require standardised cost effectiveness with reimbursements (Bosetti, 2015). An increase in the investment capital of nanomedicine R&D in Africa could facilitate the production of affordable health and pharmaceutical solutions in Africa. Additionally, finding the best model to support small and medium enterprises (SMEs) could assist towards job creation and boost economic growth in Africa.

Nanotechnology infrastructure

Lack of proper infrastructure affects the progress in nanotechnology research, especially in developing countries (Naseri & Davoodi, 2011; Mazumder et al., 2014). Although nanotechnology promises inexpensive pharmaceutical products and diagnostic and medical devices, the research in nanotechnology requires very expensive equipment.[viii] The equipment is critical for the research but it is

---

viii Examples of some of the current cutting-edge equipment for nanotechnology characterisation available in African universities, research councils, and industries are Transmission Electron Microscopes (TEM), Scanning Electron Microscopes (SEM), Focused Ion Beam Scanning Electron Microscopes (FIB-SEM), Atomic Force Microscopes (AFM), Optical microscopes, Photoluminescence Spectrometers, UV/VIS Spectrometers, Nanoparticle size analysers, Nanolog Spectro-Fluorometers, EvoVac and NexDep for thin film deposition equipment, and many more (CSIR, 2018; MAScIR, 2018). The Centre for High Resolution Transmission Electron Microscopy at Nelson Mandela University is the home of the following instruments: The JEOL JEM-ARM200F double Cs-corrected Transmission Electron Microscope (ARM-TEM); JEOL JEM 2100 LAB6 TEM, an Analytical TEM; JEOL JSM-7001F, an analytical FEG SEM, the FEI Helios NanoLab DualBeam 650, and a nanoindenter (Chrtem – Nelson Mandela University, 2018).

expensive to maintain and quickly becomes outdated. This makes it more difficult for researchers, particularly in Africa, to keep up with researchers around the world.

Although the South African government has, over the years, financially supported nanotechnology infrastructure (National Nanotechnology Equipment Programme), it is currently facing financial constraints in sustaining the investment. In 2015, DST in partnership with the Council for Scientific and Industrial Research (CSIR) launched a new nanotechnology production facility for the up-scaling, processing, and testing of plastics and cosmetics. The lack of world-class infrastructure, the centralisation of nanotechnology facilities, and laboratories that are not fully funded will delay local nanotechnology R&D from reaching the clinic and marketplace. Furthermore, lack of the nanotechnology infrastructure to support start-ups, SMEs, and entrepreneurs will continue to affect business growth in nanotechnology in Africa.

Lack of public awareness and public perception on nanomedicine

For an emerging technology to be successful, public acceptance and uptake of the technology is crucial, yet many international surveys have shown that the majority of the public has limited knowledge or no awareness about nanotechnology (Sechi et al., 2014). In an attempt to increase public awareness, nanotechnology communities around the world have established initiatives that aim for facilitation of public engagement with the science (NPEP, 2018; Jones, 2009; Nisbet & Markowitz, 2015). The American Association for the Advancement of Science (AAAS) describes public engagement with science as a great opportunity for mutual learning between both scientists and non-scientists or members of the public (Nisbet & Markowitz, 2015). Some citizens who are familiar with nanotechnology have concerns regarding the uncertainty around the potential toxicity of nanomedicine to human health and the environment. Essentially, the public is unsure about the benefits versus the risks of nanotechnology (Waldron et al., 2006; Bankole et al., 2014; Beumer, 2017). Poor communication on the benefits and risks of nanomedicine and/or negative public perception can hinder the development and diffusion of the technology.

South Africa established its own Nanotechnology Public Engagement Programme (NPEP) in 2008. NPEP is an initiative funded by the DST, and implemented and administered by the South African Agency for Science and Technology Advancement (SAASTA), a business unit of the National Research Foundation (NRF). The main objective of the NPEP is to increase the public's awareness and knowledge of nanotechnology and educate them about the benefits and risks of nanotechnology innovations to enable them to make an informed decision. To this end several programmes have been established. One of these is school debates at national level as a platform to give the public an opportunity to debate issues around nanotechnology. Another is Nano Tour, which allows members of the public to visit industries and universities where nanotechnology facilities are in place, such as the Mintek Nanotechnology Innovation Centre (NIC), the University of the Free State (UFS) nanotechnology facility, and the CSIR production facility for nanotechnology materials. Other initiatives are: a role-model campaign, where nanotechnology scientists can interact with the public and talk about their work; a variety of media platforms, like community radio stations and vernacular language newspapers; and public dialogue through symposiums and workshops. In addition, NPEP also publishes online nanotech articles on a quarterly basis on its website (www.npep.co.za) and produces fact sheets that offer the public accurate information on nanotechnology. NPEP, in partnership with Nabio Consulting (Pty) Ltd, the Swiss Embassy in South Africa, the University of Basel, Switzerland, and the DST Science Forum, has also organised symposiums aiming to facilitate public engagement on nanomedicine development in South Africa and in Switzerland (NPEP, 2017). The symposiums engage the media on the discussions on nanomedicine and ensure that the public is informed about research development in the following areas: HIV/AIDS, TB, malaria, cancer, water, and energy (NPEP, 2018).

Lack of regulation of nanomedicines

The lack of regulation of nanomedicines could delay the acceleration of nanomedicines from research laboratory to the clinic and/or marketplace. The United States Food and Drug Administration

(USFDA) recently approved the regulation of nanotechnology products (USFDA, 2018). The USFDA's approach to the regulation focuses on the understanding of interactions of nanomaterials with biological systems, safety, effectiveness, and quality of products containing nanomaterials. Pharmaceutical regulatory agencies that are based in Africa and active in nanotechnology development include the South African Health Products Regulatory Authority (SAHPRA), the National Agency for Food and Drug Administration and Control (NAFDAC, Nigeria), the Egyptian Drug Authority (EDA), the Direction du Médicament et de la Pharmacie (DMP, Morocco), and the National Laboratory for the Control of Pharmaceutical Products (LNCPP, Algeria) (Ndomondo-Sigonda et al., 2017). African regulatory agencies currently don't have regulatory frameworks/guidelines on nanomedicine and this could affect the commercialisation of nanomedicines. The approved guidelines by international agencies such as the USFDA and the European Medicines Agency (EMA, 2006) can, however, be used as reference points.

The need for the regulation of nanomedicines is due to the nature of materials at nanoscale (1–100 nm). They are highly reactive, can easily bypass biological barriers, and have the potential for high accumulation in human tissue/cells, which could have unexpected human toxicity (Senje, 2013). Some metal materials have been reported to have different properties at nanoscale. For example, gold and silver nanoparticles have been reported to have medicinal benefits at nanoscale. In the past decade, research has been conducted investigating their pharmaceutical potency using metallic nanomaterials as antimicrobial and anti-cancer agents (He et al., 2016; Ronavari et al., 2018). The impact of some of these nanomaterials on human health (and also their environmental risks) is still unknown, which necessitates the regulation of nanotechnology by African countries' regulatory authorities in order to assure that the medicines containing nanomaterial are safe for human consumption.

Currently there are many nanodrugs that have received approval status from one or more regulatory authorities for commercial use (Fornaguera & García-Celma, 2017). This approval status is used to reassure patients and citizens, as well as physicians, that the particular medicine is safe for human consumption.

Due to unknown long-term impacts on health and the environment, many countries are starting to look at the establishment of a nano code of conduct for nanotechnology R&D to protect the researchers, consumers, and the environment. South Africa's Department of Science and Technology (PSM, 2018) has this under consideration, with the following objectives:

- Proactively prevent the negative impact and/or undesired consequences of nanotechnology;
- Create an environment for safe and responsible nanotechnology R&D at university and industry;
- Deal with the potential risks of nanotechnology before they emerge; and
- Create an environment for sustainable development of nanotechnology.

COMMERCIALISATION OF NANOMEDICINE

Commercialisation of nanomedicine is necessary in order to achieve universal health care on the African continent. Pan-African and multilateral bodies are encouraging African countries to focus on producing local solutions to local problems and to commercialise their health innovation research. Singer et al. (2008) argues that African countries need to capitalise on local technology and local talent as a way to reduce international dependency for every technology they need. Local production could lead into affordable medicine. However, whether or not nanomedicine makes a significant impact on health care in the African region will depend on the success of commercialisation.

In order for African countries to commercialise their nanomedicine R&D and patents, they need to consider smart commercialisation strategies (Mufamadi, 2016). Such strategies might include:

Licensing venture: marketing technology or intellectual property (IP) in exchange for compensation.

Spin-off venture: transferring the IP to a new business venture with the equity investment from a parent company. This is often spun out from university laboratories, research councils and industry.

Start-up venture: typically born from innovative business ideas (and different to the spin-off venture), this would depend on the type of investment and technology application. With this venture there is no parent company and so its launch would be a totally new and groundbreaking nanotechnology application. Often the founder/s and/or investors make a decision regarding the mode through which the company will capture value from the technology assets.

Larger corporations venture: forming alliances with larger corporations. Partnerships of this nature are often motivated by technology application, equity, infrastructure, and manufacturing and marketing capabilities.

Alliance business venture: investors decide on which technology should be designed and the application for which it should be designed – in most cases, technology is designed to meet market need.

BRICS alliance venture: BRICS countries would collaborate with each other to enhance the economic benefits.

Africa to Africa alliance venture: two or more African countries enter into joint ventures in a selected nanotechnology application. In this way they would foster intra-Africa partnerships, enhance one other's achievements, and deliver economic benefits.

Nanomedicine and nanopharmaceuticals in the commercial market

A US health care nanotechnology (nanomedicine) 2018 market report indicated that US-based pharmaceutical companies believe that nanomedicines are the next big thing (Marketers Media, 2018). There are a few nanomedicine innovations in Africa which are currently in pre-clinical to clinical, prototype, and pre-commercialisation phases, focusing on combating communicable and non-communicable diseases (DST/Mintek NIC, 2016; Grobler, 2017; Venter et al., 2017).

The Nanotechnology Innovation Centre (NIC), established in 2007 and situated at Mintek, Johannesburg, has a few nanomedicine products that are already in a pre-commercialisation stage (DST/Mintek NIC, 2016). In the case of nanodrug delivery and/or nanopharmaceutical products, Nigeria and South Africa are showing promising results. Maduike and colleagues (2014) from Nigeria have reportedly produced nanomaterials made up of synthetic aluminium-magnesium silicate (AMS) with antiretroviral effects. The AMS nanoparticles are reported to have the potential to bypass physical barriers such as the mucous membrane of the gastrointestinal tract. In another study Maduike et al. (2017) reported that HIV-positive patients recover from HIV post-treated with Antivirt® (Medicinal synthetic Aluminium-magnesium silicate). In an interview with the *New Telegraph*, Maduike indicated that some Nigerian HIV patients showed HIV-negative results with no antigens and antibodies (Madike & Orji, 2017). In a recent clinical trial, conducted by Venter et al. (2017) from the Wits Reproductive Health and HIV Institute (Wits RHI) and OPTIMIZE consortium, researchers reported that they have developed candidate universal antiretroviral (optimised) drugs with a potential to reduce the cost of ART-HIV first line and second line drug by half. In 2010, the CSIR teams reported the development of a pre-clinical efficacy study on a TB nanodrug with the potential to change a daily dose into a weekly dose over a four-week period (Makoni, 2010b).

The high burden of drug resistance on communicable diseases and the rapid growth of NCDs such as cancer, diabetes, and cardiovascular diseases, around the world and in Africa, require urgent medical intervention – nanomedicine (Juma & Wisdom, 2018). A JRC-EURO report observed that the commercialisation of nanomedicine in Europe was seemingly being driven by start-ups and SMEs (Wagner et al., 2006) and that large pharmaceutical and medical device companies showed low interest in investing in nanomedicine. The business model of start-ups and SMEs for bringing nanomedical products to the market, however, mostly depends on big pharmaceuticals and/or medical device corporations being willing to license their established technology. Big pharmaceutical firms find it easy to invest in established technology and to then facilitate the clinical trials and to provide their distribution networks. According to Tsuzuki, the success of nanotechnology will depend on the interaction between multiple stakeholders, R&D and product development, intellectual property, health and safety, regulation and standardisation, and public engagement (Tsuzuki, 2013). Moreover, Mazzucato (2011) insists that governments should take the investment risk where there is uncertainty in areas of R&D and when the private sector is not willing. She observes that in countries where there is economic dynamism, it has been the state, and not the private sector, that has supported risky research areas and created this dynamism (Mazzucato, 2011).

The increase in the pharmaceutical efficacy, the improved bioavailability of nano-sized drugs, and targeted delivery systems were the major focus of the approved nano-enabled drugs that have gained the attention of big pharmaceutical companies in the past decade. The advantage of using nanodrugs is not only in advancing efficacy but also in the reduction of side-effects associated with the bulk counterpart therapeutics currently in use. Most of the FDA-approved nanodrugs are in oncological therapeutics (Morigi et al., 2012). These include PEGylated liposome-encapsulating doxorubicin (Doxil, FDA approved in 1995) for ovarian cancer and the albumin-bound form of paclitaxel (Abraxane, FDA approved in 2005) for various cancers (Wang et al., 2013; Fornaguera & García-Celma, 2017). At present there are few nanopharmaceutical products that are FDA approved and/or in the commercial marketplace (Table 2).

Table 2: Examples of nanomedicines that are in the commercial market

No	Product	Type of Nanoformulation	Application	Company
1	Doxil	PEGylated liposome – Doxorubicin hydrochloride	Ovarian cancer	JNJ
2	Abraxane	Albumin nanoparticles – Paclitaxel	Various cancers, e.g. breast cancer	Celgene

No	Product	Type of Nanoformulation	Application	Company
3	Rapamune	Nanocrystal – Rapamycin	Immuno -suppressive	Pfizer
4	Somavert	Polymer NPs – Pegvisomant	Acromegaly	Pfizer
5	Avinza	Nanocrystal NPs – Morphine sulfate	Psychostimulant	Pfizer
6	Focalin	Nanocrystal NPs – Dexmethylphenidate HCl	Psychostimulant	Novartis
7	Ritalin LA	Nanocrystal NPs – Methylphenidate HCl	Psychostimulant	Novartis
8	Emend	Nanocrystal – Aprepitant	Antiemetic	Merck
9	PegIntron	Pegylated IFN alpha-2b	Hepatitis C	Merck
10	Pegasys	Pegylated IFN alpha-2a	Hepatitis B and Hepatitis C	Genentech
11	Caelyx	PEGylated liposome – Doxorubicin	Solid tumors	Janssen
12	Invega sustenna	Nanocrystal – Paliperidone palmitate	Schizophrenia	Janssen
13	Copaxone	Glatiramer acetate	Multiple sclerosis	Teva Pharma
14	Myocet	Liposome – Doxorubicin	Various tumors	Teva Pharma
15	AmBisome	Liposome – Amphotericine B	Fungal infections	Astellas Pharma
16	Marqibo	Vincristine – Sphingomyelin -based liposomes	Leukemia and melanoma	Talon Therapeutics
17	Resovist	Iron oxide nanoparticles coated with carboxydextran	Liver and spleen lesion imaging	Bayer
18	Tricor	Nanocrystal – Fenofibrate	Hypercholest -erolemia	Abbott
19	Plegridy	Pegylated IFN beta-1a	Multiple sclerosis	Biogen
20	Neulasta	Polymer NPs – Pegfilgrastim	Chemotherapy-induced neutropenia	Amgen

No	Product	Type of Nanoformulation	Application	Company
21	AmBIsome	Liposomal amphotericin B	Fungal and protozoal infections	Gilead Sciences
22	Rebinyn	Polymer NPs – Coagulation factor IX	Haemophilia B	Novo Nordisk
23	Eligard	PEGylated polymeric NPs – Leuprorelina	Prostate cancer	Tolmar
24	DaunoXome	Lipid encapsulation of daunorubicin	HIV-associated Kaposi's sarcoma	Galen Ltd.
25	Rexin-G	Targeting protein/ phospholipid microRNA	Various cancers, e.g. sarcoma	Epeius Biotech-nologies
26	Estrasorb	Micellar estradiol	Menopause	Novavax
27	Abelcet	Liposomal amphotericin B lipid complex	Fungal infections	Sigma-Tau
28	DepoCyt	Liposomal cytarabine	Meningitis	Sigma-Tau
29	Oncaspar	PEGylated asparaginase	Leukemia	Enzon Pharma
30	Megace ES	Nanocrystal – Megestrol	Anti-anorexic	Par Pharma

Source: Wang et al., 2013; Fornaguera & García-Celma, 2017

Nanotechnology entrepreneurship

In Africa, despite a large number of nanotechnology research outputs, the commercialisation of nanotechnology is very slow (Makhoba & Pouris, 2017; Mboyi et al., 2017). A study by Maine (2014) showed that entrepreneurial skills can be an important tool in facilitating the commercialisation of nanotechnology in the 21st century. Although the study's focus was on academic entrepreneurs, its broader application is useful to consider. If academic researchers were to be trained in entrepreneurship – the principles, practices, and skills – and given the tools, they would be in a strong position to commercialise their university's technologies and/or patents (Wood, 2011; Pattnaik & Pandey, 2014). Traditional universities normally focus on training postgraduate students for knowledge generation, but recent trends show that many universities around the world are becoming increasingly interested in the commercial value of their research outputs and patents (Siegel & Wright, 2015; Mzekandaba, 2018).

Acquiring entrepreneurship skills would help academic nanotechnology researchers in a number of ways:

- to identify the commercial value of their nanotechnology research outputs;
- to translate their nanotechnology research work into commercial products;
- to identify the business opportunity in the optimisation of benefits and reduction of potential risks;
- to develop an appropriate business model to commercialise their prototypes;
- to navigate the funding space for nanotechnology ventures; and
- to evaluate the market potential of nanotechnology research.

Various African countries are now focusing on the technology transfer of their university innovations through their own technology enterprise for innovation support – finding licensees from the industry and/or creating spin-off ventures (De Beer, 2018). The advantage of a spin-off company from a university or research laboratory is that this will not only enable the university to commercialise their technologies, but also contribute towards economic development and job creation (Pattnaik & Pandey, 2014). In addition, university spin-offs may continue to receive support from their university enterprise until the company is able actively to sustain itself. Ghana is an example of an African country that is harnessing its science-based health innovation as a way to achieve affordable health solutions and/or to build strong health innovation systems for Ghanaians (Al-Bader et al., 2010).

According to Libaers and Wang (2012), the term 'academic entrepreneurs' refers to academics who participate in university research with a hope of commercialising their university-invented technologies. In African countries, where most nanomedicine patents originate from universities, such a strategy could be used to facilitate the commercialisation process. Whether academic researchers will make good entrepreneurs or not remains up for debate. They may be highly technically skilled and excel in inventing new technologies under the auspices of their university, but it also needs to be accepted that those technologies and patents will not necessarily be commercially viable or result in business success (Rahim et al., 2015; Siegel & Wright, 2015).

Nevertheless, having entrepreneurs in nanomedicine application could facilitate the creation of new business or start-up companies which will eventually create new jobs and benefit a large number of currently unemployed postgraduate students in nanoscience and nanotechnology. For old industries, the presence of entrepreneurs could facilitate the growth of existing companies. Incorporating nanomaterials into their current products and/or enabling those with new functionality and/or new properties could lead old industries to establishing new businesses or spin-off companies. Furthermore, the presence of entrepreneurs in the research consortium could help in capitalising on the existing nanomedicine patents and in making profit from them or creating new business ventures.

Nanotechnology cluster: a case for collaboration

If developing countries want to succeed in nanotechnology development, they need to consider clustering to create nanotechnology industries (Gkanas et al., 2013). Cluster theory was first described by the economist Alfred Marshall. In his book *Principles of Economics* (1890) he characterised clusters as a concentration of specialised industries in particular localities. The concept of industrial clusters was popularised by Michael Porter (1990) from Harvard University. African countries could use this concept to group nanotech start-up companies from similar industries and foster partnerships with one another. Nanotech clusters in Africa would create a platform for African governments to centralise or mobilise resources to finance a nanotechnology industry. In collaborating in this way a world-class infrastructure could be set in place and the commercialisation of nanotechnology realised. An opportunity could be created for local inventors to showcase their prototypes to pharmaceutical and medical device companies with a view to forming partnerships that would support prototype development. Other advantages to nanotech clusters might include: assisting inventors/start-ups to reduce the cost of production and waste management; attracting foreign direct investment; enabling job creation and the sustainable development of nanotechnology.

Nanotechnology is supported by the African Union (AU) through the Science, Technology and Innovation Strategy for Africa (STISA, 2014). Creating clusters would assist in the AU's implementation of its strategy and it would be in a position to be better informed about each country's progress in nanotechnology development. African policy-makers need to engage with organisations such as the African Science, Technology and Innovation Fund (ASTIF), Africa Health Strategy (AHS), the Accelerated Industrial Development of Africa (AIDA), Advancing Healthcare Innovation in Africa (AHIA), the African Network for Drugs and Diagnostics Innovation (ANDI), and global partners such as the Wellcome Trust and the Bill and Melinda Gates Foundation to access funding partners for health innovation solutions. Academia, inventors, and entrepreneurs should also be engaged in such policy discussion in order to accelerate the growth of nanotechnology. Africa needs an active cluster policy that promotes growth and development in a sustainable manner in the area of nanomedicine.

CONCLUSION

Despite all the health-related interventions introduced in Africa, epidemics are still prevalent on the continent. Generally weak health systems mean that quality health care remains inaccessible to the most vulnerable in many African countries. Health research, which is a component of building strong health systems, is crucial in improving the health status in Africa. However, the research capacity on the continent is insufficient.

The disease burden on African countries necessitates substantial investment in building research capacity on the continent. This includes the creation of an enabling environment for research to be conducted. Intracontinental partnerships among researchers, governments, and the private sector are important in enhancing research that is relevant to the continent. Furthermore, partnerships with the international community for research in Africa should be regulated to ensure that issues and illnesses relevant to Africa are prioritised. Research undertaken on the continent should be led by African researchers. It should be receptive to the socio-economic conditions of the African populations. African innovation is key in promoting health and economic development on the continent and should thus be prioritised. More so, technological innovation can help Africa advance into improved health care.

Nanotechnology has been used in this chapter to build a case for disruptive technology in order to challenge the status quo and introduce efficient and affordable treatments. Studies have shown that nanotechnology can improve the efficacy of the existing drugs that are used for the treatment of HIV/AIDS, TB, cancer, and other diseases by reducing their toxicity, reducing the dosage required to achieve the desired effect, and improving their solubility. These factors are pertinent when it comes to patient compliance: with fewer side-effects and less frequent dosing, patients would be more inclined to stick to regimens and thus improve the efficiency of these treatments. It has also been demonstrated how nanotechnology can be used in addressing water-borne diseases such as cholera. Nanotechnology is an efficient and decentralised solution for the provision of clean and safe water to the most vulnerable.

As an emerging technology, nanotechnology requires large investment. Big pharmaceutical companies, which have the resources and existing infrastructure, are not always willing to take the investment risk for emerging technologies. Finding an effective and sustainable way to invest in nanotechnology should thus take precedence for African governments. To advance nanotechnology research in Africa, African countries must build networks between their nanotechnology research efforts, tertiary institutions, and the private sector. Building research capacity from within African countries is how Africa can ensure the development of relevant technologies that will address the burden of disease on the continent.

REFERENCES

Adesina, S. K. & Akala, E. O. 2015. 'Nanotechnology approaches for the delivery of exogenous siRNA for HIV therapy'. *Molecular Pharmaceutics*, 12 (12), 4175–4187.

Adoga, M. P., Fatumo, S. A. & Agwale, S. M. 2014. 'H3Africa: A tipping point for a revolution in bioinformatics, genomics and health research in Africa'.

Source Code for Biology and Medicine, 9 (10), http://www.scfbm.org/content/9/1/10, accessed 21 July 2018.

Ahmad, Z., Pandey, R., Sharma, S. & Khuller, G. K. 2006. 'Alginate Nanoparticles as Antituberculosis Drug Carriers: Formulation Development, Pharmacokinetics and Therapeutic Potential'. *Indian Journal of Chest Diseases & Allied Sciences*, 48 (3), 171–176.

Al-Bader, S., Daar, A. & Singer, P. A. 2010. 'Science-based health innovation in Ghana: Health entrepreneurs point the way to a new development path'. *BMC International Health and Human Rights*, 10 (Suppl 1), S2.

Alo, B. 2017. 'Nanotechnology in a developing country: Applications and challenges'. University of Lagos. https://www.who.int/ifcs/documents/forums/forum6/ppt_nano_alo.pdf, accessed 19 July 2018.

Anjum, M., Miandad, R., Waqas, M., Gehany, F. & Barakat, M. A. 2016. 'Remediation of wastewater using various nanomaterials'. *Arabian Journal of Chemistry*. https://www.sciencedirect.com/science/article/pii/S1878535216301757. available online 17 October 2016.

Bankole, M. T., Tijani, J. O., Mohammed, I. A. & Abdulkareem, A. S. 2014. 'A review on nanotechnology as a tool change in Nigeria'. *Scientific Research and Essays*, 9 (8), 213–223.

Bawa, J. 2011. 'Regulating Nanomedicine – Can the FDA Handle It?'. *Current Drug Delivery*, 8 (3), 227–234.

Beumer, K. 2017. 'How economic assumptions constitute publics as consumers in South African nanotechnology governance'. *Science as Culture*, 26 (4), 481–490.

Bhushan, B. 2007. 'Introduction to nanotechnology', in Bhushan, B. (ed.) *Springer Handbook of Nanotechnology 2nd ed.* Berlin/New York: Springer, pp 1–12.

Bosetti, R. 2015. 'Cost-effectiveness of nanomedicine: The path to a future successful and dominant market?' *Nanomedicine*, 10 (12), 1851–1853.

Botswana Institute for Technology Research and Innovation (BITRI). 2018. *Annual Report 2016/17*. Gaborone, Botswana. http://www.bitri.co.bw/wp-content/uploads/2018/02/ANNUAL%20REPORT%202016-2017.pdf, accessed 11 December 2018.

Boum II, Y., Burns, B. F., Siedner, M., Mburu, Y., Bukusi, E. & Haberer, J. E. 2018. 'Advancing equitable global health research partnerships in Africa'. *BMJ Global Health*, e000868.

Chang, E. H., Harford, J. B., Eaton, M. A. W., Boisseau, P. M., Dube, A., Hayeshi, R., Swai, H. & Lee, D. S. 2015. 'Nanomedicine: past, present and future – a global perspective'. *Biochemical and Biophysical Research Communications*, 18, 468 (3), 511–517.

Chong, M. N., Jin, B., Chow, C. W. K. & Saint, C. 2010. 'Recent developments in photocatalytic water treatment technology: A review'. *Water Research*, 44, 2997–3027.

Chu, K. M., Jayaraman, S., Kyamanywa, P. & Ntakiyiruta, G. 2014. 'Building research capacity in Africa: equity and global health collaborations'. *PLoS Medicine*, 11 (3) e1001612.

Claassens, C. H. & Motuku, M. 2006. 'Nanoscience and nanotechnology research and development in South Africa'. *Nanotechnology Law and Business*, 3, 217–228.

COHRED. Health Research: Essential Link to Equity in Development, 1990. *Oxford University Press.*

Commissioned Annotated Bibliography in Support of the Leadership Institute American Association for the Advancement of Science, Washington, DC.

Council for Scientific and Industrial Research (CSIR). 2018. 'Available instrumentation: optical'. http://www.csirnano.co.za/ncnsm-characterisation-facility/available-instrumentation-optical/, accessed 8 October 2018.

Crane, J. 2010. 'Adverse events and placebo effects: African scientists, HIV, and ethics in the global health sciences'. *Social Studies of Science*, 40 (6) 843–870.

Curley, P., Liptrott, N. J. & Owen, A. 2017. 'Advances in nanomedicine drug delivery applications for HIV therapy'. *Future Science OA*, 4 (1), FSO230.

De Beer, C. 2018. *Improving the Efficiency of University Technology Transfer*. Doctoral dissertation, Stellenbosch: Stellenbosch University.

Din, F. U., Aman, W., Ullah, I., Qureshi, O. S., Mustapha, O., Shafique, S., & Zeb, A. 2017. 'Effective use of nanocarriers as drug delivery systems for the treatment of selected tumors'. *International Journal of Nanomedicine*, 12, 7291–7309.

Doyel, L. & Hoffman, M. 2009. 'The growing burden of chronic diseases among South African women'. *Continuing Medical Education*, 27 (10), 456–458.

DST/Mintek Nanotechnology Innovation Centre (DST/Mintek NIC) 2016. The NIC Groups. *DST/Mintek* http://www.nic.ac.za/Groups.html, accessed 17 July 2018.

Dube, A. & Ebrahim, N. 2017. 'The nanomedicine landscape of South Africa'. *Nanotechnology Reviews*, 6 (4), 339–344.

European Medicines Agency. 'Reflection paper on nanotechnology-based medicinal products for human use'. 2006. https://www.ema.europa.eu/documents/regulatory-procedural-guideline/reflection-paper-nanotechnology-based-medicinal-products-human-use_en.pdf, accessed 1 October 2018.

Ezema, I. C., Ogbobe, P. O., & Omah, A. D. 2014. 'Initiatives and strategies for development of nanotechnology in nations: A lesson for Africa and other least developed countries'. *Nanoscale Research Letters*, 9 (1), 133. doi:10.1186/1556-276X-9-133.

Farshchi, P., Sadrnezhaad, S. K., Nejad, N. M., Mahmoodi, M. & Abadi, L. I. G. 2011. 'Nanotechnology in the public eye: The case of Iran, as a developing country'. *Journal of Nanoparticle Research*, 13 (8), 3511–3519.

Fornaguera, C. & García-Celma, M. J. 2017. 'Personalized nanomedicine: A revolution at the nanoscale'. *Journal of Personalized Medicine*, 7 (4): 12. doi:10.3390/jpm7040012.

Franzen, S. R., Chandler, C. & Lang, T. 2017. 'Health research capacity development in low and middle income countries: reality or rhetoric? A systematic meta-narrative review of the qualitative literature'. *BMJ Open*, 7 (1), e012332. doi:10.1136/bmjopen-2016-012332.

Gkanas, E. I., Mogkou-Kriticou, V., Makridis, S. S., Stubos, A. K. & Bakouros, I. 2013. 'Nanotechnology and Innovation: Recent status and the strategic implication for the formation of high tech clusters in Greece, in between a global economic crisis'. *International Open Access publishing*. DOI:1303.5290.

Grobler, A. 2017. 'The use of nano and micro-delivery systems in the pharmaceutical space: Gold and beyond'. *Journal of Nanomedicine and Nanotechnology*, 8, 4. DOI: 10.4172/2157-7439-C1-048.

Gudimalla, A., Mishra, R. K. & Arora, P. 2017. 'Novel approaches to nanomedicine and nanotechnology', in Thomas, J., Thomas, S., Jose, J. & Kalarikkal, N. (eds.) *Recent Trends in Nanomedicine and Tissue Engineering*. Denmark: River Publishers, pp. 19–52.

Hashem, E. A. 2014. 'Nanotechnology in water treatment, case study: Egypt'. *Journal of Economics and Development Studies*, 2 (3), 243–259.

Havlir, D. & Gandhi, M. 2015. 'Implementation challenges for long-acting antivirals as treatment'. *Current Opinion in HIV and AIDS*, 10 (4), 282–289.

Hayeshi, R., Semete, B., Kalombo, L., Katata, L., Lemmer, Y., Melariri, P., Nyamboli, B. & Swai, H. 2012. 'Nanomedicine in the development of drugs for poverty-related diseases', in Chibale, K., Davies-Coleman, M. & Masimirembwa, C. (eds.) *Drug Discovery in Africa: Impacts of Genomics, Natural Products, Traditional Medicines, Insights into Medicinal Chemistry, and Technology Platforms in Pursuit of New Drugs*. Berlin: Springer-Verlag, pp 407–429.

He, Y., Du, Z., Ma, S., Cheng, S., Jiang, S., et al. 2016. 'Biosynthesis, Antibacterial Activity and Anticancer Effects Against Prostate Cancer (PC-3) Cells of Silver Nanoparticles Using *Dimocarpus Longan* Lour. Peel Extract'. *Nanoscale Research Letters*, 11 (1), 300.

Industrial Development Corporation (IDC). 2015. New Industries: Driving industrial development and facilitating job creation. IDC, http://staging.idc.co.za/index.php?option=com_content&view=article&id=800&Itemid=173&catid=13, accessed 14 December 2018.

Jackson, O. 7 June 2018. 'Dr. Dougbeh Nyan among Top 50 African Innovators'. *Daily Observer*. https://www.liberianobserver.com/news/dr-dougbeh-nyan-among-top-50-african-innovators/, accessed 8 October 2018.

Jones, R., 13 January 2009. 'Public Engagement and Nanotechnology – the UK experience'. *Soft Machines*, http://www.softmachines.org/wordpress/?p=443.

Juma, P. A. & Wisdom, J. 2018. 'Introduction: Non-communicable disease prevention policies in six African countries'. *BMC Public Health* 201818 (Suppl 1), 955. https://doi.org/10.1186/s12889-018-5824-8.

Kamminga, E. & Wegelin-Schuringa, M. W. 2005. 'HIV/AIDS and water, sanitation and hygiene'. IRC International Water and Sanitation Centre. Netherlands.

Kanchi, S. 2014. 'Nanotechnology for water treatment'. *Journal of Environmental Analytical Chemistry*, 1 (2), 102.

Kariuki, T. & Kay, S. 3 May 2017. 'There are not enough scientists in Africa. How can we turn this around?'. *World Economic Forum*, https://www.weforum.org/agenda/2017/05/scientists-are-the-key-to-africas-future/, accessed 1 August 2018.

Kebede, D., Zielinski, C., Mbondji, P. E., Sanou, I., Kouvividila, W. & Lusamba-Dikassa, 2014. 'Expenditures on health research in sub-Saharan African countries: Results of a questionnaire-based survey'. *Journal of the Royal Society of Medicine*, 107 (1S), 77–84.

Kunduru, K. R., Nazarkovsky, M., Farah, S., Pawar, R. P., Basu, A. & Domb, A. J. 2017. 'Nanotechnology for water purification: applications of nanotechnology methods in wastewater treatment'. *Water Purification*, 33–74.

Lane, N. & Kalil, T. 2005. 'The national nanotechnology initiative: Present at the creation.' *Issues in Science and Technology*, 21 (421), 49–54.

Lessler, J., Moore, S. M., Luquero, F. J., McKay, H. S., Grais, R., Henkens, M., Mengel, M., Dunoyer, J., M'bangombe, M., Lee, E. C., Djingarey, M. H., Sudre, B., Bompangue, D., Fraser, R. S. M., Abubakar, A., Perea, W., Legros, D. & Azman, A. S. 2018. 'Mapping the burden of cholera in sub-Saharan Africa and implications for control: An analysis of data across geographical scales'. *The Lancet*, 391 (10133), 1908–1915.

Libaers, D. & and Wang, T. 2012. 'Foreign-born academic scientists: entrepreneurial academics or academic entrepreneurs?' *R&D Management*, 42 (3), 254–272.

Madike, S. & Orji, I. 19 August 2017. 'Doctors confirm my drug cures HIV, says Ezeibe'. *New Telegraph*, https://newtelegraphonline.com/2017/08/doctors-confirm-drug-cures-hiv-says-ezeibe/, accessed 8 August 2018.

Maduike, C. O. E., Dahiru, A., Nnaemeka, K. A., Thompson, N. O., Ijeoma, J. O., Ekenma, K. & Njoku, U. N. 2017. 'Effective treatment of HIV/AIDS with the medicinal synthetic aluminum-magnesium silicate'. *SciFed AIDS & HIV Research Journal*, 1 (1), 1–6.

Maduike, C. O., Ngene, A., Idika, K. K., Ezeh, I. O., Mbuko, I. J., Ekwuruke, J. O., Anene, I., Amechi, B., Olowoniyi, P. & Ifekwe, I. 2014. 'Assessment of antiretroviral effects of a synthetic aluminum-magnesium silicate'. *British Journal of Medicine & Medical Research*, 4 (8), 1672–1679.

Maine, E. 2014. 'Scientist-entrepreneurs as the catalysts of nanotechnology commercialization'. *Reviews in Nanoscience and Nanotechnology*, 2, 1–8.

Makaudze, E., Du Preez, M. & Potgieter, N. 2012. 'How does the HIV and AIDS epidemic in South Africa impact on Water, Sanitation and Hygiene Sectors?' *Water Research Commission*, www.wrc.org.za, accessed 19 July 2018.

Makhoba, X. & Pouris, A. 2017. 'Bibliometric analysis of the development of nanoscience research in South Africa'. *South African Journal of Science*, 113 (11–12), 1–9.

Makoni, M. 2010a. 'Nano "tea bag" purifies water'. *SciDevNet*, https://www.scidev.net/global/water/news/nano-tea-bag-purifies-water.html, accessed 17 July 2018.

Makoni, M., 2010b. 'Case study: South Africa uses nanotech against TB'. *SciDevNet*, https://www.scidev.net/global/systems/feature/case-study-south-africa-uses-nanotech-against-tb-1.html, accessed 10 October 2018.

Maksimovi, M. 2017. 'The roles of nanotechnology and internet of nano things in healthcare transformation'. *TecnoLógicas*, 20 (40), 139–153.

Mallipeddi, R. & Rohan, L. C. 2010. 'Progress in antiretroviral drug delivery using nanotechnology'. *International Journal of Nanomedicine*, 5, 533–547.

Marshall, A. 1890. *Principles of Economics* (Eight edition). The Online Library of Liberty.

Mazumder, S., Sarkar, D. & Puri, I. K. 2014. 'Nanotechnology commercialization: Prospects in India'. *Journal of Materials Science & Nanotechnology*, 1 (4), 402.

Mazzucato, M. 2011. 'The entrepreneurial state'. *Demos*, www.demos.co.uk/files/Entrepreneurial_State_-_web.pdf, accessed 11 December 2018.

Mboyi, A., Ilunga, K. & Momba, B. M. N. 2017. 'Nanoscale development and its application in multidisciplinary area: An African perspective'. *African Journal of Biotechnology*, 16, 193–208.

McConnell, H., Chathoth, P., Pardy, A., Boostrom, C., Boostrom, E., Louw, K., Cuervo, L. G., & Ogawa, S. 2008. 'Leapfrog technologies for health and development'. *Global Forum Update on Research for Health*, 5, 130–135.

McDonald, T. O., Giardiello, M., Martin, P., Siccardi, M., Liptrott, N. J., Smith, D., Roberts, P., Curley, P., Schipani, A., Khoo, S. H., Long, J., Foster, A. J., Rannard, S. P. & Owen, A. 2014. 'Antiretroviral solid drug nanoparticles with enhanced oral bioavailability: Production, characterization, and in vitro-in vivo correlation'. *Advanced Healthcare Materials*, 3 (3), 400–411.

Molapisi, J. 2012. 'Nanotechnology development in South Africa', in *International Symposium on Assessing the Economic Impact of Nanotechnology: 2012* March 27–28. Washington, DC.

Montgomery, M. A. & Elimelech, M. 2007. 'Water and sanitation in developing countries: Including health in the equation'. *Environmental Science & Technology*, 17–24. https://pubs.acs.org/doi/pdf/10.1021/es072435t.

Morel, T., Maher, D., Nyirenda, T. & Olesen, O. F. 2018. 'Strengthening health research capacity in sub-Saharan Africa: Mapping the 2012–2017 landscape of externally funded international postgraduate training at institutions in the region'. *Globalization and Health*, 14 (1), 77–86.

Morigi, V., Tocchio, A., Bellavite Pellegrini, C., Sakamoto, J.H., Arnone, M. & Tasciotti, E. 2012. 'Nanotechnology in medicine: From inception to market domination'. *Journal of Drug Delivery*. http://doi.org/10.1155/2012/389485.

Moroccan Foundation for Advanced Science, Innovation and Research (MAScIR), 2005. 'Nanomaterials and Nanotechnology'. *MAScIR*, https://www.mascir.com/Nanomaterials-and-Nanotechnology_a134.html.

Mufamadi, S. 2016. 'South Africa needs to start to venture into nanotechnology commercialisation by employing sustainable models'. *Science Stars*. http://sciencestars.co.za/south-africa-needs-to-start-to-venture-into-nanotechnology-commercialisation-by-employing-sustainable-models.

Munung, N. S., Mayosi, B. M. & De Vries, J. 2017. 'Equity in international health research collaborations in Africa: Perceptions and expectations of African researchers'. *PLoS ONE* 12 (10), e0186237. https://doi.org/10.1371/journal.pone.0186237, accessed 21 July 2018.

Mzekandaba, S. 7 August 2018. 'Tuks to groom tech-skilled entrepreneurs'. *ITWeb*, https://www.itweb.co.za/content/LPp6V7r4ZRZqDKQz,ccccccc accessed 16 October 2018.

Nanotechnology Public Engagement Programme (NPEP). NPEP, https://www.npep.co.za, accessed 4 October 2018.

Nanotechnology Public Engagement Programme (NPEP). 2017. NPEP, https://www.npep.co.za/sa-swiss-nanomedicine-symposium, accessed 10 October 2018.

Nanototechnology Public Engagement Programme (NPEP). March 2016. 'DST-NRF Nanotechnology Symposium, in Gauteng on 27–28 June 2016'. *NPEP Newsletter*. https://www.npep.co.za/newsletter/issues/march-2016/dst-nrf-nanotechnology-symposium/.

Naseri, R. & Davoodi, R. 2011. 'Commercialization of nanotechnology in developing countries'. *3rd International Conference on Information and Financial Engineering* IPEDR 12 (2011), 385–389.

Nass, S. J., Levit, L. A. & Gostin, L. O. 2009. 'Beyond the HIPAA privacy rule: Enhancing privacy, improving health through research'. *Institute of Medicine (US) Committee on Health Research and the Privacy of Health Information: The HIPAA Privacy Rule*. Washington, DC: National Academies Press (US). Available from: https://www.ncbi.nlm.nih.gov/books/NBK9578/ doi: 10.17226/12458, accessed 10 October 2018.

National Nanotechnology Equipment Programme (NNEP). NNEP website: http://hicd.nrf.ac.za/?q=node/19, accessed 9 October 2018.

Ndomondo-Sigonda, M., Miot, J., Naidoo, S., Dodoo, A. & Kaale, E. 2017. 'Medicines Regulation in Africa: Current state and opportunities'. *Pharmaceutical Medicine*, 31 (6), 383–397.

Nisbet, M. C. & Markowitz, E. D. 2015. 'Public engagement research and major approaches'. https://www.aaas.org/sites/default/files/content_files/Biblio_PublicEngagement_FINAL11.25.15.pdf, accessed 9 October 2018.

NPEP Newsletter. 'The safe and responsible development of nanotechnology in South Africa'. Published 1 April 2018. https://www.npep.co.za/newsletter/issues/oct-2018/the-safe-and-responsible-development-of-nanotechnology-in-south-africa/, accessed 9 October 2018.

Nwabor, N. O., Ikechukwu, N. E., Emenike, M. P. & Christiana, A. O. 2016. 'Water and waterborne diseases: a review'. *International Journal of Tropical Disease & Health,* 12 (4), 1–14.

Obiukwu, O. 2015. 'Nanofilter: An African innovation for safe drinking water'. *How We Made It In Africa*, https://www.howwemadeitinafrica.com/nanofilter-an-african-innovation-for-safe-drinking-water/, accessed 19 July 2018.

Olu, O. 2017. 'Resilient health system as conceptual framework for strengthening public health disaster risk management: An African viewpoint'. *Frontiers in Public Health*, 5 (263), DOI: 10.3389/fpubh.2017.00263.

Online Cambridge Dictionary. https://dictionary.cambridge.org/dictionary/english/cluster, accessed 10 October 2018.

Pandey, R. & Khuller, G. K. 2004. 'Subcutaneous nanoparticle based antitubercular chemotherapy in an experimental model'. *Journal of Antimicrobial Chemotherapy*, 54 (1), 266–268.

Pandey, R., Sharma, S. & Khuller, G. K. 2005. 'Oral solid lipid nanoparticle-based antitubercular chemotherapy'. *Tuberculosis*, 85 (5–6), 415–420.

Pattnaik, P. N. & Pandey, S. C. 2014. 'University spinoffs: what, why, and how?'. *Technology Innovation Management Review,* 4 (12), 44–50.

Perrot, R. 2018. 'The dynamics of new and emerging technologies in developing countries & the new role of the state', in Mazibuko, Z. (ed.) *Beyond Imagination: The Ethics and Applications of Nanotechnology and Bio-Economics in South Africa.* Johannesburg: MISTRA, pp. 1–16.

Peters, K., Leitzke, S., Diederichs, J. E., Borner, K., Hahn, H., Müller, R. H. & Ehlers, S. 2000. 'Preparation of a clofazimine nanosuspension for intravenous use and evaluation of its therapeutic efficacy in murine Mycobacterium avium infection'. *Journal of Antimicrobial Chemotherapy*, 45 (1), 77–83.

Photopoulos, J. 2018. 'Q&A: Catalysing investment in innovation, R&D in Africa'. SciDevNet, https://www.scidev.net/sub-saharan-africa/r-d/feature/q-a-catalysing-investment-in-innovation-r-d-in-africa.html, accessed 11 December 2018.

Porter, M. E. 1990. 'Competitive advantage of nations'. *Harvard Business Review*, March–April 1990.

Pouris, A. & Ho, Y-S. 2014. 'Research emphasis and collaboration in Africa'. *Scientometrics*, 98, 2169–2184.

Public Sector Manager (PSM). 2018. 'The safe and responsible development of nanotechnology in South Africa'. https://issuu.com/topcomedia/docs/

psm_april_2018_final_issuu?e=2548535/60048837, accessed 10 October 2018.

Rahim, N. A., Mohamed, Z. B. & Amrin, A. 2015. 'Commercialization of Emerging Technology: The role of academic entrepreneur'. *Procedia – Social and Behavioral Sciences*, 169, 53–60.

Rahman, M. & Fukui, T. 2003. 'Biomedical publication – global profile and trend'. *Public Health*, 117 (4), 274–280.

Rateng, B. 2017. 'Nanotech holds promise for Africa, but not prioritised'. *SciDevNet.*.https://www.scidev.net/sub-saharan-africa/r-d/news/nanotech-africa-prioritised.html, accessed 17 October 2018.

Ronavari, A., Igaz, N., Gopisetty, M. K., Szerencses, B., Kovacs, D., Papp, C., Vagvolgyi, C., Boros, I. M., Konya, Z., Kiricsi, M. & Pfeiffer, I. 2018. 'Biosynthesized silver and gold nanoparticles are potent antimycotics against opportunistic pathogenic yeasts and dermatophyte'. *International Journal of Nanomedicine*, 13, 695–703.

Russo, P. & Adler, A. 26 July 2015. 'Health care efficiency: measuring the cost associated with quality'. *Managed Care,* https://www.managedcaremag.com/archives/2015/7/health-care-efficiency-measuring-cost-associated-quality, accessed 6 December 2018.

Sahin, N. & Ekli, E. 2013. 'Nanotechnology awareness, opinions and risk perceptions among middle school students'. *International Journal of Technology and Design Education*, 23 (4), 867–881. DOI: 10.1007/s10798-013-9233-0.

Saiyed, Z. M., Gandhi, N. H. & Nair, M. P. 2010. 'Magnetic nanoformulation of azidothymidine 5'-triphosphate for targeted delivery across the blood-brain barrier'. *International Journal of Nanomedicine,* 5, 157–166.

Science, Technology and Innovation Strategy for Africa 2024. 2014. https://au.int/sites/default/files/newsevents/workingdocuments/33178-wd-stisa-english_-_final.pdf, accessed 17 October 2018.

Sechi, G., Bedognetti, D., Sgarrella, F., Van Eperen, L., Marincola, F. M., Bianco, A. & Delogu, L. G. 2014. 'The perception of nanotechnology and nanomedicine a worldwide social media study'. *Nanomedicine*, 9 (10), 1475–1486. DOI: 10.2217/nnm.14.78.

Senje, R. 2013. 'Nanomedicine: new solutions or new problems?'. *Health Care Without Harm Europe.*

Siegel, D. S. & Wright, M. 2015. 'Academic entrepreneurship: Time for a rethink?' *British Journal of Management*, 26 (4), 582–595.

Singer, A. P., Al-Bader, S., Shah, R., Simiyu, K., Wiley, R. E., Kanellis, P., Pulandiran, M. & Heymann, M. 2008. 'Commercializing African health research: Building life science convergence platforms'. *Global Forum Update on Research for Health: Technological Innovations*, 5, 143–150.

Smit, P. 2010. 'Stellenbosch University scientists patent tea-bag-like water filter'. *Engineering News,* http://www.engineeringnews.co.za/article/stellenbosch-university-scientists-patent-tea-baglike-water-filter-2010-08-13.

South African Agency for Science and Technology (SAASTA). 2011. 'Water and nanotechnology'. SAASTA, http://www.saasta.ac.za/images/stories/National%20School%20Debates/Water%20Nanotechnology%20Purification%20-%20media%20article.pdf, accessed 19 July 2018.

Spreen, W., Ford, S. L., Chen S., Gould, E., Wilfret, D., Subich, D., Taishi, T. & Hong, Z. 2012. 'Pharmacokinetics, safety and tolerability of the HIV integrase inhibitor S/GSK1265744 long acting parenteral nanosuspension following single dose administration to healthy adults'. Presented at: *19th International AIDS Conference.* Washington, DC, USA, 22–27 July 2012 (Abstract TUPE040).

Stein, R. A. 2014. 'Nanotechnology: Is the magic bullet becoming reality?' *Genetic Engineering and Biotechnology News,* http://www.genengnews.com/insight-and-intelligence/nanotechnologyis-the-magic-bullet-becomingreality/77900016/, accessed 17 October 2018.

Sunday Standard, 13 December 2017. 'BITRI set to produce high value minerals products'. *Sunday Standard,* http://www.sundaystandard.info/bitri-set-produce-high-value-minerals-products, accessed 17 October 2018.

Tatham, L. M., Rannard, S. P. & Owen, A. 2015. 'Nanoformulation strategies for the enhanced oral bioavailability of antiretroviral therapeutics'. *Therapeutic delivery*, 6 (4), 469–490.

Temu, F., Leonhardt, M., Carter, J. & Thiam, S. 2014. 'Integration of non-communicable diseases in health care: Tackling the double burden of disease in African settings'. *Pan African Medical Journal*, 18 (202), DOI:10.11604/pamj.2014.18.202.4086.

Tiwari, G., Tiwari, R., Sriwastawa, B., Bhati, L., Pandey, S., Pandey, P., & Bannerjee, S. K. 2012. 'Drug delivery systems: An updated review'. *International Journal of Pharmaceutical Investigation*, *2* (1), 2–11.

Tsuzuki, T. 2013. *Nanotechnology Commercialisation.* Pan Stanford, New York: Taylor & Francis Group.

UNESCO. 2016. 'Green technologies a focus of innovation in Morocco'. UNESCO Office, Dhaka, http://www.unesco.org/new/en/dhaka/about-us/single-view/news/green_technologies_a_focus_of_innovation_in_morocco/, accessed 14 December 2018.

United States Food and Drug Administration. (USFDA), 2018. 'Nanotechnology fact sheet'. *US Food and Drug,* https://www.fda.gov/ScienceResearch/SpecialTopics/Nanotechnology/ucm402230.htm, accessed 17 October 2018.

United Nations Institute for Training and Research. 2012. 'Nigeria holds nanotechnology workshop as part of National Pilot Project'. UNITAR, http://www.unitar.org/nigeria-holds-nanotechnology-workshop-part-national-pilot-project, accessed 18 September 2012.

University of Nottingham. Public engagement in nanotechnology. 2013–2016. https://www.nottingham.ac.uk/nmrc/publicengagement/

publicengagementinnanotechnology.aspx
MarketersMedia. 12 April 2018. 'Healthcare Nanotechnology (Nanomedicine) – At the Forefront of a Budding New Market'. https://marketersmedia.com/healthcare-nanotechnology-nanomedicine-at-the-forefront-of-a-budding-new-market/330015.

Venter, W. D. F., Kaiser, B., Pillay, Y., Conradie, F., Gomez, G. B., Clayden, P., Matsolo, M., Amole, C., Rutter, L., Abdullah, F. & Abrams, E. J. 2017. 'Cutting the cost of South African antiretroviral therapy using newer, safer drugs'. *South African Medical Journal*, 107 (1), 28–30.

Wagner, V., Hüsing, B., Gaisser, S. & Bock, A. 2006. 'Nanomedicine: Drivers for development and possible impacts'. JRC European Commission, Joint Research.Centre,.ftp://s-jrcsvqpx101p.jrc.es/pub/EURdoc/JRC46744.pdf, accessed 10 October 2018.

Waldron, A. M., Spencer, D. & Batt, C. A. 2006. 'The current state of public understanding of nano-technology'. *Journal of Nanoparticle Research*, 8 (5), 569–575.

Wang, R., Billone, P. S. & Mullett, W. M. 2013. 'Nanomedicine in action: an overview of cancer nanomedicine on the market and in clinical trials'. *Journal of Nanomaterials*, 1–12. http://dx.doi.org/10.1155/2013/629681

Wood, M. S. 2011. 'A process model of academic entrepreneurship'. *Business Horizons*, 54 (2), 153–161.

Woodson, T. S. 2012. 'Research inequality in nanomedicine'. *Journal of Business Chemistry*, 9 (3), 133–146.

World Bank Group. 2017. 'Bringing clean, affordable water to poor communities through decentralized water treatment kiosks'. World Bank, Washington, DC.

World Health Organization (WHO). 2002. 'Genomics and world health: Report of the advisory committee on health research'. WHO, Geneva.

World Health Organization (WHO). 2010. 'Monitoring the building blocks of health systems: A handbook of indicators and their measurement strategies'. *WHO Library Cataloguing-in-Publication Data*. Geneva.

World Health Organization (WHO). 2015. 'Water sanitation hygiene'. WHO. https://www.who.int/water_sanitation_health/monitoring/jmp-2015-key-facts/en/, accessed 2 August 2018.

Zamxaka, M. & Riley, J. 2010. 'Nanotechnology's campaign for safe drinking water'. SAASTA Nanotechnology Public Engagement (NPE), Pretoria.

TEN

From Present African Health Care Systems to the Future

Health Financing in Ghana and Rwanda

SAMUEL ADU-GYAMFI

INTRODUCTION

THAT THERE IS A POSITIVE correlation between healthy populations and socio-economic and human development is not in dispute. It is in countries' interests, therefore, to aim to have healthy, productive citizens. A strong, well-functioning public health care system would go some way to realising this. In sub-Saharan Africa, the issue of how to finance health care and make it accessible to the majority of citizens is an ongoing challenge.

While the overall intention behind The Structural Adjustment Programmes (SAPs) of the 1980s and 1990s was to assist development, the inadvertent result in many African countries that subscribed to SAPs was, in fact, the deepening of poverty and inequality. The aims of the

Millennium Development Goals (MDGs) and, later, the Sustainable Development Goals (SDGs) are to reduce poverty and poverty-related diseases, increase gender equality, reduce maternal and child mortality, to address climate change and environmental degradation, and to further ensure prosperity, peace, and justice (UN, 2018).

One of the consequences of the adoption of SAPs was that governments reduced their spending on health care. In some instances (Zimbabwe, for example) the gains countries had made after independence were eroded. The targets the MDGs and the SDGs set in place created – and continue to create – the possibility for pursuing actions aimed at sustaining the health systems of these countries, despite the rising maternal and infant morbidity and mortality rates and child deaths (UN, 2018). Significantly, goal three of the SDGs aims, among other things, at focusing on providing more efficient funding of health systems, improved sanitation and hygiene, increased access to physicians, and more tips on ways to reduce ambient pollution (UN, 2018). Globally, this is directed at making strong progress to save the lives of millions.

Some African governments have attempted to bridge the gap between the rich and the poor with regard to access to health services through the introduction of different forms of public health insurance – Ghana (2003), Nigeria (2005), and Rwanda (1999) are examples. Using Ghana and Rwanda as case studies, this chapter traces the post-independence precursors to public health insurance and the impact of socio-economic and political factors on the development of health insurance schemes. The rationale for the selection of Ghana and Rwanda as case studies is that these two countries introduced a form of health insurance that sought to bridge the inequities within the social and economic spaces of their respective countries and to further render effective support in the area of tackling diseases, whether communicable or non-communicable. Organically, Ghana and Rwanda are middle-income and low- and middle-income African countries (World Bank in Ghana, 2018). They epitomise the general social and economic trajectories within the African environment. Similar socio-economic issues, alongside similar communicable and non-communicable health challenges, were the impetus for Ghana and Rwanda's governments to put systems in place, especially relating to health financing, to allow for public action in accessing health care and participating in the prevention, control, and management of diseases.

In pursuing this research, the theory of lesson-drawing has been found useful. Rose (1991) argues that '(l)esson-drawing addresses the question: under what circumstances and to what extent can a programme that is effective in one place transfer to another?' In a study describing health insurance practices, as this one does, using the separate examples of Ghana and Rwanda, lessons to be drawn can be examined and, if appropriate, tested elsewhere. If striving to shape present and future discourses and policy-related issues of health care in Africa, and specifically in sub-Saharan Africa, is the intention, these two case studies are good starting points. Thus, this study envisages that interested activists and policy-makers will draw lessons from these two countries, contingent upon prevailing circumstances in their own countries.

Methodologically, this qualitative contribution synthesises thoughts and draws lessons from multiple secondary sources covering health care financing in Ghana and Rwanda. In the main, these were pertinent journal articles, books on the subject, and specialist reports. I selected the sources based on their authenticity and relevance to the study. Sources have been corroborated and triangulated to deal with the challenges associated on occasion with single source arguments. In presenting a thematic analysis, the research deals with the issue of continuity and change within the respective two countries' strategies for health care financing aimed at ensuring universal health coverage.

The chapter is presented in five sections. The first section discusses the evolution of health care management in Africa. In the second, attention is paid to the Structural Adjustment Programmes (SAPs) and their impact on health care in sub-Saharan Africa. The third and fourth sections discuss the case studies of the National Health Insurance Scheme (NHIS) in Ghana and the community-based health insurance scheme (CBHI) in Rwanda. These two sections examine the origins, implementation and financing, socio-economic impact, and challenges facing the scheme. The final section provides a comparative narrative of the case studies, suggests lesson-learning, and offers recommendations.

THE EVOLUTION OF HEALTH CARE MANAGEMENT IN AFRICA

Health institutions serve as a useful foundation in the social, political, and economic development of every society. The positive correlation that exists between health and development underscores why health institutions in terms of importance are on a par with other central institutions of governance (Akortsu & Abor, 2011). The age-old association of disease with impediments to realising one's full human capabilities caused Africa's governments to search for ways to combat disease and encourage the health of citizens (Brenya & Adu-Gyamfi, 2014).

In the pre-colonial era, health care was managed by traditional authorities who entrusted the health of their subjects to traditional practitioners (Maier, 1979). Since payments were made in kind or through livestock, it was essentially an out-of-pocket payment system. Indigenous practitioners received respect and dignity from their patients; and this system of reward replaced the need to provide a monetary value for their services (Kale, 1995; Akortsu & Abor, 2011; Igoli et al., 2005; Yankuzo, 2014).

During colonisation, the management of health was transferred gradually to the colonial government through the introduction of a different cosmology about what caused disease and ill health – the germ theory. The expansion of biomedicine and Western ideas of disease causation went hand in hand with the entrenchment of colonial rule. Initially, biomedicine was used to treat the ailments affecting imperial settlers and colonialists. However, during the period of the 1920s to the 1960s, a time when native labour was critical to building the colonies, biomedicine became deeply rooted in treating epidemics and keeping native populations relatively healthy (Lock & Nguyen, 2010). Health care during this period was funded from both the taxation of indigenous populations and through colonial grants. Though the mode of funding was largely through cost sharing, Africans were marginalised in the colonial health system. They were often suspicious of biomedical doctors; many preferred to use traditional or indigenous medicine (Addae, 1997; Tilley, 2016).

During the period of independence (1960s–1980s), biomedicine and health care became an emblem for modernity and nation building. African governments saw health as an essential requirement for economic, social, and political development. In the post-independence era they placed the issue of cost at the centre of their efforts to bridge the health accessibility gap between the poor and the rich. Most post-independence African governments adopted a user fee-free mode of health care delivery in order to ensure that cost would not deter any individual from seeking health care. Kwame Nkrumah's Convention People's Party (CPP) in Ghana, Julius Nyerere's Chama Cha Mapinduzi (CCM) in Tanzania, and Seretse Khama's Botswana Democratic Party (BDP) in Botswana are examples of governing parties that adopted the user fee-free model of health financing (Brenya & Adu-Gyamfi, 2014; Gros, 2015).

To ensure that these policies were effectively implemented, post-independence governments developed health infrastructure and training of personnel for the health industry. These developments were possible at the time because of favourable economic variables, which offered the potential for Africa's economy to prosper. Some of the fundamentals that supported development were derived from nature's beneficence, such as oil, for example. Favourable oil prices, the high prices of export primary commodities, and sound colonial reserves, among other things, offered the promise of development and growth.

Although it unfolded gradually, user fee-free health care thrived in the immediate post-independence years and considerably larger numbers of people from impoverished communities had access to health care. These developments were short-lived, however (Ewusi, 1989; Castro-Leal et al., 1999; Saul & Leys, 1999; Barnes et al., 2015; Gros, 2015).

A series of coups between the late 1960s and 1980s, high inflation rates, a decline in primary commodity-based foreign exchange earnings, and corruption (Gros, 2015; Akortsu & Abor, 2011) all contributed to halting or reversing progress. The situation led to the introduction of the International Monetary Fund (IMF) Structural Adjustment Programmes (SAPs) and the debt burden on African countries that came with it. The impact was felt most profoundly on the health sectors of these African countries. Indebted governments, in exchange for loans to pay foreign creditors, were forced to strip their health systems of various subsidies, leading to the disparity in health services in sub-Saharan Africa. Through the SAPs, the user fee model was introduced in Africa and the gap between the poor and the rich began to widen. Although the user fee model had been introduced to encourage sustainability, efficiency, and effectiveness in the health services, its aim was lost as governments and health administrators saw user fees as a means of raising funds for day-to-day administration. In no time health care in large parts of sub-Saharan Africa had reverted to the colonial standard where one had to pay to access health care, thus reinforcing disparities and inequities. The difference in this period, however, was that the disparity was between poor and affluent Africans, rather than between colonisers and indigenous populations (Loewenson, 1993; Gilson, 1997).

Championed by the World Health Organization, universal health coverage in Africa was a priority of the 2015 Millennium Development Goals (MDG) agenda (Odeyemi & Nixon, 2013). The recent wave of democratisation of most countries in Africa has correlated positively with the development of their public health institutions (Carbone, 2011; Gros, 2015). Nevertheless, the recent adoption of universal health coverage and other re-emerging forms of social insurance by many governments in sub-Saharan Africa has once again raised the issue of the relationship between cost and access to health care. While there are other factors to take into account, the issue of cost remains a critical obstacle to universal health coverage, (Boateng et al., 2017).

HEALTH CARE FINANCING AND THE STRUCTURAL ADJUSTMENT PROGRAMMES (SAPS) IN SUB-SAHARAN AFRICA

In order to rescue African economies from their precarious state, caused by high inflation, high incidence of corruption, and low gross domestic product (GDP), Western policy-makers, the World Bank and the IMF, to name a few stakeholders, responded with a series of interventions under the SAP banner – Structural Adjustment Policies and Structural Adjustment Loans being two examples. SAPs were presented as short-term austerities that would lead to long-term growth and development (Peabody, 1996: 823). These solutions, which translated to cuts in health expenditure, have raised controversial arguments concerning Africa's socio-economic and human development. The common explanation given for cuts in expenditure was the decline in export commodities, which had initially financed most government revenues in post-independence Africa. The drugs and technology responsible for health care in most sub-Saharan states were imported and this fact, coupled with devaluing currencies, led to an inevitable rise in the cost of health care (Peabody, 1996).

The negative impacts of SAPs on the health sector of multiple African governments, a sector critical to a country's overall development, has been documented clearly. These have included cuts in public health expenses by participating governments, adverse effects on the public health workforce, reduced health accessibility and coverage for the population, conflict of interest between public health institutions and private health entities, and the decentralisation and increasing cost of health care (Kentikelenis, 2017). Concerning the cuts in public health expenditure, many governments had to reduce the subsidies that cushioned the cost of health care for the poor and vulnerable, and so they made paying a user fee compulsory for accessing health care (Stromquist, 1999). Essentially, it was the introduction of SAPs that raised the cost of health care in most African states.

The SAPs also affected the health sector indirectly through the macroeconomic policies African governments adopted. The changes in policy resulted in the income of individuals going down and the prices of goods and services going up. Included in this increase were the price of drugs and hospital services. This, in turn, had an effect on household incomes and savings, which resulted in low use of health services. In addition, the inability of public health centres to provide essential medical technologies to combat infirmities led to many individuals turning to private health institutions (Peabody, 1996). This situation placed rural dwellers at a further disadvantage because they could not afford the health care provided by these private entities. Public health institutions in rural centres were generally understaffed, and shortages of essential medications were common (Buor, 2004).

Ineffective tax collection coupled with stripping off tariffs and import duties in the name of increasing foreign direct investment saw a drastic drop in public revenue in those African states that had enrolled in the SAPs (Woodward, 1992). Governments could not fund health financing exemption programmes. The SAPs also led to workers being laid off so their ability to pay out-of-pocket for health care was reduced.

Although the SAPs had been directed toward extricating the economies of African countries from dire macroeconomic difficulties, these programmes in most instances resulted in increasing disparity and inequities.

Presenting an opposing view, one which sees the SAPs as having had some positive effect, Clements et al. (2013) argue that the SAPs increased social spending, which encouraged sustainability of the health systems in Africa. Similarly, Peabody (1996) contends that reducing government subsidies for health care made individuals work and pay for their own health, which increased the sustainability of Africa's health services. In contrast, Schatz (1994) states that the performances of African economies during the SAPs and after the programme became worse since indicators such as GDP and poverty status, among others, were either the same or increased slowly in this period.

In recent times African governments continue to consider the issue of health financing as an essential determinant of universal access to health care. Most countries have adopted national health coverage and other forms of social funding to health care in order to increase universal access. In the next two sections, the discussion focuses on two examples: the health insurance programmes in Ghana and Rwanda.

HEALTH CARE MANAGEMENT IN GHANA

Over time, the NHIS has become an essential tool in Ghana's system of health management and financing. The Ghanaian idea of access to national health care, as embodied in the NHIS, provides a legitimate, continuously evolving tool for free access to health care. It needs refinement, nevertheless, to ensure that the poor will be enrolled in ways that guarantee their protection.

Origins of the NHIS

Ghana is one of the few countries in Africa to have successfully implemented a form of social insurance health care, known locally as the National Health Insurance Scheme (Sarpong et al., 2010). Ghana's success rate stems from the zealous efforts made by previous governments to pursue universal health care for poor and vulnerable groups (see Adu-Gyamfi et al., 2015a). Political actors from Kwame Nkrumah, Kofi Busia, to John Kufuor all pushed for some form of health care financing based on the belief that health care implementation and financing is an essential tool for social and economic development.

After independence, Nkrumah, the founder of the CPP and Ghana's first president, gave the citizens hope of universal access to health care for all. However, mismanagement and corruption, which was especially rife in health centres and hospitals, thwarted the dream. In 1966 a military coup saw the National Liberation Council (NLC) seize power. This further complicated the provision of health care. By then Ghanaians had come to relish the idea of the free health care introduced by Nkrumah. Subsequently, when Busia's Progress Party, which replaced the CPP as the next civilian government in 1969, tried to introduce a nominal fee as guarantee for access to health care, there was widespread resistance. The idea that finance was a barrier to accessing health care prompted Busia to adopt a health insurance scheme of financing health care where the government paid a greater portion of the costs (Brenya & Adu-Gyamfi, 2014).

The type of health care management introduced by Nkrumah and Busia was put to the test during the 1970s and 1980s. Amidst a drastic decline in the health status of Ghanaians, and a high incidence of corruption and mismanagement at the national level, the introduction of a user fee as a compulsory tool to access health care widened the inequality gap, especially between the rural and urban centres (Ewusi, 1989).

A return to democratisation in 1992, as well as the fourth republican constitution, put the Ghanaian health system on a better path to ensuring universal health care to citizens (Carbone, 2011). Ghanaians' hope for better health care management resulted in the New Patriotic Party (NPP), led by Kufuor, promising to replace the 'dreadful cash and carry system' which had existed from 1970–2003 (Carbone, 2011;

Gros, 2015). It was during Kufuor's leadership that the National Health Insurance Scheme was introduced in October 2003 through an act of parliament. Efforts to establish universal health insurance date back to the 1970s when the Hospital Fee (Act 387 of 1971) was established. This step was later thwarted by the 1972 coup (Adu-Gyamfi et al., 2015b).

Some viewed the NHIS as a privilege, while political parties used it as political leverage (Carbone, 2011). The NHIS in Ghana is not a neutral entity but one that remains mired in politics. Besides the politics and political usefulness of a scheme like the NHIS, there is the need to understand the continuities and discontinuities – the changes – that gave birth to it. Towards this end it is important to consider the nature of the implementation and financing strategies.

Implementation and financing of NHIS

The first efforts to reintroduce the National Health Insurance Scheme were in 1997 under the auspices of the Ministry of Health (MoH), the Ghana Health Company, and the Social Security and National Insurance Trust (SSNIT). These stakeholders intended to mobilise funds to ensure a smooth implementation of health insurance. The Ghana Health Company, for example, was to provide other means of finance to fund health insurance in Ghana (Adoma-Yeboah, 2005). Although they were not wholly successful, the existence of private insurance companies, such as the Vanguard Assurance Company and the Gemini Life Insurance Company in urban centres, enabled alternative funding for health insurance (Adu-Gyamfi et al., 2015b). While the rural areas were at a disadvantage in terms of insurance companies, in places like Damango, Tano, Jaman, and the Dangme West districts support was also provided by NGOs and religious bodies, thus showing that a health insurance which incorporated the rural populace was possible.

Today the NHIS is managed by the National Health Insurance Authority, which is an autonomous body (NHIS, 2017). It is regulated through the National Health Insurance Council, which sees to a number of functions: planning, monitoring, and evaluation; registration and licensing; administration and management support; and funding and investment. Some of the functions the NHIS performs are: registering of members for the scheme, ensuring equity in health care coverage, protection of the poor against financial risk, and the drafting of proposals to the Minister of Health for the formulation of policies concerning health insurance.

The means of financing the scheme is through a cost-sharing responsibility between the participants of the scheme and the government of Ghana. Schedules made for this funding are a 2.5 per cent National Health Insurance levy on all goods and services collected under the Value Added Tax (VAT), 2.5 per cent of 17.5 per cent Social Security and National Insurance Trust (SSNIT) contributions per month, returns on National Health Insurance Fund investments, and premiums paid by those who work in the informal sector (MoH, 2004).

There are *two main groups* that use the scheme and they are differentiated by whether they work in the formal or informal sector. Those who work in the *formal sector* include employees of private entities and self-employed individuals who contribute to the SSNIT fund. Children under 18, persons in need of antenatal, delivery, and postnatal care, persons classified by the Ministry for Social Welfare as indigent under the Livelihood Empowerment Against Poverty (LEAP) programme, persons with mental disorders, pensioners of SSNIT, and persons aged 70 years and above are entitled to the benefits those in formal sector employment receive (NHIS, 2014).

SSNIT contributors, SSNIT pensioners, adults of age 70 and above, and children under 18 years old pay both renewal and card processing fees. However, pregnant women, programme beneficiaries, and persons with mental disorders are exempted from the card processing fee and renewal fees (NHIA, 2017b; 2017c). These *formal groups* constitute about 69 per cent of the NHIS membership composition (Wang et al., 2017: 19) and they are not required to pay the premium. The *second group* that uses the scheme are those in informal employment: 31 per cent of the 40 per cent of the national population covered by NIHS are from the informal sector (Wang et al., 2017: 17). Members who are informal sector workers are required to pay a premium.

The NHIS covers about 95 per cent of ailments treated in health facilities in Ghana (Wang et al., 2017). These are enshrined in the products rendered by the hospitals and health facilities. They are the Out-Patient Department (OPD) services addressing medical conditions like malaria, acute respiratory tract infection, skin diseases and ulcers, among other diseases. The In-Patient Department (IPD) delivers services such as laboratory investigations, cervical and breast cancer treatment, as well as surgical operations, including appendectomy. The oral and eye services deal with issues of dentistry and optometry respectively, while maternal service deals with antenatal and postnatal care, including child delivery (NHIA, 2014: 10).

The accredited centres of health care covered by the scheme (Table 1) are: community-based health planning and services (CHPS) health centres; clinics; polyclinics; primary hospitals, including district hospitals and private primary hospitals; and secondary hospitals, which include regional hospitals, pharmacies, licensed chemical shops, and diagnostic centres. In Ghana, there are about 3,500 public, private, and faith-based health care facilities. Of these, 57 per cent are public facilities, 33 per cent are private, and 7 per cent are facilities operated by the Christian Health Association of Ghana (CHAG) (Wang et al., 2017: 11). Table 1 shows the details of public, private, and missionary hospitals. In all, one teaching hospital is private, and the rest, which include teaching, municipal, metropolitan, regional, and district hospitals, are public facilities.

Table 1: The number of health service types in Ghana

Facility Type	Numbers
CHPS	653
Clinic	1,173
Health centre	787
Maternity home	369
Polyclinic	16
Hospital unidentified	276
Metropolitan/Municipal hospital	5
Regional hospital	3
Psychiatric hospital	3
Teaching hospital	3
Others	183

Source: Wang et al. 2017: 11

There exist two main types of health insurance under the NHIS in Ghana. These are the social-type health insurance and the private commercial health insurance. The social-type health insurance is categorised into the District Mutual Health Insurance Scheme (DMHIS) and the Private Mutual Health Insurance Scheme (PMHIS).

The DMHIS is an initiative of the government to target the poor who cannot access health care financially. Hence, packages vary according to finance status in the community. They are the core poor, very poor, poor, middle income, rich, and the very rich (Jehu-Appiah et al., 2011). In 2004, the government released 40.6 billion Ghana cedis to establish the DMHIS in all districts, metropolitan and municipal assemblies (Ghana News Agency, 2004). The DMHIS is self funded, with subsidies from the government (MoH, 2004: 11). Returns from investments or surplus cash are returned to the scheme.

The PMHIS operates on market principles. Premiums are determined based on a calculated risk of the group being insured getting sick. The PMHIS does not receive any funding from the government (MoH, 2004). Recently, 11 private insurance companies joined the NHIS (see Table 2). Because of their incentive to make profit, these companies are all based in urban areas. Rural areas are left to rely on DMHIS.

Table 2: Private insurance companies on the NHIS

Insurance Company	Location
Accra Health Insurance Limited	Accra
Apex Health Insurance Limited	Accra
Cosmopolitan Health Insurance Limited	Accra
Empire Health Insurance	Accra
Glico Health Limited	Accra
Kaiser Global Health Limited	Kumasi
Liberty Medical Health Limited	Tema
Metropolitan Nationwide Medical Insurance Scheme	Accra
NMH Nationwide Medical Insurance Scheme	Accra
Premier Health Insurance Company Limited	Accra
Universal Health Insurance Limited	Tema

Source: http://nhis.gov.gh/phis.asp, accessed 25 October 2017

Socio-economic impact of NHIS

The National Health Insurance Scheme has either impacted on or has been impacted by several factors associated with social, political, cultural, and economic spaces within which the NHIS is implemented in Ghana. In addition, global-orientated programmes, like those around the MDGs, have also had an impact on how the insurance scheme operates.

The enrolment base of the NHIS is highest among informal workers. In Ghana, 80 per cent of people who are employed work in the informal economy (Osei-Boateng & Ampratwum, 2011). These informal workers are largely grouped into two: the rural sector and the urban informal sector (Adu-Amankwah, 1999). Informal workers have to register for the NHIS, but when there is proof that they are indigent, they are exempted from the payments. However, the nature of informal work places workers at a higher risk of exposure to danger and disease, making them the ones most likely to need health care services (Gyasi et al., 2017b). To this end, most of them consider the NHIS as the safest way to assure their access to health care. This indirectly expands the enrolment base of the scheme and has the potential to bridge the inequity gap, since most informal workers – for instance, the young boys and girls, including women, who work as head porters (*kayayo*) on the streets of major cities like Accra, Kumasi, Tema, and Takoradi, farmers, market women, hawkers, labourers – are included in this category (Gyasi et al., 2017b). The NHIS has resulted in increased hospital attendance in Ghana and has increased the propensity for good health as well as an active labour force.

The idea of accessing health care at a subsidised cost has also had an impact on the number of subscribers as well as health facility utilisation (Dzakpasu et al., 2012). The NHIS has helped to remove lack of finances as an obstacle to seeking health care. In other words, it has brought health care to the doorstep of the poor (Gyasi et al., 2015).

Public education offered by the NHIS in collaboration with other statutory bodies like the National Commission for Civic Education (NCCE) has also increased the utilisation of and enrolment in the scheme. In 2008, NHIS coverage was 12.5 million (55 per cent). However, this increased by 7 per cent to 14.5 million a year later (NHIA, 2009). The chairman of the NHIS Council attributed this increase to the effort of the public education department of the National Health Insurance

Authority, which had sensitised the various Ghanaian communities about the benefits of enrolling in the scheme. The role played by public universities in the enrolment and utilisation of NHIS cannot be underestimated. Since 2009, the Kwame Nkrumah University of Science and Technology (KNUST), for instance, ensured that students who were not on the NHIS enrolled upon admission (see Osei et al., 2017).

The NHIS has been influenced by the politics of the day. Since its inception in 2003, Kufuor's government saw to it that subscribers had access to the health centres in their districts, municipal or metropolis (NHIA, 2008). This type of care provided by the NHIS was ubiquitous from 2004 to 2010. However, the 2008 general elections ushered the John Atta Mills-led National Democratic Congress (NDC) into office. The policy direction was to initiate a one-time premium contribution. This policy, which was to materialise in 2011, was put on hold. This factor notwithstanding, the existing NHIS eliminated the regional boundaries imposed on health care while emphasising the annual renewal of the insurance package. These policy interventions allowed for accessibility and equity in health care without prejudice to age, status, ethnicity, and geographical location.

The Millennium Development Goals to some extent have also impacted the NHIS in Ghana. The health component of the UN programme sought to promote maternal health, combat diseases like malaria and HIV/AIDS, and reduce child mortality by 2015. These three components have been incorporated into the scheme's packages, starting with the free maternal care adopted in 2008, which also included free postnatal care (NHIA, 2008). Even though there has not been much progress made at reducing maternal mortality, child mortality rates have been positively impacted. The infant mortality rate decreased from a previous high of 76 to 52 per 1,000 live births in 2011; there has also been significant improvement in terms of the health of women and children (Owoo & Lambon-Quayefio, 2013: 19). It can be inferred that mothers who had hitherto been unable to access health care due to out-of-pocket cost (and who had also formed the habit of not reporting their own ill-health and that of their children to doctors) have been spurred on to visit hospitals with their children due to the social change instigated by the National Health Insurance Policy. Again, it is important to emphasise that this policy has served a useful purpose in the lives of individuals, especially the poor and those living in deplorable conditions (like the migrant female head porters – *kayayo* – from the Northern and Upper regions of Ghana) by giving them the opportunity to access health care (Boateng et al., 2017) to seek largely curative care. Sometimes, through such access, some degree of counselling is offered, which has the tendency to prevent or stall the spread of contagions and also support the treatment of non-communicable diseases among the deprived population.

Challenges of the NHIS in Ghana

The dominant challenge for Ghana's NHIS is claims management (Adu-Gyamfi et al., 2015a: 54). The NHIS has gone through changes in the type of financing adopted by the National Health Insurance Authority over successive years. The claim system was the main way the NHIS worked. In this system, the costs of the health care of NHIS subscribers were presented to the district, municipal, or metropolitan assemblies for a refund. These costs were linked to the individual NHIS numbers, which were then forwarded to the Ministry of Finance for a refund (NHIS, 2017).

Claims payments to providers were often delayed for a long time, thereby denying subscribers essential services, such as drug supply and medical care. In addition, inconsistent billing systems by providers, lack of effective mechanisms for tracking claims, and the low billing the scheme had introduced undermined the idea of equity in the Ghanaian health system (Adu-Gyamfi et al., 2015a).

Given the complexities attached with claiming a refund, capitation was introduced as an alternative means of funding the NHIS. Capitation is structured on a 'per member per month' basis, where the cost of health care of an individual is paid by the NHIS monthly (NHIA, 2017a). It was launched in 2011 to reimburse primary care for OPD services. Capitation offers the subscriber the opportunity to choose a health facility from which they will seek medical service. Recent evaluation research has found capitation suitable to be considered 'a key provider payment method for primary out-patient care in order to control cost in health care delivery' provided that some aspects of design be reviewed (Andoh-Adjei et al., 2018).

The NHIA also complained of late submission of claims by service providers. This created a ripple effect of district, municipal, or metropolitan assemblies not vetting these claims properly or delaying payments (NHIA, 2010). The initial effort to release funds to settle debts in which the NHIS owed and which had been processed in 2015 only materialised when the government released 180 million Ghana cedis on 5 February 2017 to settle debts to service providers (Graphic Online, 2017). Initially, to combat such payment challenges, and to limit fraud, the NHIA made some efforts to introduce an E-Claim system (NHIA, 2013).

Financial sustainability of the scheme is another challenge (Adu-Gyamfi & Dramani, 2017). The increase in the scheme's coverage and health facility utilisation does not correlate with the funding source of the scheme. Subscribers increased from 23,238 in 2005 to 25,794 in 2006 (NHIA, 2009). Membership increased by 56 per cent in 2008 and 62 per cent in 2009, representing 12.5 and 14.5 million subscribers respectively over the two years. Membership increased continuously from 8 million subscribers in 2010, to 8.2 million in 2011, 8.8 in 2012, and 10.2 in 2013 (NHIA, 2013). As at 2013, 38 per cent of the total population had enrolled in the scheme (NHIA, 2013). These increasing subscriber figures denote an additional means of financing to the scheme. Although the government of Ghana had introduced the capitation in 2012 to ease the financial burden, ineffective piloting and planning caused its suspension in the Ashanti Region (Graphic Online, 2017), along with a plan to abolish it (Ampratwum-Mensah, 2017). In order to sustain the scheme financially, parliament on 14 July 2017 approved 2.2 billion Ghana cedis to aid in the scheme's debts payment (NHIA, 2017b).

The problem of identifying the poor in the informal sector is also a challenge. The general motive of the NHIS is to make the poor exempt from paying for health care, or at least make it affordable to them. The reality is that it is the larger sections of the population, exactly the poor the NHIS is wanting to assist, who are not covered (NHIA, 2010). Identifying the poor presents a major challenge in the scheme's dream to ensure equity in health care. In order to address this better, collaborative efforts have been made by the National Health Insurance Authority with organisations like LEAP to identify and enrol poor people at community level.

There is a tendency among some members of the scheme to abuse it by their over-utilisation of health centres (Adu-Gyamfi et al., 2015b). Subscribers report to health facilities even if their conditions do not demand the service of that type of facility. In other words, the chain of medical treatment, which should begin at a primary health centre, followed by a secondary and tertiary form of health care based on recommendations of respective health officials, is not being used (Gobah & Zhang, 2011: 90). Furthermore, some subscribers do not complete treatment at one health centre. This leads to a duplication of cost, which burdens the scheme financially (Adu-Gyamfi et al., 2015a). This moving from one centre of care to another might be attributed, in part, to how the subscriber was treated by health officials in their previous centre. To combat this, the NHIA established a clinical audit unit in 2012 to investigate how NHIS subscribers were being treated (NHIA, 2012).

Two other obstacles to the scheme achieving its objectives concern identification (ID) cards and Information Communication Technology (ICT). Issues relating to the ID cards include the delay in obtaining the card resulting from the management chain of data entry, data batching, card production, and distribution (NHIA, 2012). Members compound these issues further by changing residence, double registering, or failing to identify their location properly. The main problem of the ICT department is network jamming; this has a ripple effect on data entry, data batching, and checking subscriber eligibility at health centres.

These challenges negatively affect subscribers' perception of the quality of the health care the scheme is providing – they regard it as poor (Jehu-Appiah et al., 2011) – which has led to members changing their preference to out-of-pocket health care payment since it is perceived to be of a higher quality (Adu-Gyamfi et al., 2015a: 57). This puts the poor at a disadvantage as they are unable to afford this (NHIA, 2012); there have been occasions when subscribers have had to purchase medication that was supposed to be covered by the scheme. There are equally related questions concerning policy holders' perceptions and factors influencing renewal in different regions. This has been of particular concern in the Volta Region (Boateng & Awunyor-Vitor, 2013: 1–10).

A final challenge linked to the quality of health care is the issue of neonatal and maternal mortality. Neonatal mortality accounts for about 40 per cent of child death in Ghana, despite the introduction of free maternal health care in 2008. The NHIS does not cover all the cost of neonatal treatment, leading some parents to rely on out-of-pocket payment. In 2013, for instance, there were several media reports on the failing free maternal policy. As at 2016, pregnant women were compelled to buy antibiotics, blood tonics, disinfectants, and sanitary pads in preparation for delivery (Lambon-Quayefio & Owoo, 2017:2; Ghana News Agency, 2016).

THE RWANDAN HEALTH INSURANCE SYSTEM

Rwanda's system of community-based health insurance (CBHI) is sometimes described as unprecedented in the history of CBHIs in sub-Saharan Africa. It is further argued that it provides strong administrative and political support for the expansion and functioning of a health care system. Some countries therefore regard the Rwandan model as an alternative vehicle for health sector financing and delivery of basic health services (Shimeles, 2010).

Origins of CBHI

This section investigates the origins of Rwanda's health insurance system and the nature of its financing and implementation. It highlights some of the benefits as well as the challenges that were confronted through the implementation process.

Rwanda was one of the poorly performing economies of Africa, and the country relied heavily on foreign exchange earned from tea, banana, and coffee exportation (Abbott & Binagwaho, 2017: 103). In the 1990s Rwanda experienced unparalleled violence which took an exacting toll on the country (Gros, 2015: 223), culminating, in 1994, in the 100-day genocide. About 1 million people were killed and many more were displaced (Lemarchand, 2004). The genocide did not only affect the political, economic, and social institutions of the state. It also affected the health system (Binagwaho et al., 2014). During that time, Rwanda had the lowest life expectancy and highest infant mortality rates. Its health system was in shambles and many health workers had fled the country, fearing for their lives. A decade later, by 2005,

Rwanda remained one of Africa's ill-performing economies with GDP under USD 300 (Diop & Butera, 2005).

After the genocide, a development plan called Vision 2020 was formulated by the Rwandan Patriotic Front (RPF) led by President Paul Kagame. The overall aim was to reduce poverty and the plan included implementing universal health insurance coverage (Logie et al., 2008).

Previously, in the immediate post-independence era, Rwanda had provided free health care to its citizens, but this was short-lived, as the country went into economic decline (Kaberuka, 2000: 1–31). As part of the conditions of structural adjustment, in the 1980s user fees for health care were introduced, which increased disparities. After the genocide the situation worsened (Logie et al., 2008). In 1999, community-based health insurance (CBHI) was introduced, in line with the Vision 2020 goals (Binagwaho et al., 2014).

The term CBHI describes not-for-profit pre-payment plans for health care, with community control and voluntary membership that provide risk pooling to low-income populations. CBHI has the potential to improve access to and quality use of medicines. In Rwanda the scheme is called the *Mutuelle de Santé* (or Mutuelles).

Prior to the launch of the health insurance reforms, government health funds were used to directly support public providers, with households spending substantial amounts out-of-pocket to see private providers or for co-payments to public providers (Saksena et al., 2011). Rwanda's political structure also allowed premium collection from all but the poorest people.

Implementation and financing

Mutuelles is a key component of Rwanda's national health strategy on providing universal health care and reaching the health MDGs (Lu et al., 2012). Membership is structured into three categories, based on the level of economic status: the poor, those of middle income, and the privileged. This also determines the amount of premium to be paid. The poorest comprise 27 per cent of the total 74 per cent (per population) of the total subscribers in Rwanda. A report by the Rwanda Ministry of Health (RMoH) in 2016 indicated that the indigent pay a premium of RWF 2000 (approximately USD 2.99). Those of middle income comprised about 70 per cent of the subscribers and paid RWF 3,000 (approximately USD 4.35), and the privileged, representing 3 per cent, paid RWF 7,000 (approximately USD 10.34). Payment covers members for one Rwandan fiscal year, which is from July to June. Additionally, each subscriber pays a co-payment fee of RWF 200 per visit to the CBHI unit at the health centre; 10 per cent of this co-payment is paid to the hospital by the CBHI (WHO, 2016). Each subscriber is restricted to a health centre in their district and visits other specialised centres by referral only. The idea of issuing co-payments is to limit the abuse of health centres by subscribers (RMoH, 2010).

Despite the growing popularity of taxes as a key source of revenue for coverage programmes, Rwanda continued to attempt to collect voluntary premiums from informal-sector households, from whom taxes can be difficult to access (Saksena et al., 2011).

The major source of revenue to the CBHI from 2012 to 2013 was premiums, which accounted for 66 per cent of the contribution to the insurance. This was followed by government revenues, at 14 per cent, global funds (international aid) at 10 per cent, co-payments, at 6 per cent, plus other revenues (like investment returns, for example) of 3 per cent, and social and private health insurance of 1 per cent (WHO, 2018). Funds from the government covered referral hospital bills and premiums for indigent members (WHO, 2016). The majority of premiums came from the middle-income group, who were the largest source of revenue. Fifty-five per cent of the premium is retained by the health centre to cover claims, while 45 per cent is sent to district hospitals to cover hospital claims. Altogether 10 per cent of the latter is sent to the national hospitals to cover referral costs.

Highlighting some of the benefits of CBHI in Rwanda

By 2010 it had been reported that CBHI had a high degree of utilisation of health services, which helped to protect members from large and unforeseen, potentially catastrophic, health-related expenses (Shimeles, 2010). As a result of their insurance functions, CBHI schemes protect the income of their members against financial risks associated with illness. This happens through two mechanisms: sick members of CBHI schemes seek care earlier, resulting in efficiency gains in the consumption of health care services; and sick persons pay small out-of-pocket co-payments at the health centres (Diop & Butera, 2005). In 2005 it had been noted that the CBHI scheme's coverage also increased the use of reproductive health services, including prenatal care and delivery care. However, CBHI then had no effect on the use of family planning services.

Greater access of the poor to CBHI scheme benefits was promoted through a series of strategies. These included building on partnerships between CBHI schemes, and working with existing and newly formed grassroots associations under a financing scheme where micro-finance schemes provided small loans to the association's members to pay for their yearly contributions to the CBHI schemes. This also opened opportunities for the poor CBHI members to have greater access to larger micro-finance loans to finance income-generating activities (Diop & Butera, 2005; Schneider, 2005; Saksena et al., 2011).

This community-level social capital has fostered a sense of trust among the wider Rwandan community and has boosted the propensity of the poor to enrol in the scheme. Additionally, it has stimulated networks and business relations with local banks and agricultural co-operatives to provide access to credit and savings. The implication can be drawn that the cooperation among people through the insurance has also helped them reach other common goals outside the health sector (Diop & Butera, 2005; Schneider, 2005; Saksena et al., 2011). The increased mobilisation of domestic resources to ensure CBHI's financial independence also discourages the misappropriation of funds. The Rwandan health insurance system remains the most prominent and diversified scheme in terms of population coverage. The coverage is strongly associated with a reduction in unmet need and of risk of catastrophic expenditure (Saksena et al., 2011).

Challenges of CBHI in Rwanda

The major challenge of CBHI is its over-reliance on government and donor funds to cover the premiums. Although 66 per cent of the scheme's revenue comes from premiums, the majority of the Rwandan population is poor, and this means the government needs to pay more than the 14 per cent of the contribution (see Nzeyimana et al., 2014).

If government revenue declines, there will be a commensurate decline in revenue for the scheme. To guard against this, there is a need therefore to develop financing alternatives for the scheme. A recent attempt made by the government to move the management of the scheme from the MoH to the Rwanda Social Security Board was one such effort to help sustain the scheme financially (WHO, 2016).

In 2010 critics of the programme argued that the CBHI could be inefficient and injurious to the health service, which is heavily subsidised by funds coming from the treasury as well as international aid. Two main reasons came to the fore. First, the flat premium rate (about USD 2 per year per person) is considered to be too high for the very poor. Given a choice the poor will rather defer health care expenditure until it is vitally needed. Second, even if extremely poor people become members of CBHI, they may not fully utilise its provisions, since not everything is free. There are also other layers of expenses to be borne such as transport, prescription drugs, and the opportunity cost of time, especially for casual labourers. Therefore, the CBHI has the potential to further alienate the extremely poor and the uninsured from utilising health services (Shimeles, 2010; Saksena et al., 2011).

The abuse of the CBHI by subscribers is a further challenge. The idea of free health care rendered by health centres has increased the rate at which patients visit the centres. Though this in itself is good, it has been widely reported that they also visit for matters that do not require urgent medical attention. In a bid to limit this – the over-utilisation of the health centres – the Ministry of Health introduced the co-payment method (Carrin et al., 2005).

This challenge also cuts the other way. The right to essential health care was a new concept in Rwanda and at first patients did not always know their rights with regard to health care. Generally, they did not complain or report the matter when issues were not solved by health providers. Also, in several instances, there had been no access to certain treatments, and no access to private health providers, but the authorities were not made aware. By 2014 things had changed and reports were being received that some CBHI members were not satisfied with poor courtesy, weak customer care, and the regular stockouts of drugs in some contracted health facilities. Incapacity or a delay in the reimbursement of health care bills were also being reported. Other issues included incapacity at hospital pharmacies to serve all drug prescriptions due to stockouts.

Such situations affect quality of care for CBHI members. There is also the question of over-prescription and over-charging for health services; increases in pharmaceutical and medical surgical consumables' prices due to a high inflation rate, among other things, tend to cause poor financial management, especially weak cost control (Nyandekwe et al., 2014).

POLICY DIRECTIONS AND RECOMMENDATIONS

The bases upon which these two national health insurance schemes were introduced in the two countries differ. In Ghana, the NPP introduced their scheme on the basis of winning legitimate power from the people. The preceding cash-and-carry system had caused health service complications and challenges in the country. Individuals who could not afford health care refused to visit hospitals and this had the tendency to increase self-help approaches and self-medication. People would only go to the hospital in an emergency. The people wanted a better health financing system, which the Kufuor-led administration promised in the 2000 general election campaign. The NHIS in Ghana had come to stay through political democratisation in Ghana (Carbone, 2011).

In Rwanda, it was the evils of the genocide of 1994 which prompted the RPF to introduce the universal health insurance which was to become the Mutuelle CBHI scheme in 1999. The harsh socio-economic and political situation after the genocide had prepared the ground for Rwanda's health insurance scheme (Binagwaho et al., 2014). Although Rwanda has 60 per cent of the population living in poverty, with about 60 per cent of the population having a household income of less than USD 52 a month, as defined by the Rwandan government, the sense of commitment from the government to provide universal health care for the citizenry, rich or poor, serves as a potential model for other African countries to emulate.

Second, the mode in which health insurance is organised differs between the two countries. Rwanda's community-based approach allows for a wider chance of sustainability than its Ghanaian counterpart. The co-payment of RFW 200 which is made also prevents the abuse of health facilities (WHO, 2016). NHIS in Ghana operates currently on a national basis where a subscriber is not restricted to a health centre in their community. Also the absence of co-payment is likely to increase the rate in which NHIS in Ghana can be abused.

Gros' suggestion of the political regime of the day influencing health policy outcomes is manifested in these two states. Nkrumah had pioneered Ghana's free health care in the 1960s and Kufuor's NHIS followed suit in 2004. In Rwanda, Kagame's provision of NHIS was a military government's move to provide the democratic good of health care (Gros, 2015). The bottom line is that in both countries the political regime of the day took major decisions to implement health insurance. This shows that the right policies with respect to universal health coverage and implementation for the benefit of both urban and rural populations can emerge from diverse political regimes.

Third, international initiatives have largely shaped the content of subscribers' packages of national health insurance in both countries. The MDGs regarding health care have largely been adopted in these states. In Ghana, the free maternal policy was adopted in 2008 to buttress the MDG goal of reducing the maternal mortality ratios in African countries. The free health care for infants also stems from the wider African MDG initiative to reduce child mortality. In Rwanda, the efforts to reduce child mortality, improve maternal health, and combat diseases like malaria and HIV/AIDS have been part of the scheme. This aim is to reduce disease prevalence among Rwandans and also to fulfil the MDGs in Rwanda. Rwanda is among the developing countries in the world to achieve MDGs in health (Abbott & Binagwaho, 2017), and the *Mutuelle de Santé* had a central role in this achievement. It is important to stress that with Sustainable Development Goals (SDGs) in the mix, Rwanda would strive harder to obtain higher optimum goals in the quest to ensure goal three of the SDGs, which aims at ensuring healthy lives and promotion of wellbeing for all at all ages (see WHO, 2018).

In Ghana, considering that over 86 per cent of the population use traditional medicine (Gyasi, 2015: 1), traditional medicine needs to be covered by the NHIS. The potency of traditional medicine has raised several arguments among policy-makers in the world. In the Ghanaian setting, there have been several government attempts to incorporate traditional medicine into orthodox forms of care but the process needs to be accelerated. As most Ghanaians access these facilities (Gyasi et al., 2017a), it is important that this takes place in order to provide and enable a more certified form of holistic care. Though some question the efficacy of traditional medicine, the Ghana Psychic and Traditional Healers Association, the Food and Drug Authority (FDA), and other allied institutions, including institutions of higher learning (like KNUST, which introduced a Department of Herbal Medicine in 2002), are there to maintain standards for treatment and prevent quackery (Adu-Gyamfi, 2016).

The alternatives offered in traditional medicine could potentially help ease the cost burden of drugs that are imported by the government. More funds should therefore be made available for further research into the range of herbs on which traditional medicine draws. Furthermore, the Centre for Plant Medicine Research (CPMR) at Mampong-Akuapim (CPMR, 2017) has conducted research into herbal plants and the production of indigenous medicine to meet the local demands. The government needs to do more to facilitate the integration of traditional medicine into the existing orthodox care to encourage more Ghanaians to utilise and enrol in the NHIS. These same ideals could be emulated in those countries in Africa with larger rural settlements which are not surveyed and are unreached by biomedical care.

In this context, governments in Africa need to encourage the establishment of private herbal hospitals and clinics. In Ghana the government has issued a few licences to herbal hospitals like the Amen Scientific Herbal Hospital, the Agbeve Herbal Hospital, the Lifeman Herbal Clinic, and the Top Herbal Clinic. This notwithstanding, the government should extend this encouragement to get more private entities to go into herbal medical services – and then follow suit with NHIS. Also, because traditional medicine is more accessible, collaborative efforts between the traditional healers associations and health insurance schemes in Africa would result in wider utilisation.

More health facilities and clinics need to be built in order to help bridge the gap between individuals/communities and health centres.

Long distances to hospitals discourage individuals from using the still sparse existing facilities. On the larger African platform, Ghana included, government hospitals should give greater attention to systems that will allow access to alternatives that will reduce fiscal burdens on the provision of health care. In countries like Nigeria, Ghana, and elsewhere in Africa, the increasing population and the increase in communicable and non-communicable diseases that are not fully covered under existing insurance packages should draw the attention of policy-makers to what is doable: preventive health care strategies, enforcement of public legislation, and research into traditional and alternative health medicines which could remain cheap, accessible, and efficacious to larger populations and reduce the financial burden on individuals and the state.

Concerning the Rwandan case study, although international donor funds subsidise the cost of covering more indigents, the Rwanda Ministry of Health might reconsider its decision on the co-payment method as this is an obstacle to greater inclusivity. To prevent the possible reliance on other means of medical care, it might also engage traditional healers to provide efficient health care alongside the orthodox care in order to subsidise cost. The larger debate to use traditional medicines in countries is further enforced by the question of affordability and sustainability of health insurance in growing populations. New and emerging technologies that are enhancing or accelerating the science of herbal and alternative medicines should also be part of the debate.

The African question continues to beg for policies that are home grown rather than those that have been bequeathed to the continent by institutions like the IMF and the World Bank. With all good intents and purposes, the question of effective management of health care, including the question of health financing, seemed to have been largely left in the hands of political patrons. The issue of financial accountability by office holders and those who manage health care should not remain in the general mix. African countries that hope to develop their economies must appreciate that mismanaging health care operates in tandem with economic mismanagement. The former can grievously hurt the health of labour in African countries, especially of those who are largely in the informal sector; it will also affect those employed in the public sector, and those in the private sector whose insurance is not fully guaranteed under poor-paying jobs and harsh working conditions, such as in the mines and in the fields. Improved health status dovetails with increased productivity, educational performance, and life expectancy, as well as a propensity for a decrease in debt and expenditure on healthcare. Quality health care should be seen as an inalienable right of all human beings, and Africans in particular.

REFERENCES

Abbott, P. S. & Binagwaho, A. 2017. 'Learning from success: How Rwanda achieved the millennium development goals for health'. *World Development*, 92, 103–116.

Achime, N. H. 2005. 'Economics of health care financing mechanism in Nigeria'. *Africa: Rivista trimestrale di studi e documentazione dell'Istituto italiano per l'Africa e l'Oriente*, 60 (3/4), 494–507.

Addae, S. 1997. *History of Western Medicine in Ghana 1880-1960*. Durham: Durham Academic Press.

Adoma-Yeboah, L. 14 September 2005. 'Financing health care in Ghana since independence'. *Daily Graphic.*

Adu-Amankwah, K. 1999. 'Trade unions in the informal sector: Finding their bearings. Nine country papers'. *Labour Education Report*, 116 (3).

Adu-Gyamfi, S. 2016. 'Spiritual and indigenous healing practices among the Asante people of Ghana: A testimonial from twenty-first century practitioners and recipients in Kumase'. *Journal of Basic and Applied Research International*, 12 (1), 39–50.

Adu-Gyamfi, S. 10 July 2018. 'Public health narratives on the Asante people of Ghana'. https://ssrn.com/abstract=2975285 or http://dx.doi.org/10.2139/ssrn.2975285, accessed 12 December 2018.

Adu-Gyamfi, S., Brenya, E. & Adjei, G. N. 2016. 'Maternal and infant health section of the demographic and health survey report of Ghana, 2008: A commentary'. *Journal of Humanity*, 4 (1), 35–43.

Adu-Gyamfi, S., Brenya, E. & Adjei, G. N. 2017. 'Maternal and infant health section of the demographic and health survey report of Ghana'. *Journal of Humanity*, 5 (1), 98–105.

Adu-Gyamfi, S. & Dramani, A. 2017. 'Sustaining Ghana's national health insurance scheme through preventive healthcare strategies and legislation'. *International and Multidisciplinary Journal of Social Sciences*, 6 (1), 47–69.

Adu-Gyamfi, S., Brenya, E. & Amoah, A. 2015a. 'National health insurance scheme of Ejisu-Juaben and matters arising'. *International Journal of Social Science Studies*, 3 (5), 40–60.

Adu-Gyamfi, S., Brenya, E. & Nuako A. G. 2015b. 'National health insurance and free maternal healthcare in Ghana: Responses from women and health workers in Akropong'. *An International Journal of Humanities and Social Sciences*, 2 (4), 696–737.

Adu-Gyamfi, S., Dramani, A., Amakye-Boateng, K. & Akomeah, S. 2017. 'Public health: Socio-political history of a people'. *Journal of Arts and Humanities*, 6 (8), 12–33.

Akortsu, M. A. & Abor, P. A. 2011. 'Financing public healthcare institutions in Ghana'. *Journal of Health Organization and Management*, 25 (2), 128–141.

Akosua, A. M. & Aseweh, A. P. 2011. 'Financing public healthcare institutions in Ghana'. *Journal of Health Organization and Management*, 25 (2), 128–141.

Ampratwum-Mensah, A. 11 August 2017. 'Government pays part of debt to NHIS providers'. Graphic News, https://www.graphic.com.gh/news/general-news/government-pays-part-of-debt-to-nhis-providers.html, accessed 29 October 2017.

Andoh-Adjei, F-X., Boudewijns, B., Nsiah-Boateng, E., Asante, F. A. Van der Velden, K. & Spaan, E. 2018. 'Effects of capitation payment on utilization and claims expenditure under National Health Insurance Scheme: A cross-sectional study of three regions in Ghana'. *Health Economics Review*, 8, 17.

Anon. 2017. 'NHIA begins process to introduce capitation in 3 regions'. National Health Insurance Scheme (NHIS), http://www.nhis.gov.gh/News/nhia-begins-process-to-introduce-capitation-in-3-regions-4066, accessed 27 October 2017.

Barnes, A., Brown, G. & Harman, S. 2015. *Global Politics of Health Reform in Africa: Performance, Participation, and Policy*. Hampshire: Palgrave Macmillan.

Binagwaho, A., Farmer, P. E., Nsanzimana, S., Karema, C., Gasana, M., De Dieu Ngirabega, J., Ngabo, F., Wagner, C. M., Nutt, C. T., Nyatanyi, T. & Gatera, M. 2014. 'Rwanda 20 years on: Investing in life'. *The Lancet*, 384 (9940), 371–375.

Boateng, D. & Awunyor-Vitor, D. 2013. 'Health insurance in Ghana: Evaluation of policy holders' perceptions and factors influencing policy renewal in the Volta region'. *International Journal for Equity in Health*, 12 (1), 50.

Boateng, S., Amoako, P., Poku, A. A., Baabereyir, A. & Gyasi, R. M. 2017. 'Migrant female head porters' enrolment in and utilization and renewal of the national health insurance scheme in Kumasi, Ghana'. *Journal of Public Health*, 25 (6), 625–634.

Brenya, E. & Adu-Gyamfi, S. 2014. 'Interest groups, issue definition and the politics of healthcare in Ghana.' *Public Policy and Administration Research*, 4 (6), 88-96.

Buor, D. 2004. *Accessibility and utilisation of health services in Ghana*. Doctoral dissertation. Maastricht: University of Maastricht.

Carbone, G. 2011. 'Democratic demands and social policies: The politics of health reform in Ghana'. *The Journal of Modern African Studies*, 49 (3), 381–408.

Carrin, G., Waelkens, M. P. & Criel, B. 2005. 'Community-based health insurance in developing countries: a study of its contribution to the performance of health financing systems'. *Tropical Medicine & International Health*, 10 (8), 799–811.

Castro-Leal, F., Dayton, J., Demery, L. & Mehra, K. 1999. 'Public social spending in Africa: Do the poor benefit?' *The World Bank Research Observer*, 14 (1), 49–72.

Centre for Plant Medicine Research (CPMR). 2017. https://www.gbif.org/publisher/9d062cda-9931-4719-81a1-5a4e2d4e7457, accessed 1 December 2018.

Clements, B., Gupta, S. & Nozaki, M. 2013. 'What happens to social spending in IMF-supported programmes?' *Applied Economics*, 45 (28), 4022–4033.

Diop, F. P. & Butera, J. D. (2005). 'Community-based health insurance in Rwanda'. The World Bank, 9650 (7), 19–22.

Dzakpasu, S., Soremekun, S., Manu, A., Asbroek, G., Tawiah, C., Hurt, L., & Kirkwood, B. R. 2012. 'Impact of free delivery care on health facility delivery and insurance coverage in Ghana's Brong Ahafo region'. *PLOS ONE*, 7 (11), 49430.

Ewusi, K. 1989. *Equity and Efficiency in the Supply of Health Manpower in Ghana*. Tema Press of Ghana Publishing Corporation.

Ghana Broadcasting Corporation. 5 February 2017. 'Government directs Release of 180 million cedis to pay NHIS indebtedness'. Ghana Commercial Bank, http://www.gbcghana.com/1.3405370, accessed 30 October 2017.

Ghana News Agency. 18 March 2004. 'National Health Insurance Scheme Launched'. GhanaWeb. https://www.ghanaweb.com/GhanaHomePage/features/National-Health-Insurance-Scheme-launched-54131, accessed 27 October 2017.

Ghana News Agency. 3 April 2016. 'Free Maternal Care not working'. Ghana News Agency, http://www.ghananewsagency.org/health/free-maternal-healthcare-policy-not-working-103030, accessed 29 October 2017.

Gilson, L. 1997. 'The lessons of user fee experience in Africa'. *Health Policy and Planning*, 12 (3), 273–285.

Gobah, F. K. & Zhang, L. 2011. 'The National Health Insurance Scheme in Ghana: prospects and challenges: a cross-sectional evidence'. *Global Journal of Health Science*, 3 (2), 90–101.

Graphic Online. 26 July 2017b. 'NHIS suspends capitation in Ashanti Region'. Graphic Communications, https://www.graphic.com.gh/news/general-news/nhis-suspends-capitation-in-ashanti-region.html, accessed 24 October 2017.

Gros, J. G. 2015. *Healthcare Policy in Africa: Institutions and Politics from*

Colonialism to the Present. Lanham, Maryland: Rowman & Littlefield.

Gyasi, R. M. 2015. 'Relationship between health insurance status and the pattern of traditional medicine utilization in Ghana'. *Evidence-Based Complementary and Alternative Medicine*, 2015 (717926), 1–10.

Gyasi, M. R., Buor, D., Adu-Gyamfi, S., Adjei, P. O. W. & Amoah, P. A. 2017a. 'Sociocultural hegemony, gendered identity, and use of traditional and complementary medicine in Ghana'. *Women & Health*, 58 (5), 1–18.

Gyasi, R. M., Abass, K., Adu-Gyamfi, S. & Accam, B. T. 2017b. 'Nurses' knowledge, clinical practice and attitude towards unconventional medicine: Implications for intercultural healthcare'. *Complementary Therapies in Clinical Practice*, 29 (2017), 1–8.

Igoli, J. O., Ogaji, O. G., Tor-Ayiin, T. A. & Igoli, N. P. 2005. 'Traditional medicine practice amongst the Igede people of Nigeria. Part II'. *African Journal of Traditional, Complementary and Alternative Medicines (AJTCAM)*, 2 (2), 134–152.

Jehu-Appiah, C., Aryeetey, G., Agyepong, I., Spaan, E. & Baltussen, R. 2011. 'Household perceptions and their implications for enrolment in the national health insurance scheme in Ghana'. *Health Policy and Planning*, 27 (3), 222–233.

Kaberuka, D. 2000. Rwanda Vision 2020. Republic of Rwanda, Ministry of Finance and Economic Planning.

Kale, R. 1995. 'Traditional healers in South Africa: A parallel health care system'. *British Medical Journal*, 310 (6988), 1182–1185.

Kentikelenis, A. E. 2017. 'Structural adjustment and health: A conceptual framework and evidence on pathways'. *Social Science & Medicine*, 187 (2017), 296–305.

Lambon-Quayefio, M. & Owoo, N. S. 2017. 'Determinants and the impact of the National Health Insurance on neonatal mortality in Ghana'. *Health Economics Review*, 7 (1), 34–43.

Lemarchand, R. 2004. 'The Rwanda Genocide', in Lemarchand, R. (ed.) *The Rwanda Genocide*. London: Routledge, pp. 394–412.

Lock, M. & Nguyen, V-K. 2010. *An Anthropology of Biomedicine* (1st Edition). London: Wiley Blackwell.

Loewenson, R. 1993. 'Structural adjustment and health policy in Africa'. *International Journal of Health Services*, 23 (4), 717–730.

Logie, D. E., Rowson, M. & Ndagije, F. 2008. 'Innovations in Rwanda's health system: Looking to the future'. *The Lancet*, 372 (9634), 256–261.

Lu, C., Brian, C., Jiwon, L. L., Basinga, P., Hirschhorn, L. R., Hill, K., Murray, M. & Binagwaho, A. 2012. 'Towards universal health coverage: An evaluation of Rwanda Mutuelles in its first eight years'. *PLoS One*, 7 (6), 3982.

Maier, D. 1979. 'Nineteenth-century Asante medical practices'. *Comparative Studies in Society and History*, 21 (1), 63–81.

Mills, A., Ataguba, J. E., Akazili, J., Borghi, J. Garshong, B. Makawia, S., Mtei, G., Harris, B., Macha, J., Meheus, F. & McIntyre, D. 2012. 'Equity in financing and use of health care in Ghana, South Africa, and Tanzania: Implications for paths to universal coverage'. *The Lancet*, 380 (9837), 126–133.

Ministry of Health (MoH) Ghana. August 2004. *National Health Insurance Policy Framework for Ghana*. Revised Version. www.moh.gov.gh/wp-content/uploads/2016/02/National-Health-Insurance-Policy-framework.pdf, accessed 12 December 2018.

National Health Insurance Authority (NHIA). 2008. NHIS report 2008. National Health Insurance Authority. Ghana Health Insurance Review.

National Health Insurance Authority (NHIA). 2009. NHIS report 2009. National Health Insurance Authority. Ghana Health Insurance Review.

National Health Insurance Authority (NHIA). 2010. NHIS report 2010. National Health Insurance Authority. Ghana Health Insurance Review.

National Health Insurance Authority (NHIA). 2011. NHIS report 2011. National Health Insurance Authority. Ghana Health Insurance Review.

National Health Insurance Authority (NHIA). 2012. NHIS report 2012. National Health Insurance Authority. Ghana Health Insurance Review.

National Health Insurance Authority (NHIA). 2013. NHIS report 2013. National Health Insurance Authority. Ghana Health Insurance Review.

National Health Insurance Authority (NHIA). 2017a. 'Capitation'. National Health Insurance Scheme. http://www.nhis.gov.gh/capitation.aspx, accessed 28 October 2017.

National Health Insurance Authority (NHIA). 2017b. 'Membership'. National Health Insurance Scheme. http://www.nhis.gov.gh/membership.aspx, accessed 30 October 2017.

National Health Insurance Authority (NHIA). 2017c. 'Private Health Insurance Scheme in Ghana'. National Health Insurance Scheme. http://www.nhis.gov.gh/phis.aspx, accessed on 28 October 2017.

National Health Insurance Scheme (NHIS). 2014. Abuja, Nigeria. National Health Insurance Scheme. http://www.nhis.gov.ng/, accessed 21 November 2014.

Nyandekwe, M., Nzayirambaho, M., & Kakoma, J. B. 2014. 'Universal health coverage in Rwanda: Dream or Reality'. *The Pan African Medical Journal*, 17.

Nzeyimana, D., Nzayirambaho, M. & Nzakirutimana, J. 2014. 'The behaviour of the low income genocide survivors in case of illness'. *Rwanda Medical Journal*, 71 (3), 5–13. www.bioline.org.br/pdf?rw14010.

Odeyemi, I. & Nixon, J. 2013. 'Assessing equity in health care through the national health insurance schemes of Nigeria and Ghana: A review-based comparative analysis'. *International Journal for Equity in Health*, 12 (1), 9–10.

Osei-Boateng, C. & Ampratwum, E. 2011. *The Informal Sector in Ghana.* Accra: Friedrich Ebert Stiftung.

Osei, C., Otchere, K. G., Banunle, A. & Dontwi, I. K. 2017. 'Trend analysis of students' admission, enrolment and completion in KNUST distance learning postgraduate programmes'. *Journal of Education and Human Development*, 6 (2). DOI: 10.15640/jehd.v6n1a17.

Owoo, N. S. & Lambon-Quayefio, M. P. 2013. 'National health insurance, social influence and antenatal care use in Ghana'. *Health Economics Review*, 3 (1), 19.

Peabody, J. W. 1996. 'Economic reform and health sector policy: Lessons from structural adjustment programs'. *Social Science & Medicine*, 43 (5), 823–835.

Rose, R. 1991. 'What is lesson-drawing?' *Journal of Public Policy*, 11 (1), 3–30.

Rwanda Ministry of Health (RMoH). 2009. Health Financing Policy.

Rwanda Ministry of Health (RMoH). 2010. Rwanda Community Based Health Insurance Policy.

Rwanda Ministry of Health (RMoH). 2018. *Rwanda Health Resource Tracking Output Report.* http://www.moh.gov.rw/index.php?id=512, accessed 12 December 2018.

Saksena, P., Antunes, A. F., Xu, K., Musango, L. & Carrin, G. 2011. 'Mutual health insurance in Rwanda: Evidence on access to care and financial risk protection'. *Health Policy*, 99 (3), 203–209.

Sarpong, N., Loag, W., Fobil, J., Meyer, C. G., Adu-Sarkodie, Y., May, J. & Schwarz, N. G. 2010. 'National health insurance coverage and socio-economic status in a rural district of Ghana'. *Tropical Medicine & International Health*, 15 (2), 191–197.

Saul, J. J. & Leys, C. 1999. 'Sub-Saharan Africa in global capitalism'. *Monthly Review*, 51 (3), 13–30.

Schatz, S. P. 1994. 'Structural adjustment in Africa: A failing grade so far'. *The Journal of Modern African Studies*, 32 (4), 679–692.

Schneider, P. 2005. 'Trust in micro-health insurance: An exploratory study in Rwanda'. *Social Science & Medicine*, 61 (7), 1430–1438.

Shimeles, A. 2010. Community based health insurance schemes in Africa: The case of Rwanda. University of Gothenburg, School of Business, Economics and Law, 463 (1403–2465), 1–10.

Stromquist, N. P. 1999. 'The impact of structural adjustment programmes in Africa and Latin America'. *Gender, education and development: Beyond access to empowerment*, 98 (4), 25–30.

Tilley, H. 2016. 'Medicine, Empires, and Ethics in Colonial Africa'. *AMA Journal of Ethics*, 12 (7), 743–753.

United Nations (UN). 2018. 'Goal 3: Ensure healthy lives and promote well-being for all at all ages'. https://www.un.org/sustainabledevelopment/health/, accessed 27 October 2017.

Wang, H., Otoo, N. & Dsane-Selby, L. 2017. 'Ghana National Health

Insurance Scheme: Improving financial sustainability based on expenditure review'. World Bank Study. http://documents.worldbank.org/curated/en/493641501663722238/Ghana-national-health-insurance-scheme-improving-financial-sustainability-based-on-expenditure-review, accessed 2 November 2018.

Woodward, D. 1992. *'Present pain, future hope'? Debt, adjustment and poverty in developing countries.* Overseas Department, Working paper No. 1, Save the Children.

World Health Organization (WHO) Regional Office for Africa. 2016. *Assessment of medicine pricing and reimbursements systems in health insurance.* WHO. apps.who.int/iris/bitstream/10665/246416/1/9789290233145-eng.pdf, accessed 12 December 2018.

World Bank in Ghana, 2018. http://www.worldbank.org/en/country/ghana/overview, accessed 1 November 2018.

Yankuzo, K. I. 2014. 'Impact of globalization on the traditional African cultures'. *International Letters of Social and Humanities Sciences*, 15 (8), 1–8.

ELEVEN

Preparedness for Epidemics in South Africa

The Health System and Proposals for National Health Insurance

Alex Van Der Heever

INTRODUCTION

An epidemic occurs when (typically) an infectious disease becomes widespread. This therefore excludes many health conditions that are not infectious. In fact, most prevalent health conditions in South Africa today are not infectious, or at least not thought to be. A health system must, however, cater for all conditions, including emergency care, conditions associated with lifestyle, ageing, maternity, and all the associated support services and functions. A health system encompasses multiple subsystems which have complex interactions and requirements. Responding to epidemics forms only a part of the large range of its functions.

An *epidemic* is considered to have occurred when a particular disease demonstrates a significant increase in prevalence (or ratio of existing occurrences) over and above some stable baseline (which can be zero occurrences). This can be distinguished from an *outbreak*, which typically refers to a limited (both in terms of geography and time) change in prevalence. A *pandemic*, by way of contrast, refers to an epidemic that stretches over wide geographic areas (multiple countries and continents). Although an epidemic is typically associated with infectious diseases, it refers equally to any significant change in the prevalence of any disease.[i]

Epidemics therefore reflect significant health threats with many potential causes, not all of them predictable or even preventable. A health system must also focus on reducing pre-existing stable prevalence rates for all diseases, the only difference being that in the former instance the health system needs to respond to a change in the threat levels while in the latter it must focus resources on minimising an existing or known threat.

A health system that responds poorly to known threats can reasonably be expected to respond poorly to unexpected changes in circumstances with complex response requirements. More straightforward threats can, however, be addressed through focused one-off interventions that are not as reliant on a resilient health system. This is where the distinction between an outbreak and an epidemic is important. Whereas the latter may be addressed through a limited and focused intervention, the former may only be mitigated through integrated support from a working health system.

To better understand a country's ability to respond to epidemics, rather than outbreaks, first requires an assessment of the capabilities of the health system as a whole. This chapter begins with a review of the current health system in South Africa through the use of proxy indicators of general capability. This is followed by a review of the extent to which the National Health Insurance (NHI) proposals, as presented to date (early 2019), are likely to influence the responsiveness of the health system to a general systemic threat such as an epidemic. This is followed by a discussion on the implications of the two assessments.

---

i For a discussion of the distinction between outbreaks, epidemics, and pandemics see Centers for Disease Control and Prevention (CDC), 2006, 1-72.

METHODOLOGY

Two assessments are offered in this chapter. The first reviews the capabilities of South Africa's health system, while the second examines the extent to which the capabilities of the health system will be improved by the proposed NHI framework under consideration for the country. The assumption made is that indicators of capability are suggestive of the likely level of preparedness for any change in the health risks facing South Africa. Specific public health arrangements for responding to epidemics are therefore not assessed.

Capabilities of the health system

South Africa usefully generates a fair amount of data and information on the health system each year. While the various sources of data and information are not integrated, it is nevertheless possible to structure the information to provide a picture of the capabilities of the health system.

To avoid errors in attribution this analysis focuses on health indicators that are attributable principally to the capabilities of the health system rather than those that may derive from wider socio-economic conditions. Whereas the latter reflect challenges for the health system, the former relate to the responsiveness of the health system to challenges, whether known or unknown. To avoid distortions that may arise from historical high or low health performance, indicators will in certain instances be compared to benchmarks taken from peer countries rather than from baseline data.

Performance-related indicators could take the following forms: *inputs*, suggestive of the adequacy of resourcing; *outputs*, which could provide an indication of aspects of system efficiency; and *outcomes*, which offer a picture of what the system is able to achieve in relation to existing health challenges. Due to weaknesses in the usefulness of output data generated in South Africa, at least for the purposes of this analysis, the focus in this chapter is on input and outcome data of various forms.[ii]

ii For an assessment of health data availability for hospitals in South Africa see Ranchod et al., 2017. (For a general discussion on indicators used to evaluate health systems performance see Cylus et al., 2016.

Input information will rely on the most recent information (that for 2016/17) supplied by South Africa's Office of Health Standards Compliance (OHSC) which provides evaluations of process-related indicators that may be suggestive of performance (OHSC, 2016/17). This information is based on inspections of public health facilities carried out over a period of time, resulting in scores which can be used both for comparison between facilities (league tables) and against a performance benchmark. In the latter instance this is set by the OHSC in its report at 80 per cent of the maximum possible score (OHSC, 2016/17). Data is available by facility and can also be weighted up to a provincial score.

Two outcome measures are considered: maternal mortality ratios (MMRs) (or the number of women per 100,000 live births who die as a result of childbearing during the pregnancy or within 42 days of delivery or termination of pregnancy during a given year) at a particular facility (Health Systems Trust, 2012: 1); and Auditor-General findings on financial performance.[iii] Both measures are regarded as objective (i.e. measures that are not susceptible to manipulation by public health facility managers) proxy indicators of managerial capability within the health sector. While there are potentially more accurate indicators for facility-based performance, when applied at a provincial and national level they are regarded as appropriate measures for provincial-level performance.

The assumption is that poor facility-based outcomes in maternity services are strongly suggestive of overall managerial capability, rather than just a weakness specific to maternity services. This is consistent with the use of mortality indicators for elective services used in other settings with better data. Similar assumptions have been made using 30-day acute myocardial infarction rates (Cooper et al., 2011).

While financial performance is technically an input indicator, it is assumed in this chapter that an inability to properly manage finances is an outcome indicator indicative of managerial (in)competence. This

iii The Auditor-General of South Africa has the power to examine and report on the financial activities of government. The office of the Auditor-General audits national and provincial government departments, identified public entities, municipalities, and municipal entities. The Auditor-General is accountable to the National Assembly.

data is used principally to determine whether there is any consistency with the MMR results at a provincial level and for the country as a whole. The data source is the most recent Auditor-General report published in 2018 for provincial and national government (Auditor-General, 2018).

National Health Insurance

Although South Africa's NHI proposals have been circulating for over ten years (Van den Heever, 2016), no implementation of any form has occurred to date. The review of NHI will consequently assess whether any of the proposals will address any of the system weaknesses identified through the analysis of capabilities. This assessment will rely on official texts, grey literature published on the NHI, and relevant scholarly literature. An important constraint in this review is the limited extent of any literature of substance on the NHI proposals. The Department of Health (DoH) has only produced superficial proposals, while National Treasury has published no financial analysis.

CONTEXT

This section provides a contextual overview of the South African health system for the more specific analyses that follow. Two features are covered: first, the organisation of the health system; and second, the burden of disease. The former offers an overview of the formal decision-making structures of the health system, and its expenditure levels and trends. The latter offers a profile of the prevailing disease patterns in South Africa at a national level, with an additional focus on the two most rapidly changing metropolitan regions, Johannesburg and Cape Town.

Organisation of the health system

South Africa's health system has evolved over the past 100 years into two distinct sub-systems. The first is the public health sector which effectively provides coverage for around 84 per cent of the population (in 2016) (Council for Medical Schemes, 1980 to 2016; Statistics South Africa, 1980 to 2017) and which is largely provided and managed at a provincial level, with strategic aspects the responsibility of the DoH.

The constitution establishes health services as a concurrent function of national and provincial governments (Republic of South Africa, 1996). While local government does play a role in public health, this is not mandated by the constitution and occurs only when provincial health departments make use of local authorities on an agency basis. These mainly involve primary care services and emergency medical services in the major metropolitan areas (Van den Heever, 2016).

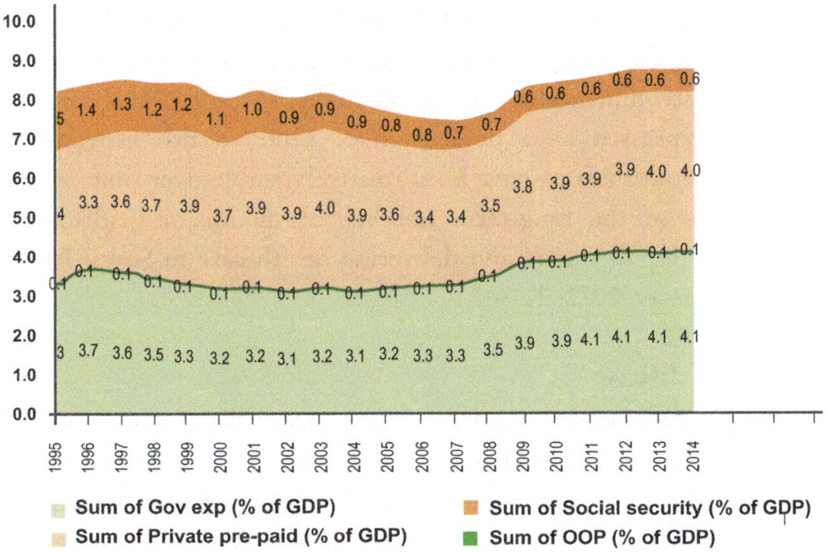

Figure 1: Health expenditure in South Africa expressed as a percentage of Gross Domestic Product 1995 to 2014

Source: World Health Organization, 1995 to 2014

Sum of government expenditure: Total general tax funded expenditure by general government departments.
Sum of social security: Total contributory social insurance coverage for medical expenses (inter alia, the Compensation Fund for Occupational Injuries and Disease and the Road Accident Fund).
Sum of private pre-paid: Total contribution income to private medical schemes.
Sum of OOP: Total out-of-pocket expenditure.

The second sub-system is the regulated medical schemes which cover families (on an individual basis – often referred to as beneficiaries) with relatively high income earners, encompassing roughly 16 per cent of the national population (Council for Medical Schemes, 1980 to 2016;

Statistics South Africa, 1980 to 2017). A relatively minor source of coverage occurs through the Compensation Fund for Occupational Injuries and Diseases and the Road Accident Fund; these are indicated as 'social security' in Figure 1. However, both these schemes combined are responsible for less than 1 per cent of GDP in expenditure, compared to 4.1 per cent for the public sector and 4 per cent for medical schemes (see Figure 1; Department of Social Development et al., 2017). Out-of-pocket expenditure, a sign of coverage failure in health systems, forms a relatively minor 0.6 per cent of GDP and is mainly incurred by higher income groups on medical schemes and overall does not substantially involve catastrophic health expenses (Van den Heever, 2016).

When expressed as a percentage of GDP, health expenditure patterns in South Africa have been relatively stable over time, which is indicative of the long-term stability of the major institutional frameworks for financing and delivering health care in South Africa (Van den Heever, 2012; 2016).

Burden of disease

South Africa has faced a number of health care challenges over the past 30 years. Consistent with international trends, South Africa was facing declines in the prevalence of infectious diseases, together with increases in non-communicable disease. Both trends could be attributed to increased urbanisation, which tends to improve access to health services and population-based prevention programmes (i.e. vaccinations), but negatively alters lifestyles, which increases morbidity due to smoking, alcoholism, motor vehicle accidents, and obesity. However, prevalence rates for infectious diseases such as HIV/AIDS and tuberculosis (TB) began to increase substantially from 1997 (Coovadia et al., 2009; Development Bank of South Africa, 2008; Karim et al., 2009). This was largely due to the HIV/AIDS epidemic which, through attacking the immune system of infected individuals, caused TB infections to rise. From 2009, however, a downward trend in the burden of disease, measured as potential years of life lost (YLLs) due to premature deaths, can be observed for HIV and TB (Figure 2). It should be noted that prior to 2000 the YLL due to HIV/AIDS was negligible and TB was in decline (Karim et al., 2009).

While there are slow structural declines in the burden of disease from 'social' (communicable, maternal, perinatal, and nutritional) causes and 'HIV/TB' from 2009, both are from a very high, arguably unacceptably high, base. Maternal and child deaths, which form part of the 'social' category, are at unusual levels for a country with South Africa's per capita income and health infrastructure (Schaay et al., 2011; National Planning Commission, 2011; Development Bank of South Africa, 2008). South Africa in fact failed to achieve any of its health-related Millennium Development Goals (MDGs) (WHO, 2018).

The very high HIV/AIDS and TB infection and prevalence rates in South Africa could also reasonably be attributed to the general failure of the HIV prevention programmes in the 1990s, for which both the pre- and post-apartheid governments are accountable through poor leadership and stewardship of the health system (Coovadia et al., 2009; Karim et al., 2009). Post-2000 the failure rapidly to introduce treatment programmes affected both mortality and new infections. The latter was because treatment with antiretroviral drugs reduces the viral load in infected individuals, thereby reducing their probability of infecting other individuals (Attia et al., 2009). A structurally lower HIV prevalence rate would, by reasonable inference, have had important implications for the burden of disease and the burden on the public health system. The actual trajectory of the disease into the 2000s as measured in the Actuarial Society of South Africa's AIDS model (Actuarial Society of South Africa, 2008) in fact follows the 'non-intervention' scenario (i.e. where government does nothing) of the modelling analysis published early on in the epidemic in 1991 (Doyle et al., 1991). Whatever the South African health system implemented in the 1990s had no apparent effect on the worst epidemic to face South Africa in the 20th and 21st centuries. Related to these trends is the increase in drug-resistant TB which results from the poor management of TB treatment programmes, i.e. when patients do not complete their drug therapy (Karim et al., 2009).

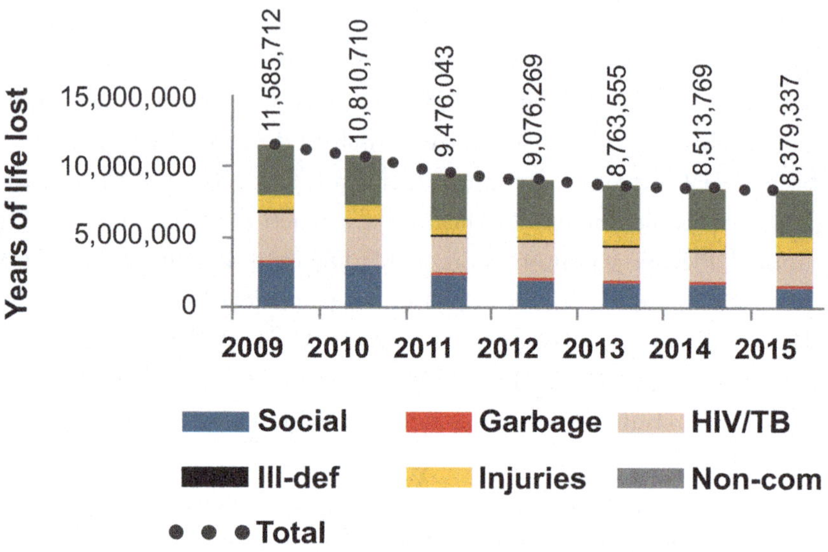

Figure 2: Burden of disease for South Africa from 2009 to 2015

Source: Analysis used data from Health Systems Trust, 2017

Social	YLLs due to communicable, maternal, perinatal, nutrition causes.
Garbage	YLLs due to garbage code deaths (not attributable).
HIV/TB	YLLs due to HIV and TB.
Ill-defined	YLLs due to ill-defined deaths.
Injuries	YLLs due to injuries.
Non-com	YLLs due to non-communicable diseases.[iv]

The increased YLL due to non-communicable diseases also represents an emergent epidemic that South Africa is not yet effectively able to address. While the YLLs expressed at a national level are relatively unchanged over time (Figure 2), those for fast-growing cities such as Johannesburg (Figure 3) and Cape Town (Figure 4) show that early mortality for NCDs is high and rising (although Johannesburg shows a decline to 2012 and then a sharp rise again to 2015). The very rapid population growth in provinces such as the Western Cape and Gauteng i[iv]mply a moving target from a population health perspective.

iv Note that this includes all the diseases of lifestyle, e.g. diabetes and hypertension, which result from poor eating habits.

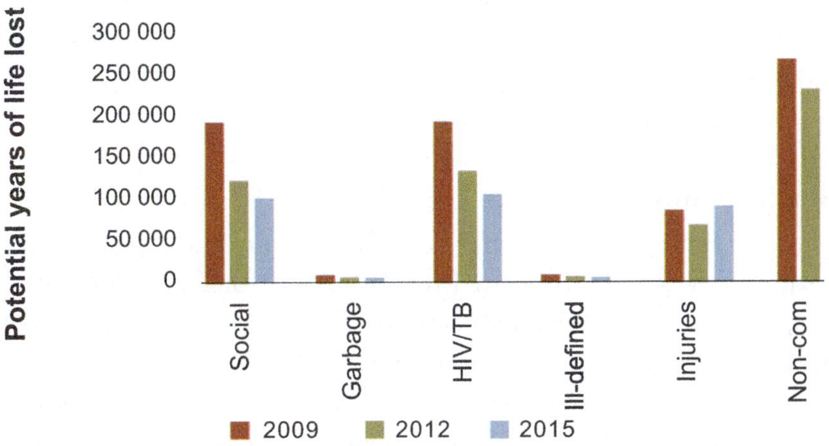

Figure 3: Burden of disease trend for Johannesburg from 2009 to 2015

Source: Analysis used data from Health Systems Trust, 2017

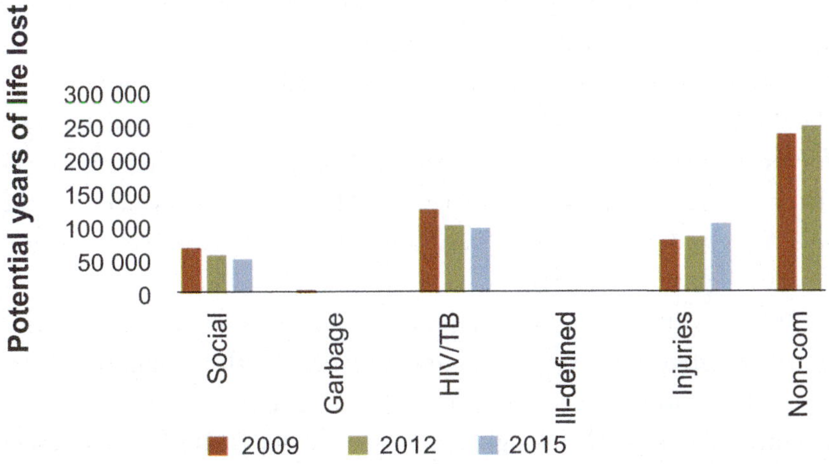

Figure 4: Burden of disease trend for Cape Town from 2009 to 2015

Source: Analysis used data from Health Systems Trust, 2017

HEALTH SYSTEM CAPABILITIES

This section provides insights into the capabilities of the South African health system using three approaches. Maternity mortality ratios contrasted with benchmarks of appropriate performance; the quality assurance assessments of health facilities as performed by the OHSC; and the audit outcomes produced by the Auditor-General. All three indicators offer insights into the general capabilities of the health system, seen individually and in combination.

Maternal mortality ratios

Maternal mortality ratios offer some insight into the capabilities of health services when compared to reasonable benchmarks based on the performances of other peer countries. South Africa's facility-based MMRs at both a provincial and national level are far in excess of what occurs elsewhere for countries with a similar or lower level of economic development (Development Bank of South Africa, 2008; WHO, 2015). Figure 5 provides provincial averages of MMRs for three time periods: 2000–2004, 2005–2009, and 2010–2012.

These show that South Africa performs poorly relative to the appropriate benchmark of 19 (roughly consistent with the lowest estimate of performance by Chile, as indicated in Table 1). Apart from the Western Cape, which is slightly higher than international averages for peer developing countries, South Africa's eight other provinces demonstrate very poor performances. The worst performers are the Free State and the Northern Cape, both of which have MMRs in excess of 200 (Figure 5).

When South Africa is compared to other countries it performs poorly relative both to peer countries (those with a roughly similar level of economic development) in general, and against benchmark countries (those with a roughly similar or lower level of development with good achievements in lowering MMRs) in particular (Table 1).

Chile, for instance, has an average MMR of 22 compared to 138 for South Africa, as reflected in Table 1. China and Costa Rica are 27 and 25 respectively. Even poorly performing peer countries such as Brazil (44), Colombia (64), and Ecuador (64) perform better than the best performing province in South Africa, which is the Western Cape at 77.

Industrialised countries have MMRs that are below 10, except for the United States of America (Table 1). It is worth noting that the health systems arrangements in these countries vary widely. For instance, Brazil, Chile (Velasco et al., 2018), Argentina (Cotlear et al.,

2015), Colombia (Bauhoff et al., 2018), Belgium (Schokkaert et al., 2018), Israel (Brammli-Greenberg et al., 2018), and the Netherlands (Schut and Varkevisser, 2017) have regulated private insurance systems that either form the basis of their universal coverage model or a substantial part of it. All the developing country health systems have mixed private and public sector regimes with industrialised countries either dominated by regulated private markets (most of the instances in Table 1) or a public regime, e.g. United Kingdom (Böhm et al., 2013), Australia (Paolucci et al., 2018).

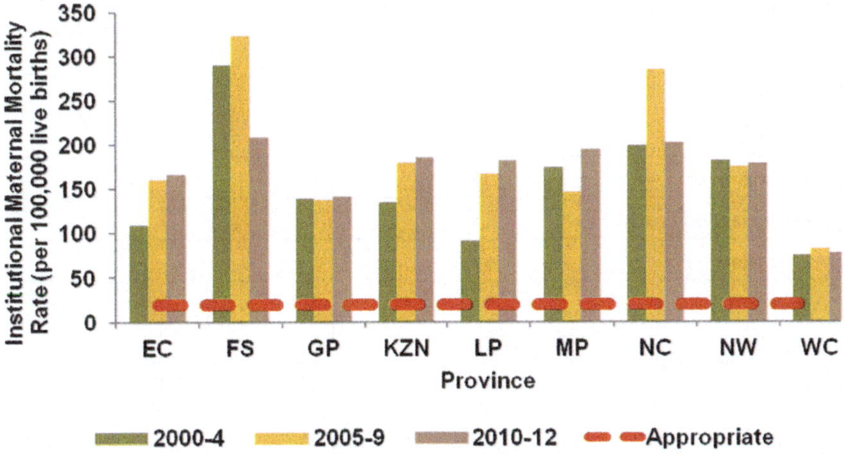

Figure 5: Facility-based maternal mortality ratios by province compared to international benchmarks for countries at an equivalent level of development to South Africa

Source: Based on Health Systems Trust indicators, http://www.hst.org.za/healthindicators; accessed 28 May 2018

Legend: EC = Eastern Cape; FS = Free State; GP = Gauteng; KZN = KwaZulu-Natal; LP = Limpopo; MP = Mpumalanga; NC = Northern Cape; NW = North West; WC = Western Cape.

Table 1: Maternal mortality ratio estimates for South Africa and relevant comparator countries (2015)

Country	MMR	Lower	Upper
Developing countries			
South Africa	138	124	154
Argentina	52	44	63

Country	MMR	Lower	Upper
Developing countries			
Brazil	44	36	54
Chile	22	18	26
China	27	22	32
Colombia	64	56	81
Costa Rica	25	20	29
Cuba	39	33	47
Ecuador	64	57	71
El Salvador	54	40	69
Malaysia	40	32	53
Romania	31	22	44
Sri Lanka	30	26	38
Vietnam	54	41	74
Industrialised countries			
Australia	6	5	7
Austria	4	3	5
Belgium	7	5	10
Canada	7	5	9
Israel	5	4	6
Netherlands	7	5	9
Spain	5	4	6
United Kingdom	9	8	11
United States of America	14	12	16

Source: WHO, 2015

SOUTH AFRICA'S UNDERPERFORMANCE

The data presented here would suggest that the South African public sector is poorly managed relative to other developing countries, with the strongest management performance in the Western Cape and the weakest in the Free State and Northern Cape. The consistency of the results over time suggests that management weaknesses are structural and unresponsive to existing accountability regimes, whether administrative or ultimately political in nature. An analysis of the confidential enquiry maternal mortality data reports that while HIV-related mortality has seen a slight downward trend, haemorrhage-related facility-based mortality rates are increasing (Moodley et al., 2014), which is indicative of a worsening of service provision. They also identify the following preventable aspects of maternal mortality, most of which fall within the domain of the health services to resolve: 49 per cent of maternal deaths are patient related

> *'and include delays in seeking care, problems with transport to facilities, and also some women who accessed unsafe termination of pregnancy by unregistered providers. Administrative problems occurred in 35% of maternal deaths. This included problems with transport between facilities; access to intensive care units; availability of blood and inadequate staff numbers/competence. Healthcare provider problems occurred in 14–38% of maternal deaths with more episodes at district and regional hospitals than tertiary. This included not assessing patients properly, delays in referral, failure to recognise the problem; not following standard protocols and poor monitoring.' (Moodley et al., 2014: 58).*

Office of Health Standards Compliance and the achievement of core quality assurance norms and standards

The Office of Health Standards Compliance (OHSC) is a statutory body established at the national level of government to audit the quality assurance levels of all health facilities. To date it has focused only on public facilities and will eventually expand to private facilities. Its functions include:

- *'Monitoring and enforcing compliance by health establishments with norms and standards prescribed by the Minister of Health in relation to the national health system';*
- *'Ensuring consideration, investigation and disposal of complaints relating to non-compliance with prescribed norms and standards for health establishments in a procedurally fair, economical and expeditious manner.'*
- *'The term health establishment refers to both public and private healthcare services and facilities.'*

- *'It includes hospitals and primary healthcare clinics and extends to emergency medical services, hospices, private medical practices and institutions offering frail care.'* (OHSC, 2018).

To assess capabilities of the South African health system the data from the 2016/17 audit of the OHSC has been weighted provincially using hospital bed data provided by the DoH (DoH, 2013). Table 2 presents the results and compares them to the MMR provincial averages for the period 2010–2012. Although the data is from two different time periods, they are regarded as sufficiently close in time to draw meaningful conclusions.

Table 2: Office of Health Standards Compliance scores for hospital facilities weighted up to a provincial level compared to provincial MMRs for 2010–2012

Province	Weighted average quality score from the OHSC (2016/17) (highest score = 100)(benchmark = 80)	MMR (2010–2012)
Western Cape	74.52	77.13
Gauteng	72.23	141.07
Eastern Cape	59.00	167.23
North West	73.57	179.23
Limpopo	61.43	182.67
KwaZulu-Natal	71.25	185.23
Mpumalanga	58.40	194.17
Northern Cape	46.28	202.60
Free State	63.00	209.37

Source: The OHSC data is based on the OHSC Annual Report 2016/2017. The MMR data is from Table 1 and repeated for comparison with the OHSC. Usable public hospital bed data by province was sourced from the NDOH, 2013.

While the results show a degree of consistency between the two proxy indicators of managerial capability, it appears that the OHSC potentially overstates the capabilities in some provinces, assuming that the MMR is a better indicator of performance. Western Cape scores best on the OHSC and the MMR, and Northern Cape and Free State score very low on the OHSC and the lowest on the MMR.

Outliers in the scoring are Gauteng, North West, and KwaZulu-Natal, all of which score above 70 on the OHSC (suggesting they are in the same range of performance as the Western Cape) but very poorly on the MMR (much lower than the Western Cape MMR).

The two forms of analysis shown in Table 2 are, however, potentially incompatible as the features of hospital performance are too distant (or upstream) from health outcome measures, as argued by Van Biljon (2018). This facility-based study that compared perinatal mortality rates with the OHSC assessments found very poor correlations, consistent with the general picture reflected in Table 2, as the OHSC reviews are effectively not measuring factors important to outcomes. Another finding was that of no improvements in perinatal mortality linked to the accreditation process. It is therefore argued that the OHSC is not truly measuring quality, raising the possibility that hospitals may improve their OHSC scores while facing worsening outcomes.

Even with the potential over-estimate of expected performance in some provinces, the OHSC results are consistent with a poorly performing public health system, with all provinces, barring Western Cape, considerably below the benchmark requirement of 80. Only 16 hospitals out of a total of 135 assessed scored 80 and above, i.e. are at an acceptable standard of performance. This equates to 11.9 per cent of all public hospitals and 18.8 per cent of all public hospital beds. Overall this is suggestive of a poorly performing public health sector even with the potential overstatement of performance in some provinces by the OHSC.

Auditor-General

The most recent Auditor-General report applies to the 2016/17 financial year (Auditor-General, 2018) and offers overview results by province and for major government functions. As the health function forms roughly 30 per cent of overall provincial spending, the performances of the provincial governments is broadly indicative of the capabilities of the health functions. This section provides two results: first, the summarised provincial results (Table 3); and second, by assessments of the health departments (Table 4).

The 'clean audit' results ('where the financial statements are free from material misstatements and there are no material findings on reporting on performance objectives or non-compliance with legislation' (Auditor-General, 2012: 4), by province are broadly consistent with the MMR and the OHSC results. The Western Cape achieves an 83 per cent result, with the next nearest province Gauteng at a relatively poor 52 per cent. No other province achieves more than 24 per cent. Irregular expenditure also stands at a relatively minor R44 million for Western Cape while the other provinces range from R860 million to R9.917 billion. Although these results are not health department specific, they suggest that the management weaknesses are influenced by governance at the wider provincial level. The Free State, KwaZulu-Natal, and North West all have irregular expenditure in excess of 8 per cent of their levels of expenditure – at 11.9 per cent, 9.0 per cent, and 8.2 per cent respectively.

Table 3: Provincial overview of findings by province (2016/17)

Province	Clean audits (%)	Financially unqualified financial statements (%)	No findings on performance reports (%)	No findings on compliance with legislation (%)	Irregular expenditure with the percentage of expenditure in brackets
Western Cape	83	94	89	94	R44 million (0.1%)
Gauteng	52	100	68	57	R6.367 billion (5.9%)
Mpumalanga	24	76	71	24	R2.218 billion (5.3%)
Northern Cape	23	85	69	23	R1.050 billion (6.7%)
Eastern Cape	19	86	57	19	R860 million (1.2%)
Free State	13	47	36	0	R3.860 billion (11.9%)

Province	Clean audits (%)	Financially unqualified financial statements (%)	No findings on performance reports (%)	No findings on compliance with legislation (%)	Irregular expenditure with the percentage of expenditure in brackets
KwaZulu-Natal	12	79	64	12	R9.917 billion (9.0%)
North West	5	37	35	5	R3.065 billion (8.2%)
Limpopo	5	60	45	10	R2.471 billion (4.1%)

Source: Auditor General, 2018; National Treasury, 2018

When the Auditor General compared the financial health of the health and education departments with other departments it is clear that while both health and education perform poorly, health departments stand out as the worst performing. Overall only one health and one education department achieve a 'good' result, defined as having fewer than 30 per cent unfavourable indicators. For health departments 37 per cent raises concerns, and 50 per cent requires an intervention. Other departments achieve a 'good' result in 42 per cent of cases, with 8 per cent requiring an intervention. The Auditor General in fact notes that urgent action is required to prevent a collapse of health services:

> *The financial health of provincial departments of health and education needs urgent intervention to prevent the collapse of these key service delivery departments. In comparison with the other departments, these sectors (particularly the health sector) are in a bad state. (Auditor General, 2018: 76).*

Table 4: Financial health and unauthorised expenditure for health, education, and other departments at a provincial level (number of departments relevant to the outcome in brackets)

Departments	Good	Of concern	Intervention required
Health departments	13% (1)	37% (3)	50% (4)
Education departments	11% (1)	78% (7)	11% (1)
Other departments	42% (60)	50% (72)	8% (12)

Source: Auditor-General, 2018: 76

Note: Explanation of headings in Table 4:

Good	Fewer than 30% unfavourable indicators.
Of concern	30% or more unfavourable indicators.
Intervention required	Significant doubt that can continue in future (vulnerable position) and/or where auditees received a disclaimed or adverse opinion, which meant that the financial statements were not reliable enough for analysis.

Source: Auditor-General, 2018: 72

Discussion of results

All three sets of indicators presented in this section support the finding that the South African public health system is poorly managed and is operating below its potential. The health outcome indicator, in the form of facility-based MMRs, directly implicates the health services, rather than wider socio-economic factors, as the source of higher than normal mortality. Countries of a similar level of development to South Africa and with comparable or lower levels of fiscal support for public health services achieve better MMR results (also see Development Bank of South Africa, 2008). There is no evidence that suggests that South Africa's public health services are improving. The contrary appears to be more accurate.

When these results are compared with the weak responses to the HIV/AIDS and TB epidemics from 1994 to 2002, the evidence supports the view that the public health system is in a fragile state and is suggestive of systemic governance failures. The failure of the health system adequately to prevent both HIV and TB during the 1990s has resulted in a more severe AIDS and TB epidemic than would otherwise have been the case. This has added to the strains on an already fragile system, diverting resources away from the emergent epidemics in non-communicable diseases.

An important indicator of governance failure is the evidence of endemic corruption that has been widely reflected in almost every sphere and organisation of the public sector. Evidence of this can be found in the high levels of irregular expenditure identified by the Auditor General as well as in the extensive moonlighting by key public sector staff such as nurses (Rispel et al., 2014). The causes of governance failure in the public health sector have not, however, been systematically researched to date. As with other state institutions, institutionalised systems of patronage (networks based on familial relationships and quid pro quos) operating through incumbent political parties represents the most reliable explanation of failure (Public Protector, 2016; Von Holdt, 2013).

When patronage is combined with centralised decision-making, the capture of strategic functions such as staff appointments, the issuing of licences and associated regulation of various entities both public and private, and procurement is potentially inevitable. Governance reform within the public health system therefore needs to consider all avenues to eliminate the structural occurrence of systems of patronage while implementing institutional frameworks that incentivise good performance and responsiveness to the served community. These systems weaknesses are structural because they derive from the current institutional framework; they can only be removed through an adjustment to the institutional framework.

While the relatively devolved nature of the public health system offers opportunities for increased accountability to the served population, in the absence of institutional frameworks that address conflicts of interest and that localise accountability, it is inevitable that principal-agent problems will arise (i.e. where the *principal* in the form of the served community will not be able to steer the conduct of the *agent* in the form of health service providers and administrators). As far as possible, therefore, principal-agent problems must be addressed structurally to address any misalignment of incentives by agents. However, governance redesign through the distribution of mandates and accountability structures is complex and needs to consider carefully existing structures in designing the way forward (Contandriopoulos et al., 2004; Barnett et al., 2009; Smith et al., 2012; Walker et al., 2001; Hayes, 2006).

Emerging health systems designs involve the following key features consistent with a multi-level governance framework (Abimbola et al., 2014; Maino et al., 2007; Ostergren et al., 2007): the separation of political decision-making from operational decision-making; the centralisation of strategic resource allocation decisions to ensure the equitable distribution of resources; the distribution of health service decision-making to the most appropriate level (with strategic decisions more central, and operational decisions closest to the ground); and the introduction of accountability frameworks such that each level of decision-making is accountable to the most relevant role-players and stakeholders such that the public interest is served. A careful mix of mandates, accountability regimes, institutional flexibility, financing mechanisms, and quasi and actual contracting approaches is an inevitable feature of a well-functioning health system.

It is within the context of South Africa's health system weaknesses and reform imperatives that consideration must be given to the adequacy of the proposed NHI as a means to improve the system's capabilities.

ADEQUACY OF REFORM PROPOSALS – NATIONAL HEALTH INSURANCE

Overview

The government process to consider a NHI began in 2009 with the establishment of a ministerial advisory committee with Dr Olive Shisana as the chairperson (DoH, 2009). Various reports have outlined the NHI policy framework to date. These include a Green Paper and two White Papers (DoH, 2011; DoH, 2015; DoH, 2017).

The official government processes have therefore run from November 2009 to 2019 (the present) – a period of 10 years. During this period all incremental structural reforms of the health system were halted until such time as the NHI policy could be finalised and implemented (Van den Heever, 2016). This included the halting and withdrawal of all structural reforms of the private health system which were in the process of implementation during 2008 (Van den Heever,

2016; Beresford, 2008). Furthermore, no consideration was given to achieve governance reforms of the public system.

The apparent reason for blocking incremental reforms was due to the assumption that the complete NHI framework could be implemented in a single year, i.e. over the period 2009 to 2010 (Van den Heever, 2011). However, even when it became clear that this was not possible, the de-prioritisation of incremental reforms remained in place.

While there has been an extensive public discourse on the NHI over this period, research papers, technical reports, implemented systems, or even a business case have not been taken into account. Most proposals are descriptive in form with no systematic evaluations forming the basis for technical reforms.

Some research was attempted through the implementation of 11 NHI pilot projects from 2012. However, there is no evidence of what they were meant to research or what they achieved (Section 27, 2016; Khan, 2016; Magubane, 2017; Botha, 2018). In fact, no independent evaluation has ever been made public on the pilot project outcomes.

What is proposed?

The main motivation for the NHI framework can be reduced to a simple statement indicating that South Africa has a two-tier health system and must implement a single-tier health system (DoH, 2011). The general narrative argues that South Africa must implement universal health coverage (UHC) on the implied (but never stated) assumption that universal coverage does not exist.

> *NHI will provide coverage to the whole population and minimize the burden carried by individuals of [sic] paying directly out of pocket for healthcare services. This model of delivering health and healthcare services to the population is well accepted, described and widely promoted by the World Health Organization as universal coverage. (DoH, 2011: 5)*

The NHI is motivated as a financing scheme in which the functions of 'pooling' (which is the achievement of cross-subsidies from rich to poor and from those who don't need health care today to those who do) and 'purchasing' (which refers to contracting or buying health services) are consolidated into a single national organisation, the National Health Insurance Fund (NHIF). Combining pooling and purchasing involves a considerable departure from the current health system where (what can be regarded as) purchasing is the function of provincial governments and medical schemes.

Although somewhat unclear between the various government papers, the NHI proposals involve the introduction of general tax increases roughly equal to 3 per cent of GDP (DoH, 2011) in an attempt to redirect all health spending through the NHIF. As the central idea behind the NHI is to establish a single-tier system, inter alia the feasibility of such a tax increase is therefore a cornerstone of the entire scheme. However, to date no official analysis has been produced of the viability of such a proposal and the Minister of Health has announced to the media that no such analysis will be produced (*Mail & Guardian*, 2012).

Government already achieves a substantial degree of pooling via the tax system and the prevailing system of unconditional and conditional transfers to provincial governments and medical schemes (via the tax credit that can be claimed for medical scheme contributions). However, pooling is considerably less onerous as a function than purchasing, which requires a combination of administration, regulation, and contracting. The idea that the purchasing function will in future be consolidated in a single organisation, the NHIF, therefore has significant institutional and governance implications which have not been officially assessed. It is questionable whether a superior degree of pooling will be achievable relative to the current framework. A substantial transfer from rich to poor is implicit in the public health system as high-income earners are removed from coverage (i.e. they are either covered by medical schemes or must pay for public hospital services).

A key thematic idea arising in the NHI proposals is the (assumed) superior purchasing efficiencies that will be derived from the introduction of a 'purchaser–provider split'. This institutional approach distinguishes between the organisation that *buys* and those that *offer* health care services. The present public health system, by way of contrast, is characterised by vertical integration, where the purchaser is also the provider of health services. For instance, a public hospital merely forms part of the provincial administrative hierarchy, falling ultimately under a single accounting officer in the form of a provincial head of department (HOD). The shift to a purchaser-provider approach consequently requires the full decentralisation of health services so that they can be contracted individually, together with private sector services. The (constitutional) role of provincial health administrations in organising context-specific health strategies is not discussed or evaluated in the various official papers or in the draft NHI bill (DoH, 2018). No strategy to decentralise health service decision-making has to date been articulated, evaluated, or initiated.

The proposals also envisage that the entire population of South Africa would need explicitly to enrol as beneficiaries of the system, along the lines of medical scheme members. In addition, individuals would need to choose actively a primary health care provider to be pre-funded by the NHIF on their behalf. Therefore, not only would the NHIF need to administer 56 million enrolees, who could technically not receive benefits without being enrolled, but also manage their self-assignment to health facilities. At present, however, to receive free public services no one needs to enrol. Enrolment with an insurer is typically only required where a need exists to determine an entitlement to benefits (i.e. exclude non-contributors) in exchange for a contribution – such as a social insurance fund and a private medical scheme. This proposal is therefore a considerable undertaking for which no precedent exists in South Africa.

It is also proposed that the financing of hospitals be activity based (i.e. payment per individual medical activity), using diagnostic related groupers (DRGs) (a grouper is a group of diagnoses with a similar average cost). This would require that patient utilisation be matched with enrolee information so that reimbursable admissions can be validated against a diagnostic code (i.e. a hospital admission associated with a diagnostic code triggers a payment based on the cost associated with the group of diagnoses into which a diagnosis falls). This form of reimbursement would also require authentication against service use to prevent hospitals from misrepresenting the diagnostic codes to increase their revenues. Treatment validation would require the universal (public and private sector) implementation of electronic patient records and associated business processes at a very high standard at all levels of care. Some form of ongoing costing analysis would need to be maintained constantly to re-weight the DRGs. To date the DoH has not managed to produce a domestically costed DRG schedule or to establish a system to institutionalise it.

To prevent the excessive use of private sector hospitals (proposed to form part of the NHI network of provider services), which are perceived to be of a higher standard than public hospitals, public sector hospitals would need to be governed, managed, staffed, and equipped at similar levels to private hospitals before the implementation of the overall system. This would require more than the achievement of OHSC core standards, which only 18.8 per cent of public hospital beds by 2018 were able to attain. By early 2019 no strategy to upgrade the public hospital system has been evaluated or proposed.

The NHI proposals envisage that an internal market be created for hospital services as in the English National Health Service in the United Kingdom. Here funding follows patients (consistent with the DRG approach). However, this results in the systemic underfunding of smaller hospitals and the risk of closure or public hospital mergers (Gaynor et al., 2012). The proposals, however, do not elaborate on this complex reliance on competition as a governance and accountability regime or how it would form part of a complete system of governance and accountability. No technical report or assessment of how this could be applied in the South African context has ever been presented.

The policy framework also envisages the implementation of a standard minimum package of health services. This would require the statutory specification of some package of services, diagnoses and/or treatment protocols that are guaranteed as a right. By early 2019 no such package has yet been articulated or costed. While measures such as an essential drugs list (EDL) are relatively straightforward to determine, and already exist, to specify a positive set of hospital and out-of-hospital services (which includes all clinic-based primary care and public health interventions) would require considerable effort if attempted as a national top-down process. To date no technical report has ever been presented on how this approach may be implemented.

The NHI proposals also propose the central (national) determination of referral networks, with possible bypass fees. As with a number of NHI proposals, the legal framework already exists to allow this with existing public services. It has, however, never been implemented due to the systemic unfairness that would exist if low-income communities were penalised for bypassing poorly performing public services in their area (from personal experience of the author as the finance director of the Gauteng Department of Health in 1998 to 2000). It is worth noting that the DOH has up to early 2019 not been able to establish an organised system of referrals in the public sector.

The governance model for the NHIF, which is intended (at least as stated) to procure all health services in South Africa for the entire population (including those currently on medical schemes), is effectively appointed and removed by one person, the Minister of Health (MOH). The board members are recommended by the MOH and appointed by cabinet and also removed by the MOH (DoH, 2018: Section 14). The MOH also has wide discretion to appoint acting board members and to remove them.

While the NHIF board gets to shortlist and nominate a candidate for the position of chief executive, the actions must be approved by the MOH. Although the bill refers to an independent board, ample scope exists for the MOH to influence the membership and tenure of the board (in particular concerning acting members), and thereby the board's material decisions, including the shortlist of chief executive candidates.

This approach to governance leaves wide scope for extracting patronage, through the person in the position of MOH. Such practices have resulted in the failure of provincial health services and in South Africa's state-owned enterprises (SOEs). No technical review has been performed to justify the governance approach and explain how it will appropriately align incentives throughout the health system. No justification is provided for why the MOH should have such powers of appointment and removal within a domestic context where the experience demonstrates that it runs counter to the public interest.

It is also proposed that sub-regional contracting structures will be implemented by the NHIF. However, these appear to be subordinate structures within the NHIF administrative hierarchy. It is worth noting that this is quite different to the NHS in the United Kingdom (Vrangbaek, 2007) and the Canadian health system (Martin et al., 2018), both of which have established fully decentralised and genuinely independent regional structures (trusts) that organise the services and purchasing for their areas.

The NHIF is proposed as a national structure in which no structural decentralisation is envisaged. It is not specified how the NHIF will hold the massive administration accountable or how it will cooperate with provinces on spatial and public health strategies. It merely states that they should coordinate. No guiding vision has been provided. Therefore, it is unclear how the transition will be affected from what exists to an untested and sparsely articulated institutional framework.

A complaints and appeals regime is also proposed, with a tribunal that is appointed by the MOH with a secretariat provided by the chief executive of the NHI (an MOH appointee). The bill also allocates powers to this tribunal equivalent to those of the high court. By early 2019 no policy document or evaluation has been produced to demonstrate why this approach was adopted and why a truly independent structure was not preferred.

Discussion of proposals

With a few qualifications, South Africa does have a system of UHC, although, as discussed above, it is plainly degrading in both the public and private systems due to structural weaknesses which are likely to weaken coverage and the quality of services further over time (Van den Heever, 2016; Health Market Inquiry (South Africa), 2018).

However, South Africa has one of the lowest levels of out-of-pocket expenditure in both the developing and developed world (Van den Heever, 2016) (also see Figure 1), which suggests that the coverage problem is not serious. The rationale for NHI and UHC appears to have been *lifted* from contexts where UHC strategies are needed to close gaps in coverage rather than to address weaknesses in the institutional framework and governance. As South Africa has a free public service for those who cannot contribute to their own health care, coverage is less of a problem than the quality and sustainability of coverage. All three major government reports on NHI are in fact silent on the extremely complex questions of governance and institutional coherence and their relationship to the alignment of incentives, the key areas essential to addressing the quality of coverage (National Department of Health, 2011; 2015; 2017).

The three major government reports furthermore blur the lines between the concepts of NHI and UHC. While the former is merely a mechanism to achieve UHC, there are in fact multiple approaches (mechanisms) for achieving the objective of UHC (Kutzin, 2001; McPake and Hanson, 2016) and all but a handful of industrialised countries involve some form of single-tier centralised insurance model. Countries do not adopt particular models. Rather, their systems evolve in accordance with the opportunities offered from their institutional context. The conflation of the ideas of UHC and NHI was explicit in the Green Paper stating that '*this model of delivering health and healthcare services to the population* [NHI] *is well accepted, described and widely promoted by the World Health Organization as universal coverage*' (DoH, 2011: 5). The choice of mechanism to achieve UHC is a complex reform with the result that changes are invariably incremental, path-dependent (or significantly constrained by past decisions) and context-specific.[v]

The NHI proposals do not offer an answer to the failures of either the public or private health systems, while not actually demonstrating concretely that the key features of the system are in fact implementable. The draft bill offers no certainty that any aspect of the NHI will be operational in the foreseeable future. Even if the NHI were to be fully implemented, it still does not address the systemic weaknesses of the public and private health systems which have been identified to date in numerous inquiries and official processes (DoH, 1995; DoH, 1997; DoH, 2002; Taylor Committee, 2002; Armstrong et al., 2004; Ministerial Task Team on Social Health Insurance, 2005; Council for Medical Schemes, 2006; Health Market Inquiry (South Africa), 2018).

On the grounds of feasibility the following proposals, which are critical to the success of NHI, are also unlikely ever to be implemented:

- The financing of the NHI at a level that would result in coverage

v See Hayes, 2006: for an extensive discussion on the limits to non-incremental policy reform when faced with complexity.

for the full population within a single scheme, with the proposal for general tax increases of up to 3 per cent of GDP.

- The substitution of existing 'purchasing' functions from provinces and private medical schemes into a single national public entity.
- The enrolment of the entire national population onto a single registry, which also administers beneficiary allocations to primary care providers.
- The implementation of a purchaser-provider split in the public health system.

The most concerning aspect of the NHI reforms, however, has been the obstruction of incremental reforms to long-existing systems in both the public and private sectors that would enhance the capabilities of the health system to deal with major health-related threats, such as epidemics. No legislative development of any substance has occurred from 2004 to the present day in either the public or private sectors. As a consequence basic systems of governance have not been upgraded nor resource allocation mechanisms updated, despite accumulating evidence of system weaknesses that are amenable to intervention. The flawed governance frameworks that are exposed to patronage have been retained and, furthermore, in the NHI framework it is proposed that they be maintained.

Given the above, the most probable scenario for the South African health system going forward involves the maintenance of the status quo with the possible implementation of an NHIF which is unlikely to become fully operational. As a consequence all the weaknesses in the public and private systems apparent to date are likely to persist and thereby continue incrementally to weaken health coverage in South Africa. The ability of the health system to both anticipate and address complex health-related threats such as epidemics is therefore likely to deteriorate rather than improve.

CONCLUSIONS

This chapter sought to review the current capabilities of the South African health system with a view to forming a view on its readiness to address epidemics. The results suggest that the health system is fragile and is weakening over time. Three major epidemics have impacted on the system from the 1990s to the present, HIV/AIDS, TB, and non-communicable diseases. The initial weaknesses of the health system have allowed the epidemics to stabilise at very high levels, further increasing the fragility of the health system. Evidence of public health system capabilities through input and outcome indicators suggests considerable underperformance relative to reasonable benchmarks. This can largely be attributed to the prevailing governance framework which exposes health services to patronage systems and the resulting institutionalised corruption. Presently there are no proposals emanating from the South African government to address these weaknesses. In the absence of meaningful reforms to the governance framework, health coverage is likely to deteriorate incrementally. Not only does this imply that existing epidemics will not be adequately addressed, but that new epidemics will be poorly managed.

While the NHI proposals could be argued to address the structural weaknesses of the health system, when the detail is examined, all the prevailing systemic weaknesses are retained, with the added confusion of an attempt to implement an untested reform that is not evidence based. Based on the failure to implement incremental reforms over the past 10 years, it is quite likely that the pursuit of the NHI policy framework will continue to obstruct the consideration of workable reforms that address the fundamental challenges in the health system. It is a well-understood feature of policy change over time that non-incremental complex policies rarely succeed (Pierson, 2000; Hayes, 2006) and that most policy change is incremental and of necessity acknowledges existing implemented policy as the starting point. The NHI reforms, however, presume a blank sheet and ignore all existing implemented policies. The overtly political nature of the proposals (Van den Heever, 2016) has removed the checks and balances that normally constrain unrealistic policy proposals and has allowed them to obstruct real reform. If permitted to continue, the capabilities of the health system will further deteriorate and reduce its capacity to respond to complex threats – which include epidemics.

REFERENCES

Abimbola S., Negin J., & Jan S. 2014, Towards people-centred health systems: a multi-level framework for analysing primary health care governance in low- and middle-income countries, *Health Policy and Planning*, 29, ii29–ii39.

Actuarial Society of South Africa. 2008. 'HIV Model', in Actuarial Society of South Africa (ed).

Armstrong J., Deeble J., & Dror, D. 2004. Report to the South African Risk Equalization Fund Task Group by the International Review Panel.

Attia S., Egger, M., & Müller, M. 2009. 'Sexual transmission of HIV according to viral load and antiretroviral therapy: Systematic review and meta-analysis'. *AIDS*, 23, 1397–1404.

Auditor-General. 2018. *Consolidated General Report on National and Provincial Audit Outcomes: PFMA 2017-18*, Pretoria: Auditor General.

Auditor-General. 2012. Background to the three aspects we audit.

Barnett, P., Tenbensel, T., & Cumming, J. 2009. 'Implementing new modes of governance in the New Zealand health system: An empirical study'. *Health Policy*, 93, 118–127.

Bauhoff, S., Rodriguez-Bernate, I., & Gopffarth, D. 2018. 'Health plan payment in Columbia', in McGuire, T. G. & Van Kleef, C. (eds.) *Risk Adjustment, Risk Sharing and Premium Regulation in Health Insurance Markets: Theory and practice. (*1st Edition). London: Candice Janco, 279–294.

Beresford, B. 2008. 'War over healthcare'. *Mail & Guardian.*

Böhm, K., Schmid, A., & Götze, R. 2013. 'Five types of OECD healthcare systems: Empirical results of a deductive classification'. *Health Policy*, 113, 258–269.

Botha, C. 2018. 'NHI: Why an objective reassessment of the pilot phase is needed (II)'. *Politicsweb.* South Africa: Politicsweb.

Brammli-Greenberg, S., Glazer, J. & Shmueli, A. 2018. 'Regulated competition and health plan payment under the National Health Insurance Law in Israel - The unfinished story', in McGuire, T. G. & Van Kleef, C. (eds.) *Risk Adjustment, Risk Sharing and Premium Regulation in Health Insurance Markets: Theory and practice. (*1st Edition). London: Candice Janco, pp 365–398.

Centers for Disease Control and Prevention (CDC). 2006. *Principles of Epidemiology in Public Health Practice: An Introduction to Applied Epidemiology and Biostatistics.* Atlanta: Department of Health and Human Services.

Contandriopoulos, D., Denis, J-L., & Langley, A. 2004. Governance Structures and Political Processes in a Public System: Lessons from Quebec. *Public Administration*, 82, 627–655.

Cooper, Z., Gibbons, S., & Jones, S. 2011. 'Does hospital competition save lives? Evidence from the English NHS Patient Choice Reforms'. *Economic Journal (London, England)*, 121, F228–F260.

Coovadia, H., Jewkes, R., & Barron, P. 2009. 'The health and health system of South Africa: Historical roots of current public health challenges'. *The Lancet*, 374, 817–834.

Cotlear, D., Gómez-Dantés, O. & Knaul, F. 2015. 'Overcoming social segregation in health care in Latin America'. *The Lancet*, 385, 1248–1259.

Council for Medical Schemes. 1980-2016. 'Data based on the Annual Reports of the Council for Medical Schemes from 1980 to 2016', in Schemes CfM (ed), Pretoria.

Council for Medical Schemes. 2006. 'Circular 8 of 2008: Consultation on a revised benefit design structure for medical schemes', in Schemes CfM (ed). Council for Medical Schemes.

Cylus, J., Papanicolas, I. & Smith, P. C. 2016. 'A Framework for Thinking about Health System Efficiency' in Cylus, J., Papanicolas, I. & Smith, P. C. (eds.) *Health system efficiency: How to make measurement matter for policy and management.* United Kingdom: World Health Organization, 1–20.

Department of Health (DoH). 1995. 'Restructuring the national health system for universal access to primary health care', in Health NDo (ed). Pretoria: Department of Health.

Department of Health (DoH). 1997. 'A Social Health Insurance Scheme for South Africa: Policy Document', in Health NDo (ed). Pretoria: Department of Health (unpublished), 16.

Department of Health (DoH). 2002. Inquiry into various social security aspects of the South African Health system: Based on the health subcommittee findings of the Committee of Inquiry into a Comprehensive System of Social Security (Taylor Committee).

Department of Health (DoH). 2009. 'Establishment of the National Health Insurance Advisory Committee' in Health NDo (ed), Government Gazette 32564, Pretoria: Government Gazette.

Department of Health (DoH). 2011. 'Policy on National Health Insurance' (Green Paper), in Health NDo (ed). Pretoria: Government Gazette.

Department of Health (DoH). 2013. Public hospital beds. Data provided on request to A. M. van den Heever (ed).

Department of Health (DoH). 2015. ' National Health Insurance for South Africa: Towards universal health coverage' in Health NDo (ed). Pretoria: Government Gazette.

Department of Health (DoH). 2017. 'Towards a national health insurance policy' (White Paper). Pretoria: Government Gazette.

Department of Health. 2018. National Health Insurance Bill. South Africa: Government Gazette.

Department of Social Development, Wits School of Governance and Oxford

Policy Management. 2017. *Social Budget Bulletin*, Pretoria.

Development Bank of South Africa. 2008. A roadmap for the reform of the South African Health System. Development Bank of South Africa.

Doyle, P. R., Broomberg, J., & Steinberg, M. 1991. *AIDS in South Africa: The Demographic and Economic Implications*: Centre for Health Policy, University of the Witwatersrand.

Gaynor, M., Laudicella, M. & Propper, C. 2012. 'Can governments do it better? Merger mania and hospital outcomes in the English NHS'. *Journal of Health Economics*, 31, 528–543.

Hayes, M.T. 2006. *Incrementalism and Public Policy*. Lanham, Maryland: University Press of America.

Health Market Inquiry (South Africa). 2018. Provisional findings and recommendations report. Pretoria: Competition Commission (South Africa).

Health Systems Trust. 2012. District Health Barometer 2012/3: Focus on Maternal Mortality. *DHB Supplementary Series 1.* Durban: Health Systems Trust.

Karim, S. S. A., Churchyard, G. J., & Karim, Q. A. 2009. 'HIV infection and tuberculosis in South Africa: An urgent need to escalate the public health response'. *The Lancet*, 374, 921–933.

Khan, T. 2016. 'NHI pilot projects fail to reach targets'. *Business Day.*

Kutzin, J. 2001. 'A descriptive framework for country-level analysis of health care financing arrangements'. *Health Policy*, 56, 171–204.

Magubane, K. 2017. 'Committee hears of NHI pilot problems'. *Business Day.*

Mail & Guardian 2012. 'Motsoaledi launches NHI pilot programme'. *Mail & Guardian.*

Maino, F., Blomqvist, P., & Bertinato, L. 2007. 'Effects of decentralization and recentralization on political dimensions of health systems' in Saltman, R. B., Bankauskaite, V. & Vrangbaek. K. (eds.) *Decentralization in Health Care: Strategies and Outcomes.* (1st Edition). Berkshire: McGraw-Hill, Open University Press, 120–140.

Martin, D., Miller, A. P., & Quesnel-Vallée, A. 2018. 'Canada's universal health-care system: achieving its potential'. *The Lancet*, 391, 1718–1735.

McPake, B. & Hanson, K. 2016. 'Managing the public-private mix to achieve universal health coverage'. *The Lancet*, 388, 622–630.

Ministerial Task Team on Social Health Insurance. 2005. 'Social Health Insurance Options: Financial and fiscal impact assessment' in Health NDo (ed). Pretoria: National Department of Health.

Moodley, J. Pattinson, R., & Fawcus, S. 2014. 'The confidential enquiry into maternal deaths in South Africa: A case study'. *BJOG: An International Journal of Obstetrics & Gynaecology*, 121, 53–60.

National Planning Commission. 2011. National Development Plan 2030, our future, make it work. Pretoria: Sherino Printers.

National Treasury. 2018. Tabled Provincial Budgets 2018 MTEF, in Treasury N (ed).

Office of Health Standards Compliance (OHSC). 2016/17. *Annual Inspection Report 2016/17,* Pretoria: Office of Health Standards Compliance.

Office of Health Standards Compliance (OHSC). 2018. *Mandate of the Office of Health Standards Compliance.* Available at: http://ohsc.org.za/who-we-are/#mandate.

Ostergren, K., Boni, S., & Danishevski, K. 2007. 'Implementation of health care decentralisation', in Saltman, R. B., Bankauskaite, V. & Vrangbaek, K. (eds.) *Decentralization in Health Care: Strategies and Outcomes.* 1st edn. Berkshire: McGraw-Hill, Open University Press, 225–245.

Paolucci, F., Sequeira, A. R., & Fouda, A. 2018. ' Health plan payment in Australia', in McGuire, T. G. & Van Kleef, R. C. (eds.) *Risk Adjustment, Risk Sharing and Premium Regulation in Health Insurance Markets: Theory and practice. (*1st Edition). London: Candice Janco, 181–207.

Pierson, P. 2000. 'The limits of design: Explaining institutional origins and change'. *Governance*, 13, 475–499.

Public Protector. 2016. State of Capture. Public Protector.

Ranchod, S., Adams, C., & Burger, R. 2017. 'South Africa's hospital sector: Old divisions and new developments', in Padarath, A. & Barron, P. (eds.) *South African Health Review 2017*, Durban, 101–110.

Republic of South Africa. 1996. Constitution of the Republic of South Africa.

Rispel, L. C., Blaauw, D., & Chirwa, T. 2014. 'Factors influencing agency nursing and moonlighting among nurses in South Africa'. *Global Health Action*, 7: 10.3402/gha.v3407.23585.

Schaay, N., Sanders, D. & Kruger, V. 2011. Overview of health sector reforms in South Africa. DFID Human Development Resource Centre.

Schokkaert, E., Guillaume, J. & Van de Voorde, C. 2018. 'Risk Adjustment in Belgium: Why and how to introduce socioeconomic variables in health plan payment', in McGuire, T. G. & Van Kleef, R. C. (eds.) *Risk Adjustment, Risk Sharing and Premium Regulation in Health Insurance Markets: Theory and practice. (*1st Edition). London: Candice Janco, 209–233.

Schut, F. T. & Varkevisser, M. 2017. 'Competition policy for health care provision in the Netherlands'. *Health Policy*, 121, 126–133.

Section 27. 2016. Section 27 submission on the NHI White Paper.

Smith, P. C., Anell, A., & Busse, R. 2012. ' Leadership and governance in seven developed health systems' . *Health Policy*, 106, 37–49.

Statistics South Africa. 1980–2017. Mid-year population estimates. 31 July 2017 ed. Pretoria: Statistics South Africa.

Taylor Committee. 2002. Transforming the present – protecting the future: Report of the Committee of Inquiry into a Comprehensive System of Social Security for South Africa, 1st edn.

Van Biljon, C. 2018. 'Hospital behaviour in South Africa: The role of an accreditation programme in the context of health outcomes'. *Economics*, Stellenbosch: University of Stellenbosch.

Van den Heever, A. M. 2011. Evaluation of the Green Paper on National Health Insurance: Submission to the National Department of Health. Wits School of Governance.

Van den Heever, A. M. 2012. 'The role of insurance in the achievement of universal coverage within a developing country context: South Africa as a case study'. *BMC Public Health*, 12, 1–13.

Van den Heever, A. M. 2016. 'South Africa's universal health coverage reforms in the post-apartheid period'. *Health Policy*, 120, 1420–1428.

Velasco, C., Henriquez, J. & Paolucci, F. 2018. 'Health plan payment in Chile', in McGuire, T. G. & Van Kleef, C. (eds.) *Risk Adjustment, Risk Sharing and Premium Regulation in Health Insurance Markets: Theory and practice. (*1st Edition). London: Candice Janco, 235–262.

Von Holdt, K. 2013. 'South Africa: The transition to violent democracy'. *Review of African Political Economy*, 40, 589–604.

Vrangbaek, K. 2007. 'Key factors in assessing decentralization and recentralization in health systems', in Saltman, R. B., Bankauskaite, V. & Vrangbaek, K. (eds.) *Decentralization in Health Care: Strategies and Outcomes.* (1st Edition). Berkshire: McGraw-Hill, Open University Press, 63–76.

Walker, W. E., Rahman, S. A. & Cave, J. 2001. 'Adaptive policies, policy analysis, and policy-making'. *European Journal of Operational Research*, 128, 282–289.

World Health Organization (WHO). 2015. *Trends in maternal mortality: 1990 to 2015*, Geneva: World Health Organization.

World Health Organization (WHO). 2018. South Africa, fact sheets of health statistics. Geneva: World Health Organization.

TWELVE

Conclusion

ZAMANZIMA MAZIBUKO

THE ABILITY OF NATIONAL HEALTH systems to detect and respond to disease threats is the difference between containing an outbreak and facing a calamity. Strong systems for the monitoring and detection of diseases are crucial as they provide countries with the necessary mechanisms to effectively manage disease outbreaks. Yet in many African countries, which shoulder a disproportionate burden of disease, the systems required to enable decisive action are on the brink of collapse or are accessible only to some population groups.

The International Health Regulations (IHR)[i] (2005) state that countries should be able to detect, assess, and respond to all incidents that may lead to public health emergencies of international concern (PHEICs) and report them to the World Health Organization (WHO, 2008).

i The IHR are an international legal instrument that is binding on 196 countries across the globe, including all the Member States of WHO. Their aim is to help the international community prevent and respond to acute public health risks that have the potential to cross borders and threaten people worldwide.

Throughout this volume, a case has been made for the fact that an effective health system is comprised of many components. These include service delivery; health information; health workforce; medical products and technologies; financing; leadership and governance. These all need to function efficiently to ensure that diagnostics, drugs, vaccines, information, and other methods of prevention, care, or treatment are delivered on time, affordably and in sufficient quantities (WHO, 2017a). In addition to the above factors, the availability of a health workforce of sufficient numbers, motivation and skill – a workforce that is responsive and productive – is critical in offering good quality care. For this care to translate into universal health coverage, sound infrastructure, that is efficient and properly maintained, is required. Other factors to consider are the affordability of this care, and access to it for all, so that individuals seeking medical treatment are able to receive it without incurring financial devastation.

TOWARDS THE BIGGER PICTURE OF PREVENTION AND CONTROL OF EPIDEMICS IN AFRICA

Central to arguments in this volume is the understanding that health challenges do not exist outside of a socio-economic environment. An overarching theme is that in order to fully appreciate the prevalence of epidemics in Africa, and to build the systems that will counter the scourge definitively, a systematic and multifaceted approach is required. It is important to consider the foundational agents that create an environment conducive to diseases that can cause epidemics. These are captured systematically in this volume. The syndemics model of analysing disease pervasiveness recognises these diverse factors and proposes an all-encompassing approach to truly understanding disease. Furthermore, the book emphasises the crucial role that health systems play in determining the health outcomes in countries. Authors emphasise that weak and under-resourced health systems are typically found in African countries and are at the core of the dire state of health in Africa.

The introductory chapter contextualises the emergence of epidemics on the continent, arguing that the prevalence of disease and epidemics in Africa does not occur in isolation. The chapter points to some of the conditions that make certain populations more vulnerable to disease, such as urbanisation, poverty, low status and inequality. It stresses the importance of understanding the pathogenesis of diseases in order to determine the best possible methods for prevention, including vaccines and treatment. The ensuing chapters in the volume build on this foundation and provide examples of and lessons for understanding the structural and/or political-economic drivers of disease, for strengthening health systems, and for taking initiatives in pharmaceutical innovation.

The chapter also addresses one of Africa's major health challenges of the future: zoonotic diseases, i.e. those transmitted between humans and animals. It argues that these emerging zoonotic diseases emphasise the need for the syndemic approach supported by authors throughout this volume. This syndemic approach is based on the idea that disease must be firmly situated within the socio-economic and environmental factors affecting a population, and that attempts to understand or counter disease are futile without this framework. The author shows how the 2014 outbreak of Ebola illustrates the value of this framework. She analyses Ebola in relation to the conditions that lead to vulnerability to disease, in this case infection resulting from contact with animals. This chapter shows the important role that animal clinicians also have in the fight against epidemics and the significance of an interconnected system of role-players and information sharing.

The authors in the book do well to unearth the structural drivers of disease in Africa and eloquently demonstrate how diseases and epidemics require deeper understanding for them to be managed. Where the diseases occur, and who the diseases affect, have implications for their management. The book examines three epidemic diseases (cholera, ebola, and malaria), their relationship to health systems in Africa, and the complex lessons that may be extracted from these experiences. The impact of political interference, collapse in governance, and neglect of essential services and infrastructure have been shown by authors to result in disastrous outbreaks of preventable diseases.

Health outcomes depend on a network of players, many of them in positions of power. Authors show that health is not only determined by the actions of a health department, but also by the departments responsible for water and sanitation; waste and environmental management; finance;

housing and human settlement; agriculture and so on. Neglect of services by any of these departments can breed conditions ripe for an epidemic. Furthermore, cross-border and regional collaboration has been shown to facilitate the capacity to manage persistent disease and epidemics. The requirements for the efficient implementation of strategies to strengthen health systems, in particular the building of efficient surveillance systems designed to detect outbreaks timeously, is discussed in the book.

The authors concede the desperate state of health systems in Africa; however, they also point to low-hanging fruit that can assist in improving health outcomes. Factors like a medical staff that can offer both a high level of skill and decisive management can result in the prevention of an outbreak. In delving into the Nigerian success story of Ebola containment, the book systematically presents the steps that were taken to prevent the disease from spreading; starting from Dr Adadevoh's quick response and accurate diagnosis of the index patient, to the timely releasing of necessary funds, and the deployment of a health care workforce. Even though Nigeria's health system was not particularly prepared for the outbreak, the timely and unambiguous response to the outbreak was the difference between Nigeria's experience and that of Liberia, Guinea, and Sierra Leone.

Over the years, the persistent issue of epidemics in Africa has expanded to include more than infectious diseases. Non-communicable diseases, which present more chronically, are on the rise and are projected to continue on that trajectory – in many instances constituting or approximating epidemics. Authors show how this further burdens already weak and under-resourced health systems in Africa and argue that there is an urgent need to rethink long-term care within the African setting. Additionally, the way in which health professionals caring for long-term patients are managed, including enabling them to perform at their best without overwhelming them with administrative tasks, is crucial in determining the quality of care and epidemics preparedness.

The book also encourages consideration of the role of technological innovations in strengthening health systems. Innovation is a driver of economic growth and development and these impact on countries' health systems. Importantly, African countries need to establish partnerships to develop research capacity to explore emerging technologies that have the potential to improve health outcomes. In many ways, financing and resources play a big role in determining whether strong health systems and indeed quality health care and epidemic preparedness can be achieved. Consequently the book also addresses the financing of health care in Africa and explores whether it is possible to have a reliable health insurance system that supports all sections of the population.

The continent's population is expected to increase dramatically by 2030 which has major implications for health on the continent. The authors discuss these implications for disease and epidemics in Africa and offer ways of thinking about solutions. Essentially, this research is sounding a warning about the diseases of the present and future as population increase; urbanisation; climate change and deforestation change the African ecology and environment.

IMPLICATIONS FOR HEALTH SYSTEMS IN AFRICA

All components need to work in optimal alignment if a health system is to achieve positive health outcomes. From the initial infection of a pathogen reservoir to a patient needing treatment and care, there are various points in the progression of a disease at which interventions need to be implemented. Thus, to emphasise: *health systems need to be able to intervene at any point in disease progression in order to mitigate the spread of the disease.* To begin with, it has been shown how, in the absence of strong surveillance and response systems, infectious disease outbreaks can rapidly overwhelm a country's health system. Therefore, national and regional surveillance of diseases that pose a risk for epidemic outbreaks are important for ensuring quick responses. In regions where zoonotic diseases are endemic, awareness of changes in environment, climate, and animal behaviour will assist in monitoring (and averting) potential outbreaks. Citizens in close proximity to known virus reservoirs should be made aware of the dangers associated with interacting with these reservoirs. Health campaigns around handling wild animals (using protective gear, etc.) and taking cognizance of animal migration patterns would help equip the health system to develop strategies to counter potential outbreaks of zoonotic disease.

In this regard, clinicians for animal as well as human health need to share information and cooperate in identifying and preventing disease spillover. The sharing of information should go beyond national systems, as diseases spread rapidly across regions. The sharing of information will also help strengthen health systems as countries will have the necessary intelligence to prepare for disasters timeously. The living conditions of refugees, displaced populations, and victims of natural disasters should be improved, not only to protect human dignity but also to prevent conditions conducive to the rapid spread of disease.

Diagnostics, vaccines, and drugs need to be made available to counter diseases that pose the risk of epidemic outbreak. In 2018 an investigational vaccine called rVSV-ZEBOV, developed in the United States of America, which was shown to be safe and protective against the Zaire strain of the Ebola virus, was used in the Ebola outbreak in North Kivu in the Democratic Republic of Congo (WHO, 2018). However, because more research still needs to be conducted on it (WHO, 2018), the vaccine is unlicensed and could only be employed under the principles of 'compassionate use' or 'expanded access'.[ii] The question has been legitimately posed as to why African countries, which shoulder much of the burden of disease, are not at the forefront of the research and development of such groundbreaking initiatives. Currently, research capacity in Africa is lacking. Building this capacity and creating an enabling environment for African scientists to conduct research needs to be prioritised. Further, once these medical technologies have been developed, they need to be able to reach the people who need them – in time and reliably. All these interventions, with the end goal of delivering quality health care to a country's citizens, require a well-trained and motivated workforce, from capable scientists to skilled medical staff. Critically, good leadership and good governance, backed by adequate funding, need to be in place so that all aspects of the health system are well managed and can operate efficiently.

The key message of the book is that a robust and well-functioning health system is at the core of a country's capacity to provide quality health

ii Although several studies have shown that the vaccine is safe and protective against the Ebola virus, more scientific research is needed before the vaccine can be licensed. The vaccine is therefore being used on compassionate basis, to protect persons at highest risk of the Ebola outbreak, under a 'ring vaccination', which is the tracking of the epidemic, recruiting individuals at raised risk of infection due to their connection to a patient confirmed with the virus.

care and to counter the threat of an epidemic. Urgent attention should therefore be given to strengthening health systems in Africa. In the long term, it would be far more productive to be proactive about mobilising resources to build a strong health system than mobilising in a panicked response to an outbreak. Alongside this, and equally important for the prevention and/or control of diseases, is the need to address the structural drivers of vulnerability to diseases. It is futile to treat patients who will return home to poor nutrition and inadequate water services which will expose them again to disease. Essentially, the 'One Health' approach, which is a multidisciplinary and transdisciplinary approach endorsed by the World Health Organization, should be implemented. One Health promotes bringing together multiple sectors to communicate and work together to achieve better public health outcomes. These various sectors are encouraged to collaborate in designing and implementing programmes, policies, legislation, and research (WHO, 2017b).

Fundamentally, the authors, who are from across sub-Saharan Africa, compel the reader to think more broadly about the current state of epidemics in Africa and indeed about the solutions. The recurring themes in the book, and the insights and lessons offered, all build to the conclusion that Africans need to be thinking about how to prevent diseases and outbreaks through building strong health systems and adopting a cohesive, inclusive, and transdisciplinary approach to health. The message comes from Africans themselves who are looking to better the continent with solutions relevant to Africa.

REFERENCES

World Health Organization (WHO). 2008. *International Health Regulations* (2005). WHO, https://www.who.int/ihr/publications/9789241596664/en/, accessed 22 January 2019.

World Health Organization (WHO). 2017a. 'Health systems strengthening'. WHO Regional Office for Africa, Brazzaville.

World Health Organization (WHO). 2017b. 'One Health'. WHO, https://www.who.int/features/qa/one-health/en/, accessed 22 January 2019.

World Health Organization (WHO). 2018. 'Ebola virus disease frequently asked questions: compassionate use of Ebola vaccine in the context of the Ebola outbreak in North Kivu, Democratic Republic of the Congo'. WHO, https://www.who.int/ebola/drc-2018/faq-vaccine/en/, accessed 27 January 2019.

Index

Page numbers in *italics* indicate figures and tables. The letter 'n' followed by a Roman numeral indicates a footnote.

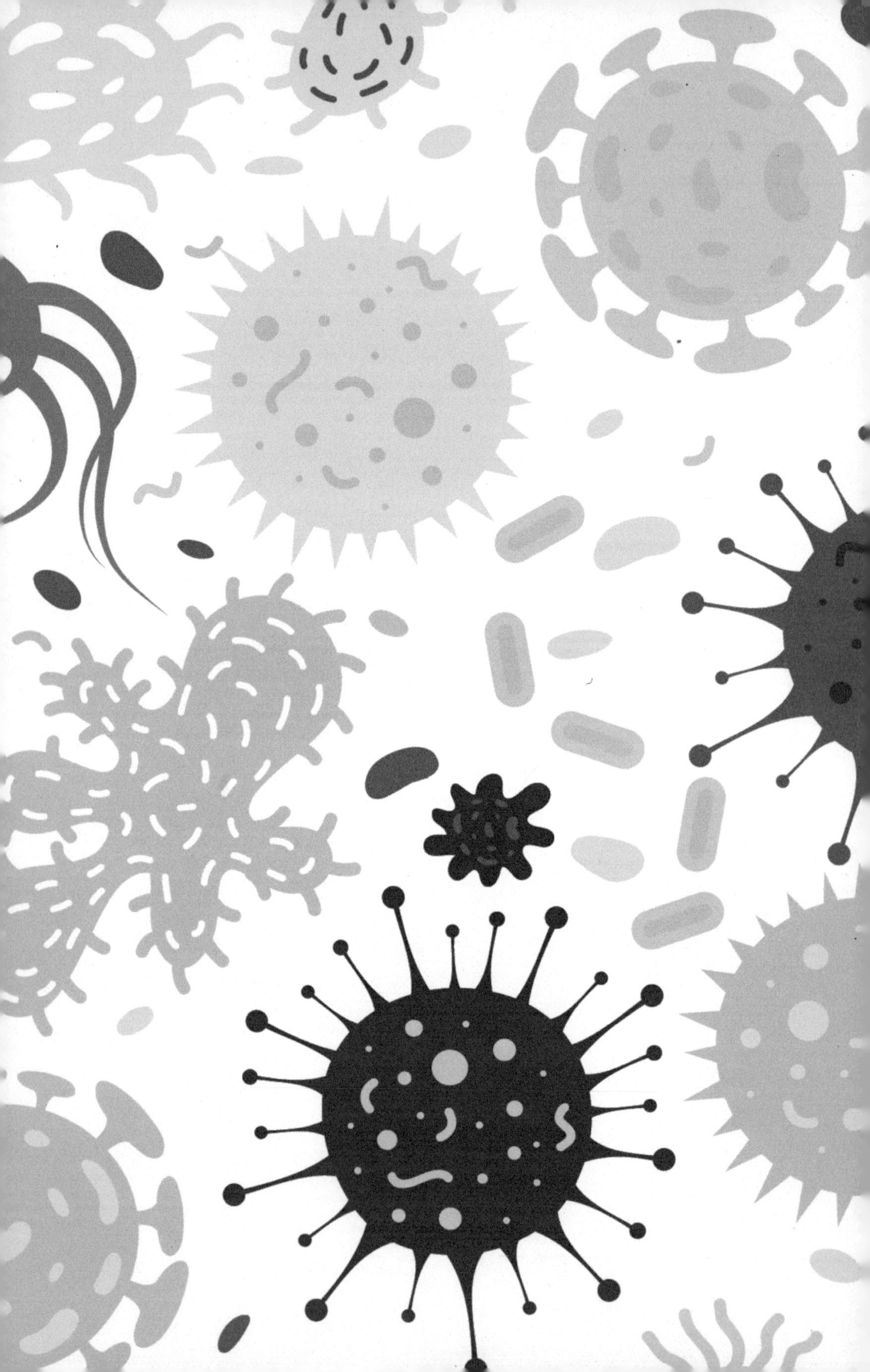